CHANGE YOUR
BRAIN
CHANGE YOUR
BODY

CHANGE YOUR
BRAIN
CHANGE YOUR
BODY

Use Your Brain to Get and
Keep the Body You Have Always Wanted

DANIEL G. AMEN, M.D.

**BOOST YOUR BRAIN TO IMPROVE YOUR
WEIGHT, SKIN, HEART, ENERGY, AND FOCUS**

HARMONY BOOKS ◁◎▷ New York

Copyright © 2010 by Daniel G. Amen, M.D.

All rights reserved.
Published in the United States by Harmony Books, an imprint of the Crown Publishing Group, a division of Random House, Inc., New York.
www.crownpublishing.com

Harmony Books is a registered trademark and the Harmony Books colophon is a trademark of Random House, Inc.

Library of Congress Cataloging-in-Publication Data is available upon request.

ISBN 978-0-307-46357-9

Printed in the United States of America

Design by Leonard Henderson

10 9 8 7 6 5 4

For my grandfather, Daniel Ara, who has directed my heart

and

for Elias, my grandson, who provides continuing inspiration.

CONTENTS

PART ONE
BRAIN BASICS

Introduction: The Missing Link
Boost Your Brain to Get and Keep the Body You Have Always Wanted   3

1. *The Brain-Body Solution*
Ten Basic Principles to Change Your Brain and Your Body   13

PART TWO
CHANGE YOUR BRAIN, CHANGE YOUR WEIGHT

2. *The Craving Solution*
Use Your Brain to Increase Your Willpower and Calm
the Urges That Prevent You From Achieving Your Goals   37

3. *The Weight Solution*
Use Your Brain to Achieve Your Optimal Weight   53

4. *The Nutrition Solution*
Feed Your Brain to Look and Feel Younger   81

5. *The Exercise Solution*
Exercise Your Body to Strengthen Your Brain   109

PART THREE
CHANGE YOUR BRAIN, BEAUTIFY AND STRENGTHEN YOUR BODY

6. *The Skin Solution*
Brain Signals to Soothe and Smooth Your Skin   129

7. *The Hormone Solution*
Balance Your Hormones to Turn Back the Clock   140

8. *The Heart Solution*
Use Your Brain to Strengthen and Soothe Your Heart   164

9. *The Focus and Energy Solution*
Boost Your Energy to Stay on Track Toward Your Goals   179

PART FOUR
CHANGE YOUR BRAIN, INCREASE LOVE AND VITALITY

10. *The Sleep Solution*
Rest Your Brain for a Slimmer Shape and Smoother Skin   195

11. *The Stress Solution*
Relax Your Brain to Reduce Your Wrinkles and
Improve Your Immune System   213

12. *The Memory Solution*
Remember What You Need to Do Every Day   236

13. *The ANT Solution*
Think Your Way to Being Thinner, Younger, and Happier   256

14. *The Passion Solution*
Make Love to Recharge Your Brain and Body   272

15. *The Brain Health Solution*
Treat Brain Disorders to Protect Against Physical Illnesses   287

16. *Change Your Brain, Change Your Body,*
Change Other People's Bodies
How Your Brain Influences the Physical and Mental Health
of Others   306

APPENDIX A: 15 IMPORTANT NUMBERS I NEED TO KNOW   311

APPENDIX B: AMEN CLINICS ABBREVIATED BRAIN SYSTEMS QUESTIONNAIRE   314

APPENDIX C: THE SUPPLEMENT SOLUTION   320

NOTE ON REFERENCES AND FURTHER READING   351

ACKNOWLEDGMENTS   353

INDEX   355

See www.amenclinics.com/cybcyb for more information.

CHANGE YOUR
BRAIN
CHANGE YOUR
BODY

PART ONE

BRAIN BASICS

THE MISSING LINK

Boost Your Brain to Get and Keep the Body You Have Always Wanted

Fifty percent of the brain is dedicated to vision.

How you look plays a large role in how you feel. Both matter to your success at work and in your relationships.

It is not just vanity, it is about health.

To look and feel your best, you must first think about and optimize your brain.

I live in Newport Beach, California. We have often been called the plastic society, because we have more plastic walking around our streets and beaches than almost anywhere else in the world. One of my friends says that God will never flood Newport Beach because all of the women will float. Most people throughout the world, not just in Newport Beach, care more about their faces, their boobs, their bellies, their butts, and their abs than they do their brains. But it is your brain that is the key to having the face, the breasts, the belly, the butt, the abs, and the overall health you have always wanted; and it is brain dysfunction, in large part, that ruins our bodies and causes premature aging.

It is your brain that decides to get you out of bed in the morning to exercise, to give you a stronger, leaner body, or to cause you to hit the snooze button and procrastinate your workout. It is your brain that pushes you away from the table telling you that you have had enough, or that gives you permission to have the second bowl of Rocky Road ice cream, making you look and feel like a blob. It is your brain that manages the stress in your life and relaxes you so that you look vibrant, or, when left unchecked, sends stress signals to the rest of your body and wrinkles your skin. And it is your brain that turns away cigarettes, too much caffeine, and alcohol, helping you look and feel healthy, or that gives you permission to smoke, to have that third cup of coffee, or to drink that third glass of wine, thus making every system in your body look and feel older.

> *Your brain is the command and control center of your body. If you want a better body, the first place to ALWAYS start is by having a better brain.*

My interest in the brain-body connection started more than thirty years ago. As a college student, my thinking was influenced by the work of O. Carl Simonton, the oncologist who taught people to use visualization to boost their immune system in order to fight cancer. In medical school, I became trained in the use of medical hypnosis and began to see the powerful effect it can have on healing the body. I personally saw that it was helpful for treating headaches, irritable bowel syndrome, pain, weight loss, insomnia, a Parkinsonian tremor, and heart arrhythmias. I then became trained in a treatment technique called biofeedback and found that when I taught my patients to use their brains to warm their hands or breathe with their bellies, their whole body went into a relaxed state, which was helpful in decreasing stress, lowering blood pressure, and combating headaches.

THE MISSING LINK

It wasn't until 1991 that I truly started to understand the brain-body connection. That was the year I started the brain imaging work we do now at the Amen Clinics. We do a study called brain SPECT imaging that looks at blood flow and activity patterns. SPECT stands for single photon emission computed tomography. Unlike MRI and CAT scans, which show the anatomy of the brain, SPECT scans look at how the brain functions.

Looking at the brain has made an enormous difference in both my professional and personal life. At the time I ordered my first scan I had been a psychiatrist for nearly a decade, and I realized that I didn't have all the information I needed to provide the very best treatment for my patients. When I scanned my first patient I was excited to discover that the SPECT scans gave me critical information about brain function that I could not ascertain just by talking to the patient. The scans helped me and my colleagues be better healers.

Since 1991, the Amen Clinics have performed more than 55,000 brain scans, more than any organization in the world. Analyzing scans in the context of individual patient histories has helped us better diagnose and treat our patients for a wide variety of problems, such as ADD, depression, anxiety, anger, learning problems, memory problems, brain injuries, and addictions. In addition, I have discovered that when I improved my patients' brain functions, I also helped to improve their bodies and overall life.

I saw dramatic evidence of this a few years ago when I created a home study course for treating anxiety and depression. To test the course, we enlisted the help of ninety people to take part in the pilot program. The results were astounding. As I expected, most of the individuals experienced significant improvement in their levels of anxiety and depression. But that's not all. A number of the people told us that by following the twelve-week program, they also lost twenty to thirty pounds. This surprising result showed us that when people help their brains, they help their bodies, and they were finally able to lose the weight they had been trying to shed for years.

> *Our brain imaging work opened a new window into*
> *why people do what they do.*
> *It provided the missing link and allowed people to see*
> *what was going on in their brains, so they could do*
> *things to improve their brain and their bodies.*

Take a close look at yourself in the mirror. If your skin seems dry, you reach for the moisturizer. Spot a pimple and you dab it with a bit of acne medication. Notice a few split ends and you call the hairdresser for a haircut. If you live in Newport Beach and you detect a few wrinkles, you call a doctor and make an appointment for Botox. Basically, whenever you see a problem with your body, you try to fix it yourself or get professional help to take care of it. But most people never even think about the health of their own brain, because they cannot see it. Many of us are walking around with brains that could use some serious help, but we don't know it, so we don't do anything to address the issue. This is at the heart, or should I say brain, of the problem. Let's look at an example of a healthy brain and a troubled brain.

In a healthy brain, there is full, even, symmetrical activity, with the most intensity in the back of the brain, in an area called the cerebellum. In troubled brains, you will see areas that are working too hard or areas that aren't working hard enough. In Image I.1, see Anna's eighty-two-year-old brain. It is very healthy and looks like a brain of someone thirty years younger. Anna was very

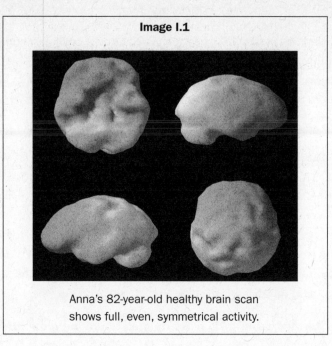

Image I.1

Anna's 82-year-old healthy brain scan
shows full, even, symmetrical activity.

healthy, not on any medications, and was a loving wife of fifty-eight years, mother, and grandmother. She was sharp, energetic, had a lot of intellectual curiosity, and was active in her community and church.

By contrast, Becca, age forty-four, came to see me for impulsiveness and obesity. She supported two hundred pounds on her five-foot frame and had tried many times without success to lose weight. When we scanned her, she had very low activity in the prefrontal cortex, located in the front part of her brain (Image I.2), likely from a car accident in childhood. The prefrontal cortex is the part of her brain responsible for planning, decision making, and impulse control. On treatment to enhance activity in her prefrontal cortex (Image I.3), her impulsiveness significantly diminished and she was able to stay on a brain and body healthy program that helped her lose eighty pounds over two years.

Our brain imaging work taught me that impulsiveness is not just a lack of willpower or a bad attitude, which is the belief shared by 95 percent of the population. We could actually see that many people had low activity in the front part of their brain, whether it was from a brain injury, toxic exposure, or an inherited problem like attention deficit disorder (ADD). And when we fixed the problem, we found that these people were better able to stay on the diet and health plans they needed for a better body.

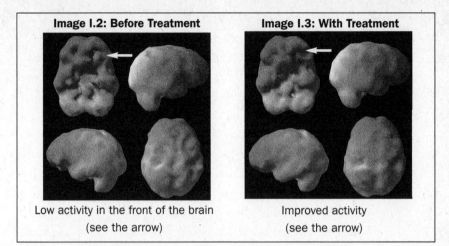

Image I.2: Before Treatment

Image I.3: With Treatment

Low activity in the front of the brain
(see the arrow)

Improved activity
(see the arrow)

Additionally, after looking at the brain, I no longer thought that compulsiveness was just from rigid people who were overcontrolling. I could see that the front part of their brain worked too hard. When we calmed down this part of the brain with supplements or medications, people were less likely to overeat or be under chronic stress.

Looking at the brain changed everything I did and taught me that in order to change your body, you MUST first change your brain. Understanding and optimizing your brain is often the missing link to being successful in your quest for a better body.

YOUR BRAIN CAN CHANGE YOUR BODY

The connection between your brain and body is truly amazing. Here are three examples.

1. My first wife, Robbin, and I tried for several years to have our third child. Robbin had a child from a previous marriage, Antony, whom I adopted, and we had already had a child together, Breanne. But this time it just wasn't happening. She even sent me to the urologist with the little plastic cup to get checked out. Not my idea of fun.

   Then one day, I was at home with Breanne, age four, and Antony, nine, while Robbin was away at school. It was about 6 p.m. when Breanne heard the sound of something crying. We looked all around the house but couldn't find anything. Then I noticed that the lonely cries were coming from the attic. I got the ladder and a flashlight and crawled into the attic where I found a kitten just a few hours old, abandoned by her mother, with her eyes still sticky shut, crying weakly.

When I brought the kitten down, the children were so excited. I called the local vet, who told me the baby was not likely to live and I should just drown her in a bucket of water. With two young children looking up at me with excited faces, I told the vet that he needed to give me another plan or I was going to be in big trouble. Reluctantly, he told me how to stimulate her to go to the bathroom with a warm, wet cotton swab (that was a new one for me), gave me the name of a baby kitten formula I could get at the pet store, and told me to keep her warm under a lamp—but there was no hope.

When Robbin got home, all of her maternal instincts went into overdrive. She cared for the kitten, dreamed about her, and got up frequently at night to check on her. Ipo, the kitten, thrived, and within three weeks Robbin was pregnant! Her maternal instincts changed the receptivity of her body.

2. Larry and I both worked together at my father's grocery store chain when we were teenagers. I have seen him again periodically through the years at various business and family functions. On the last occasion, my father's eightieth-birthday celebration, Larry looked twenty years older than his age of fifty-four. His hair was stark white, his skin was wrinkled, and had an ashen tone. His daughter had died of cancer ten years earlier and his wife had died of the same cancer the year before. The mountain of stress he had been under took a noticeably negative toll on his body.

3. On a recent trip for my public television show *Change Your Brain, Change Your Life,* I went back to the station in Atlanta where I had been a number of times before. The fund-raising director, Alicia Steele, picked me up at the hotel for an on-air appearance. This time Alicia looked different. She looked younger and more vibrant. When I asked her what she was doing, she said that since she had met me she was eating right, taking fish oil, drinking less alcohol, and was better at handling the stresses in her life. She had taken the extended version of my brain system questionnaire, found on our website, and discovered that her prefrontal cortex was likely low in activity, so she started taking the supplement SAMe with great effect. In fact, she told me that she had also dropped fifteen pounds. And she was getting her husband to exercise. That week at her station there had been a death in the

family of her producer, which had really upset the schedule; usually, she told me, an event like that would have made her cry; now, she knew she could adapt to the changes and get rid of any automatic negative thoughts (ANTs) that tried to steal her happiness. As she changed her brain, her body, her life, and even her family were much improved.

The story of our kitten highlights that when a woman acts maternal, chemical changes in the brain send signals to the body making it more likely for her to conceive. Larry's story illustrates that when someone is under a mountain of stress, it will likely have a very negative impact on his body. And Alicia's story teaches us that when you combat stress and get on a brain-healthy program specific to your own brain, you will look and feel younger. Think about this concept for a moment. You can change your brain and subsequently change your body. You can harness the power of your brain to create the body you want!

ONE PRESCRIPTION DOES NOT WORK FOR EVERYONE

Alicia's story highlights a very important point that will be a major theme throughout the rest of this book. One prescription does not fit everyone. This is why most weight-loss programs don't work. All of us need individualized or personalized prescriptions based on our own brain types and needs. Since Alicia likely had low activity in her prefrontal cortex, in the front part of her brain, she needed more stimulating interventions, such as the supplement SAMe. People who have too much activity in the front part of the brain tend to do better with interventions that are calming and boost the neurotransmitter serotonin, such as using the supplement 5-HTP. Using SAMe with people who have high prefrontal cortex activity usually makes them more anxious. Knowing how your own specific brain works is critical to getting the help that will work for you. Of course, as we will see, there are interventions that apply to all of us, such as a healthy diet and adequate sleep, but to get the most out of this book, note the interventions that apply to your individual type.

WELCOME TO THE BRAIN–BODY CONNECTION

In the past few decades, scientists and medical professionals have been exploring and researching what they've termed the *mind-body connection*. A mounting body of scientific evidence supports the concept that your mind has a very

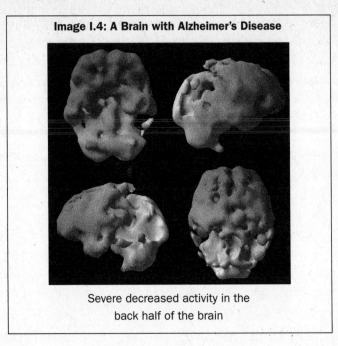

Image I.4: A Brain with Alzheimer's Disease

Severe decreased activity in the
back half of the brain

powerful influence on your appearance, your mood, your stress levels, and your overall health. In fact, a whole new branch of alternative medicine has emerged that focuses on the interactions of the mind and body.

One question people often ask me is whether the mind is separate from the brain. The answer, after looking at more than 55,000 brain scans over the past twenty years, is *no. The mind and the brain are completely dependent upon each other.* Just think about Alzheimer's disease, which is clearly a brain illness. Do people with Alzheimer's disease lose their minds? Yes, they do as the disease progresses. When you lose brain tissue (see Image I.4), you lose your memory and your ability to think rationally.

Or let's consider brain trauma. Becca's scan above showed damage to her prefrontal cortex. *Damage the brain, and you damage the mind and most everything else in your life, including your body.* When I improved Becca's brain, her mind and body were so much better.

TAKE ADVANTAGE OF THE BRAIN–BODY CONNECTION

If you are reading this book, I'm assuming there are things you'd like to change about your body. Maybe you'd like to tighten your tummy, have younger-looking skin, boost your energy level, stop getting so many colds, reduce the number of headaches you get, or lower your blood pressure without having to take medicine. Like most people, you probably know what you have to do in order to achieve your goals, but you simply don't do it. Why not? Because you aren't taking care of your brain. If you want to lose the love handles, you need to improve the function of your frontal lobes. If you want to say good-bye to all those headaches, you have to calm your brain. And if you want to turn back the clock on your skin's appearance, you have to start by rejuvenating your brain.

In this book, I will give you fifteen solutions to help you boost your brain so you can get and keep the body you have always wanted. It all begins by learning to love your brain and understanding how it affects your body. These easy-to-follow solutions also focus on using your brain to improve your willpower and eliminate the cravings that sabotage your efforts for a better body. You will see that weight-management issues, although rampant, are definitely not a single or simple problem. Based on our research, it is at least six different problems, and knowing your type of issue is the first key to being at the weight you want. You will also find ways to improve your skin and your heart by boosting your brain. Plus, you will learn how to increase your focus and energy, calm your stress, and improve your memory to keep your body in tip-top shape. You will learn how to feed your brain so you will look and feel younger, and you'll discover how adequate sleep can help prevent you from packing on pounds as well as take years off your appearance. Among the many prescriptions within these pages, you will see how balancing your hormones can give you a more youthful brain and body. One of the most effective solutions for improving every aspect of your body is learning to use new thinking skills to help you reach your weight, health, beauty, and fitness goals. You may be surprised and delighted to find out that sex is a great brain booster that's good medicine for your body, too. Plus, you will learn how your mental health is a major key to having your best body possible. Perhaps the most astounding thing you will find here is that when you change your brain and your body, you can also change other people's bodies too. Within the pages of the book I will tell you which tailored natural supplements help to ameliorate the problems we discuss, along with specific medications that may apply. You can find detailed information on these supplements in Appendix C, "The Supplement Solution."

This book is organized in four parts. Here, in Part One, you will be introduced to the ten basic principles to change your brain and body. In Part Two, you will discover how to use your brain to help you achieve something millions of us struggle with on a daily basis—lasting weight loss. Part Three focuses on the many ways your brain can help you beautify your body and improve your overall health and well-being. In Part Four, among the many brain-body strategies you will find are antiaging secrets that will help keep your brain and body young.

With the solutions in this book, you can learn to harness the power of your brain to get and keep the body you always wanted. I think you deserve to have a brain and body you love. Don't you?

1

THE BRAIN-BODY SOLUTION

Ten Basic Principles to Change
Your Brain and Your Body

Develop brain envy.
Loving your brain is the first step
toward getting the body you want.

Over the years, I have personally had ten brain SPECT scans to check on the health of my own brain. Looking back, my earliest scan, taken when I was thirty-seven, showed a toxic, bumpy appearance that was definitely not consistent with great brain function. Initially, I didn't understand why. All my life, I have been someone who rarely drank alcohol, never smoked, and never used an illegal drug. So why did my brain look so bad? Before I understood about brain health, I had many bad brain habits. I practically lived on fast food and diet sodas, worked like a nut, rarely got more than four or five hours of sleep at night, and didn't exercise much. My weight was fifteen pounds above where I wanted it, and I struggled with arthritis and had trouble getting off the floor when I played with my children. At thirty-seven, I just thought I was getting older.

My most recent brain scan at age fifty-two looks healthier and much younger than my first scan, even though brains typically become less active with age. Why? Seeing other people's scans, I developed "brain envy" and wanted mine to be better. As I learned about brain health, I put into practice what I'm teaching you and what I've been preaching to my patients for years. In doing so, I got more than just a better-looking brain. I also feel more energetic, look healthier, have lost weight, and have better body tone, no arthritis, and smoother-looking skin.

In this chapter, you will find ten basic principles that explain why it is

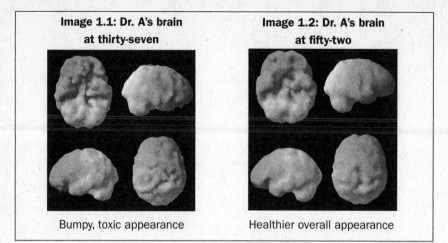

Image 1.1: Dr. A's brain at thirty-seven — Bumpy, toxic appearance

Image 1.2: Dr. A's brain at fifty-two — Healthier overall appearance

essential to love and nurture your brain in order to have your best body possible. These are the same principles that underlie our work at the Amen Clinics, where we have helped thousands of people learn to love their brains in order to improve their bodies.

TEN PRINCIPLES TO CHANGE YOUR BRAIN AND YOUR BODY

1. Your brain is involved in everything you do.
2. When your brain works right, your body looks and feels better. When your brain is troubled, you have trouble with how you look and feel.
3. The brain is the most complex organ in the universe. Respect it.
4. Your brain is very soft and housed in a really hard skull. Protect it.
5. The brain has only so much reserve. The more reserve you have, the healthier you are. The less reserve, the more vulnerable you are.
6. Specific parts of your brain are involved in certain behaviors. Trouble in specific parts of your brain tends to cause certain behavior problems. Understanding your brain can help you optimize it.
7. Many things hurt the brain and make it harder for you to get the body you've always wanted. Many things help the brain and make it easier to get and keep a body you love.
8. Brain imaging gives great insight into healing the brain so you can have a better body.
9. One prescription does not work for everyone—we are all unique, and you need to understand how your own personal brain functions.
10. Yes, you can change your brain and body!

PRINCIPLE #1

Your brain is involved in everything you do.

Your brain controls everything you do, feel, and think. When you look in the mirror, you can thank your brain for what you see. Ultimately, it is your brain that determines whether your belly bulges over your belt buckle or your waistline is trim and toned. Your brain plays the central role in whether your skin looks fresh and dewy or is etched with wrinkles. Whether you wake up feeling energetic or groggy depends on your brain. When you head to the kitchen to make breakfast, it is your brain that determines whether you go for the leftover pizza or the low-fat yogurt and fruit. Your brain controls whether you hit the gym or sit at the computer to check your Facebook page. If you feel the need to light up a cigarette or drink a couple cups of java, that's also your brain's doing.

The moment-by-moment functioning of your brain is responsible for the way you think, feel, eat, exercise, and even for the way you make love. The impact of the brain on your body goes even deeper than that. It is at the core of your very health and well-being. Whether you live a long healthy life, suffer from a debilitating condition, or have your days cut short by a terrible disease, your brain is at the center of it all. In fact, researchers from the Univer-

> ### ACTION STEP
> Remember that your brain is involved in everything you do, every decision you make, every bite of food you take, every cigarette you smoke, every worrisome thought you have, every workout you skip, every alcoholic beverage you drink, and more.

sity of Cambridge, England, found that when people made bad decisions with their brains, they took fourteen years off their life spans. People who drank heavily, smoked, didn't exercise, and had poor diets at the age of sixty had the same risk of dying as someone with a healthy lifestyle who was seventy-four. The decisions your brain makes can steal or add many years to your life!

PRINCIPLE #2

When your brain works right, your body looks and feels better.
When your brain is troubled, you have trouble with how you look and feel.

A healthy brain makes it so much easier for you to have your best body possible. When your brain is working at optimal levels, you are more likely to stick to a diet, follow an exercise routine, and adopt healthy lifestyle behaviors. That adds up to a slimmer, trimmer body, a more youthful appearance, brighter skin, better immunity, fewer headaches, less back pain, and improved health.

On the other hand, a troubled brain often leads to trouble with your body. That's right, extra pounds, wrinkles, chronic pain, and health conditions can be linked to the way your brain functions. Making poor food choices, blowing off the gym, and engaging in unhealthy behaviors are more common when your brain isn't working at its best.

Jack, a fifty-two-year-old divorced engineer, is five feet ten inches tall and weighs close to 260 pounds. He tries to diet, but just can't stick to it. Every morning, Jack wakes up with the intention of eating healthfully that day, but he never gets around to planning his day's meals or stocking the refrigerator. When lunchtime rolls around, he's starving and stops at the first fast-food restaurant he can find, where he orders a cheeseburger and fries. After coming home from work, he gazes into an empty refrigerator and then calls the local pizza delivery place for dinner.

With three young children, a demanding job, and a strained marriage, Megan appears older than her forty-three years. She'd love to recapture a more youthful look, but hasn't been able to do it with the creams and lotions from the cosmetics counter. She rarely gets more than a few hours of sleep at night and whenever she's depressed, stressed, mad, or sad, she seeks refuge in a cigarette and a glass of wine—or two or three or four glasses of wine, or maybe even the whole bottle. Smoking and drinking calms down her nerves and makes her feel better—temporarily.

Sarah is twenty-eight years old and would love to have a better body. Although she isn't technically overweight, she wants to tone and tighten the 135 pounds she carries on her five-foot-six-inch frame. She knows that exercise could help her achieve her goals, but she just can't seem to muster up enough energy or motivation to hit the gym. Sarah also struggles with feelings of anxiety and nervousness and is constantly thinking of what can go wrong in her life.

For years, Jack, Megan, and Sarah have been chalking up their problems to a simple lack of willpower or laziness, but that isn't necessarily the case. Their inability to get the body they want lies within their brains. Jack's lack of planning and poor follow-through are common signs of low activity in an area of the brain known as the prefrontal cortex (PFC). This is the part of the brain that is involved with planning, goal setting, forethought, impulse control, and follow-through. When this area isn't functioning at the proper level, it makes it very hard to be successful.

Smoking or drinking to calm emotions, which is keeping Megan from getting the youthful look she wants, may signal excessive activity in the deep limbic system of the brain. This part of the brain is involved in setting your emotional tone. When it is less active, there is generally a positive, hopeful state of mind. When it is heated up or overactive, negativity and feelings of

> **ACTION STEP**
>
> If you have trouble following a diet or exercise plan, if you have chronic pain, if you have low energy, or if you have health conditions, improving the health of your brain will help.

depression or sadness can take over, making you look for solace in nicotine, alcohol, or drugs.

Sarah's energy is drained by anxiety and worry, which may indicate a problem in an area of the brain called the basal ganglia. Located toward the center of the brain, the basal ganglia are involved with integrating feelings, thoughts, and motivation. When there is high activity in this area, it can cause problems with anxiety and may drain people of their energy and get-up-and-go.

What Jack, Megan, and Sarah show us is that your brain heavily influences your behavior and your body. Your brain can either help you have a better body or make it more difficult for you to have a body you love.

PRINCIPLE #3

The brain is the most complex organ in the universe. Respect it.

The brain is the most complicated, amazing, special organ in the universe. Your brain weighs only about three pounds, but it is more powerful than even the most sophisticated supercomputer. Even though it represents only about 2 percent of your body's weight, your brain uses about 25 percent of the calories you consume, 25 percent of the total blood flow in your body, and 20 percent of the oxygen you breathe. The calories, blood flow, and oxygen feed the cells inside your brain.

It is estimated that the brain contains more than one hundred billion nerve cells, which is about the number of stars in the Milky Way. Each nerve cell is connected to other nerve cells by thousands of individual connections between cells. In fact, it is estimated that there are more connections in your brain than there are stars in the universe! If you take a single piece of brain tissue the size of a grain of sand, it contains a hundred thousand nerve cells and a billion connections—all "talking" to one another. Information in your brain travels at speeds of up to 268 miles per hour, faster than the race cars in the Indy 500, unless of course you are drunk—then things really slow down. When we do full-body scans, the brain is lit up like a little heater while the rest of the body appears ghostlike. Your brain is the organ of your personality, character, and intelligence and is heavily involved in making you who you are.

PRINCIPLE #4

Your brain is very soft and housed in a really hard skull. Protect it.

If you are like most people, you probably think your brain is firm and rubbery. In reality, your brain is very soft. Composed of about 80 percent water, its consistency can be compared to soft butter, custard, or tofu—somewhere between raw egg whites and Jell-O. To protect your soft brain, it is housed in a really hard skull filled with fluid. Inside your skull are a number of bony edges and ridges. Some of these ridges are as sharp as knives and in the event of a head injury or trauma can damage your soft brain. Your brain was not meant for your head to be hitting soccer balls, playing tackle football, boxing, or participating in Ultimate Fighting Championships. Brain trauma is much more common than you think. Each year, two million new brain injuries are reported, and millions more go unreported. Brain injuries not only damage your brain, they can ruin your body.

If you think *brain injury* means only serious injuries like flying through the windshield of a car or falling off the roof onto your head, you are wrong. It doesn't have to be a "serious" injury to have serious consequences for your body and your health. After viewing more than 55,000 brain scans, it has become very clear to me that what many people think of as mild trauma can have a significantly negative effect on people's brains and can significantly change their lives and their ability to look and feel their best. Many times, these injuries go unnoticed, in part because mental health professionals never look at brain function.

Studies show that people who have suffered brain injuries, even mild ones, often experience emotional, behavioral, or cognitive problems. When you have trouble thinking or reasoning, you can't

---

ACTION STEP

To keep your brain and body in tip-top shape, protect your brain from injury. Don't hit soccer balls with your head or ride a bicycle, ski, or snowboard without a helmet that fits.

make the best decisions for your body. Suffering a brain injury is also associated with a higher incidence of alcoholism and drug abuse—both of which lead to premature aging, possible weight problems, potentially devastating health conditions, and homelessness. Protect your brain.

PRINCIPLE #5

The brain has only so much reserve.
The more reserve you have, the healthier you are.
The less reserve, the more vulnerable you are.

Think about your family, friends, and coworkers. When there's a crisis, do some of them completely fall apart—racing for the candy bowl, reaching for a pack of cigarettes, or searching for solace in drugs and alcohol—while others manage to soldier on with their lives in a healthy way? Have you ever wondered why that is? I have. In my work, I have noticed that stressful events, such as the loss of a loved one, layoffs at work, or divorce can lead to depression, changes in weight, a lack of motivation to exercise, and bad daily habits in some people but not in others.

After looking at brain scans for nearly twenty years, I have come to believe that these differences have to do with a concept I call brain reserve. Brain reserve is the cushion of healthy brain function we have to deal with stressful events or injuries. The more reserve you have, the better you can cope with the unexpected. The less you have, the harder it is for you to handle tough times and injuries, and the more likely you are to gobble up a bag of Oreo cookies or swig alcohol as a coping mechanism.

Mary and Katie are identical twins. They share the same genes, the same parents, and the same upbringing. Yet their lives—and looks—are very different. Mary, who is very fit, is a successful journalist in a long-term happy marriage with three great children. Katie, who is overweight, barely finished high school, suffered with depression and a bad temper, and went from job to job and relationship to relationship. Their lives and looks are nothing alike.

When I scanned them, Mary had a very healthy brain (Image 1.3), while Katie had clear evidence of a brain injury, affecting her prefrontal cortex and temporal lobes (Image 1.4). At first, when I talked with the twins together, Katie didn't remember a head injury. Then Mary spoke up, saying, "Don't you remember the time when we were ten years old and you fell off the top bunk bed onto your head? You got knocked out and we had to rush you to

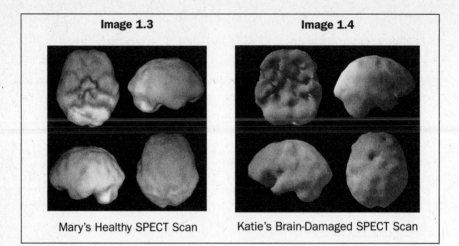

Image 1.3	Image 1.4
Mary's Healthy SPECT Scan	Katie's Brain-Damaged SPECT Scan

the hospital." The injury likely caused Katie to have less brain reserve, which may be why she was always more vulnerable to stress than her sister.

At conception, most of us have the same amount of brain reserve. From that point on, though, many things can boost or reduce the level of reserve. For example, if your mother smoked marijuana and drank a lot of Jack Daniel's while she was pregnant with you, it is likely that she lowered your level of brain reserve. If you fell off the roof as a teenager, were the victim of domestic violence as a child, or abused drugs and alcohol in high school, you probably decreased your own reserve. Basically, any behavior that harms the brain erodes your brain's reserve.

On the other hand, if your mother ate a healthy diet, took a daily multivitamin, and meditated every day, she probably pumped up your reserve. Your reserve likely got a boost if you were raised in a loving home, were exposed to a wide variety of learning as a child, and steered clear of drugs and alcohol.

When you have ample brain reserve, it builds resilience and makes it easier for you to deal with life's unexpected twists and turns without turning to Ben & Jerry's ice cream, alcohol, or drugs.

PRINCIPLE #6

Specific parts of your brain are involved in certain behaviors.
Trouble in specific parts of your brain tends to cause certain behavior problems. Understanding your brain can help you optimize it.

Here's a very simple crash course in the brain systems that play a major role in your ability to get a body you love. All of these systems can influence your behavior and either help or hurt your ability to have your best body possible.

Prefrontal cortex (PFC) Think of the PFC as the CEO of your brain. Situated at the front third of your brain, it acts like a supervisor for the rest of your brain and body. It is involved with attention, judgment, planning, impulse control, follow-through, and empathy. Low activity in the PFC is linked to a short attention span, impulsivity, a lack of clear goals, and procrastination. Alcohol lowers activity in the PFC, which is why people do such stupid things when they get drunk.

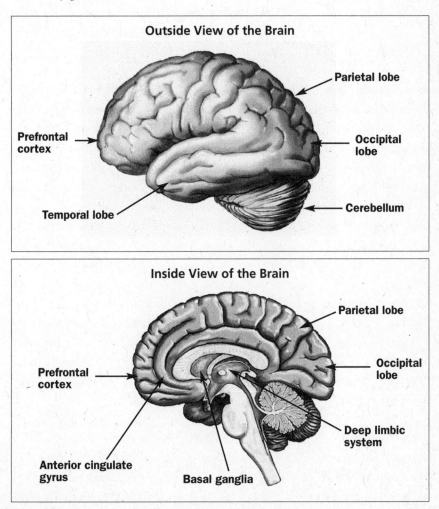

Outside View of the Brain

Parietal lobe

Prefrontal cortex

Occipital lobe

Temporal lobe

Cerebellum

Inside View of the Brain

Parietal lobe

Prefrontal cortex

Occipital lobe

Anterior cingulate gyrus

Basal ganglia

Deep limbic system

Anterior cingulate gyrus (ACG) I like to call the ACG the brain's gear shifter. It runs lengthwise through the deep parts of the frontal lobes and allows us to shift our attention and be flexible and adaptable and to change when needed. When there is too much activity in this area, people tend to become stuck on negative thoughts or actions; they tend to worry, hold grudges, and be oppositional or argumentative. It also may make them more vulnerable to being obsessive or struggle with compulsive behaviors, and has been linked to eating disorders, such as anorexia.

Deep limbic system (DLS) Lying near the center of the brain, the deep limbic system is involved in setting a person's emotional tone. When this area is less active, people tend to be more positive and hopeful. When it is overactive, negativity can take over and lower motivation and drive, decrease self-esteem, and increase feelings of guilt and helplessness. Abnormalities in the limbic brain have been associated with mood disorders.

Basal ganglia Surrounding the deep limbic system, the basal ganglia are involved with integrating thoughts, feelings, and movements. This part of the brain is also involved in setting a person's anxiety level. When there is too much activity in the basal ganglia, people tend to struggle with anxiety and physical stress symptoms, such as headaches, stomachaches, and muscle tension. With low activity here, people tend to lack motivation. This area is also involved with feelings of pleasure and ecstasy. Cocaine works in this part of the brain. Cookies, cakes, and other treats also activate this area, according to a fascinating new book called *The End of Overeating* by Dr. David Kessler, the former commissioner of the U.S. Food and Drug Administration.

Temporal lobes The temporal lobes, located underneath your temples and behind your eyes, are involved with language, short-term memory, mood stability, and temper issues. They are part of the brain's "what pathway," because they help you recognize and name what things are. Trouble in the temporal lobes often leads to memory problems, mood instability, and temper problems.

Parietal lobes The parietal lobes toward the top back part of the brain are involved with sensory processing and direction sense. The "where pathway" in the brain, they help you know where things are in space, such as navigating your way to the kitchen at night in the dark. The parietal lobes are one of the first areas damaged by Alzheimer's disease, which is why people with this condition tend to get lost. They have also been implicated in eating disorders and body-distortion syndromes, such as with anorexics who think they are fat.

Occipital lobes Located at the back of the brain, the occipital lobes are involved with vision and visual processing.

Cerebellum (CB) Located at the back-bottom part of the brain, the cerebellum is involved with physical coordination, thought coordination, and processing speed. There are large connections between the PFC and the cerebellum, which is why many scientists think that the cerebellum is also associated with judgment and impulse control. When there are problems in the cerebellum, people tend to struggle with physical coordination, slow processing, and trouble learning. Alcohol is directly toxic to this part of the brain. Improving the cerebellum through coordination exercises can improve your prefrontal cortex and also help your judgment and your body.

BRIEF BRAIN SYSTEM SUMMARY

- Prefrontal cortex—judgment, forethought, planning, and impulse control
- Anterior cingulate gyrus—shifting attention
- Deep limbic system—sets emotional tone; involved with mood and bonding
- Basal ganglia—integrates thoughts, feelings, and movements; involved with pleasure
- Temporal lobes—memory, mood stability, and temper issues; "what pathway"
- Parietal lobes—sensory processing and direction sense; "where pathway"
- Occipital lobes—vision and visual processing
- Cerebellum—motor coordination, thought coordination, processing speed, and judgment

---

PRINCIPLE #7

Many things hurt the brain and make it harder for you to get and keep the body you've always wanted. Many things help the brain and make it easier to get and keep a body you love.

You may be surprised to find out that common, everyday activities and behaviors are often the source of brain drain, which makes it more of a challenge to have a body you love. Here are some common things that can hurt your brain and body. Many of these behaviors and activities will be mentioned again in the upcoming solutions throughout this book. They are so vital to your brain and body health that they are worth repeating.

Physical trauma Severe injuries, concussions, and even mild trauma can affect every aspect of your health and well-being.

Drugs Marijuana, cocaine, ecstasy, methamphetamines, inhalants, and heroin seriously decrease brain function. Illegal drugs aren't the only culprits. Abusing prescription medications, such as Vicodin, OxyContin, and Xanax, can also hurt the brain. Drug abuse may make you feel better in the short term, but in the long term it may be a disaster for you, your looks, and your health. Drugs can drastically increase or decrease appetite, causing weight gain or weight loss, can sap your motivation and energy, and can lead to problems with your skin, teeth, and hair. Search www.youtube.com for before-and-after pictures of people on methamphetamines. The images will horrify you.

Alcohol You don't have to be a heavy drinker to hurt your brain. Even moderate amounts of alcohol can affect brain function. Studies show that people who drink every day have smaller brains than nondrinkers. When it comes to the brain, size matters! Excess drinking lowers activity in the PFC, the area responsible for judgment, forethought, and planning. That's why people make such stupid decisions when they have had a few too many—like stopping at the burger joint at three o'clock in the morning when they're trying to lose weight, having unprotected sex with someone they just met at a bar, or driving when they've had too much to drink.

Obesity Fat stores toxic materials. The more fat you have on your body, the worse for your brain. Obesity doubles the risk for Alzheimer's disease and has been associated with decreased brain tissue.

Hormonal abnormalities Abnormalities with your thyroid, estrogen, progesterone, testosterone, DHEA, or cortisol have all been implicated in both brain and body problems.

Malnutrition Your body renews all the cells in your body every few months. These new cells draw on all the foods you consume, so you literally are what you eat. If you eat a junk-food diet, you will have a junk-food brain and a junk-food body. As we will see throughout the book, low levels of vitamins, especially vitamin D, minerals, and omega-3 fatty acids are also harmful to brain tissue and your body.

Chronic inflammation in the body Chronic inflammation constricts blood flow to the brain and heart and is now thought to be at the center of many diseases, including diabetes, heart disease, obesity, and Alzheimer's disease.

Low blood flow Blood flow is important because it carries oxygen, sugar, vitamins, and nutrients to the brain, and it gets rid of toxins. Anything that decreases blood flow to an organ, such as nicotine, too much caffeine, or a lack of exercise, prematurely ages it. Nowhere is this more true than for your brain.

Chronic stress Difficult marriages, demanding jobs, and financial problems all cause chronic stress. When you constantly feel stressed, your brain tells your body to secrete higher amounts of the stress hormone cortisol. At elevated levels, cortisol increases your appetite and cravings for sugar, making you fat, bumps up your skin's oil production, making you more prone to pimples, increases muscle tension and chronic pain, increases blood pressure, and raises your risk for many serious health conditions.

Sleep deprivation Getting less than six hours of sleep a night lowers overall brain function and causes your brain to release hormones that increase your appetite and cravings for high-sugar snacks like candy, cakes, and cookies. People who don't get enough sleep tend to eat more calories and gain weight. Skimping on shut-eye also prematurely ages your skin and leaves you with dark, puffy circles under your eyes.

Smoking Smoking constricts blood flow to the brain and all the organs in your body, including your skin. Most people can tell if a person is a smoker because his skin looks older than he is. I can tell you that their brains look that way too. Smoking is linked with many serious brain and health problems.

Too much caffeine Drinking too much caffeinated coffee, tea, sodas, or energy beverages restricts blood flow to the brain, dehydrates the brain, body, and skin, and fools the brain into thinking it does not need to sleep, which are all bad things for your brain and body.

Too much TV Watching too much TV can be harmful for your brain and body. Excessive TV watching has been associated with ADD in children and Alzheimer's disease in adults. Watching more than two hours of TV a day also significantly increases your risk for obesity.

Violent video games Playing violent video games has led to an increased rate of violence and learning problems. With brain imaging, we see that video games work in the same area as cocaine, and kids and adults tend to get hooked on them like a drug. Spending more than two hours a day playing video games increases the risk of being overweight.

Dehydration Your body consists of 70 percent water, and your brain is 80 percent water. If you aren't drinking enough water, you reduce brain function. You can also expect to see thinner skin and more fine lines and wrinkles.

Lack of exercise When you don't exercise, you decrease blood flow to your brain, your body, and your genitals. It is well documented that a lack of physical activity can negatively affect your weight and overall health; it can also decrease sexual performance.

Negative thinking We have conducted studies that show that focusing on the things you don't like lowers brain activity, causes your heart to beat faster, increases blood pressure, and negatively affects many systems in your body. Negative thinking can also sabotage your efforts to lose weight, start an exercise program, or quit smoking.

Excessive texting and social networking on the Internet Neuroscientists have shown that spending too much time texting and social networking leads to attention problems and may cause difficulties communicating face-to-face. It also takes time away from physical activities, making you more prone to an uptick in your weight and a decrease in your general health.

I developed a high school course about practical brain science to teach teenagers how to love and care for their brains. It is being used in forty states and seven countries. Every time we talk about the things that hurt the brain, some sarcastic student pipes up and asks, "How can I have any fun if I have to avoid all of these things?" Our response is simple. Who has more fun—the person with the good brain or the person with the bad brain? No matter what your age, the person who has more fun is the one with the healthy brain.

The guy with the good brain is better at sticking to a diet and exercise plan, which keeps him fit and healthy and gives him lots of energy to play golf with potential clients or go dancing with his wife. The guy with the bad brain might impulsively overeat, which leads to an expanding waistline, type 2 diabetes, and less enjoyment of life. Who is having more fun? The woman with the healthy brain is more likely to sleep well and wake up feeling and looking refreshed, which gives her more confidence in her relationship and keeps her alert at work. The woman with lower brain function might skimp on snoozing, making her feel tired, which affects her job performance and prevents her from getting promoted. It also makes her look tired, which lowers her self-esteem and causes her to withdraw from her romantic partner. Who is having more fun?

I have great news for you! After years of analyzing brain scans and treating patients, I have discovered that there are many simple things you can do on a daily basis to boost your brain function. These daily prescriptions can also be the key to a better body. The rest of the book will contain many ideas for enhancing brain function. Here are just a few things you can do to start.

Protect your brain. Be conscious of how precious it is to you and your loved ones.

Eat a good diet. Getting good nutrition is essential to good brain function and to a better body. A healthy diet includes lean protein, fruits, vegetables, nuts, and healthy fats like olive oil. Studies show that your brain works better if you eat nine servings of fruits and vegetables a day.

Take daily vitamins, minerals, and fish oil. Because most of us do not get all the nutrients we need from the foods we eat, I recommend that everybody take a daily multivitamin and mineral supplement. I also urge people to take a daily fish oil supplement, which can decrease inflammation and boost blood flow to the brain and can help to combat depression, which has been associated with being obese as well as many other health conditions.

Exercise. When it comes to the brain, exercise acts like the fountain of youth. It boosts blood flow, increases the brain's use of oxygen, and improves your brain's response to stress. It is the single most important thing you can do to keep your brain healthy and is one of the best ways to change your shape and improve your mood, energy level, sexual performance, and overall health.

Get enough sleep. Getting at least seven hours of sleep at night has been shown to help keep your brain functioning at optimal levels, keeps your appetite in check, and helps your skin look younger.

Meditate. Meditation activates the most thoughtful part of the brain, so you can make better and more intelligent decisions.

Relax. Learning how to counteract stress and calm your body helps your brain work better, puts you in a better mood, reduces high blood pressure, and protects you from disease.

Practice gratitude. When you focus on what you love, your brain works better, you are more coordinated, and you feel better. Write down five things you are grateful for every day. In just three weeks you will notice a significant positive difference in your level of happiness.

Have more sex. Safe sex, and especially sex in a loving committed relationship, is good medicine for your brain and your body, helping you reduce stress, boost immunity, live longer, and more.

Balance your hormones. Hormones, such as estrogen and testosterone, play a key role in maintaining the health and vitality of your brain and body.

Treat mental disorders. A strong link between mental disorders and physical illnesses and conditions has been well established. Treating mental conditions improves brain function and general health and well-being.

As you can see, the way you live day to day is making your brain and body either better or worse. Every day you need to ask yourself which brain and which body you want. Do you want the unhealthy brain that makes you struggle with weight problems, bad moods, and health conditions? Or do you want the healthy brain that makes it easier for you to look and feel your best? The choice is yours.

PRINCIPLE #8

Brain imaging gives great insight into healing
the brain so you can have a better body.

In my practice, I do a lot of couples work. Rob and his wife came to see me because they weren't getting along. Like many men, he thought he was fine and that his wife just needed to relax and be more accepting. But when I looked at his fifty-six-year-old brain (Image 1.5), it looked like he was eighty years old. Surprised, I asked him what he was doing to hurt his brain.

"Nothing," he said.

"Really?" I replied. "How much do you drink?"

"Not very much." (In my experience as a psychiatrist, I've learned that whenever I get the answer "not very much," I always have to ask the follow-up question.)

"What's not very much?"

"Oh, maybe I have three or four drinks a day."

"Every day?"

"Yeah, every day. But it is never a problem. I never get drunk."

His brain told me that it was a huge problem. Frightened by his scan, he followed my instructions to stay away from alcohol. Plus, he developed brain envy and wanted a better brain, so he started on our brain-healthy program. Four months later I did a follow-up scan, which looked much better. By then, his relationship with his wife was stronger than ever, and he felt like he was thirty years younger.

Brain imaging helped me figure out what was troubling Rob. It has also taught us that when your brain looks old, your body often does, too. If you have decreased blood flow to your brain, odds are you have decreased blood flow to your skin, making it dull and wrinkled. You also likely have decreased blood flow to your organs, making them less functional, and to your genitals, making sexual function and enjoyment much more difficult.

Scanning the brain also helps us detect trouble within specific brain systems. For example, if you have poor PFC activity, chances are you are going to be more impulsive. Having high ACG activity means you are likely to be more compulsive. When your basal ganglia are overactive, you may be anxious and might eat to calm anxiety. With too much activity in your deep limbic system, you may feel sad and blue and might eat to medicate your sadness. If you have low cerebellar activity, your processing speed is

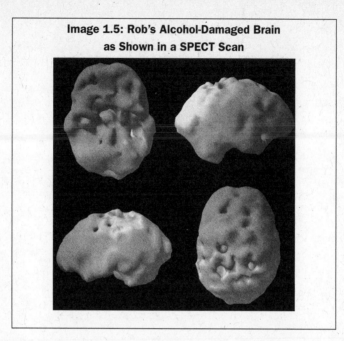

Image 1.5: Rob's Alcohol-Damaged Brain as Shown in a SPECT Scan

reduced and you will have trouble organizing and following through on your health plans.

With the help of imaging, we have learned that conditions such as obesity, depression, anxiety, and addictions are not single or simple disorders and that one treatment plan does not fit everyone. Imaging helps us understand individual patients so that we can develop treatment plans specifically tailored to you. Depending on your individual situation, your brain may need to be stimulated or it may need to be calmed down. If we never looked at the brain, how would we know the best way to treat you?

Does this mean that you have to get a brain scan in order to change your brain and change your body? No! My books have been translated into more than thirty languages, and I realize that not everyone is able to get a brain scan. That's why I have developed a series of checklists to help you predict areas of strength and weakness in your brain. The Amen Clinics Abbreviated Brain Systems Questionnaire can be found in

ACTION STEP

Remember that having a beautiful brain clearly connects to having a beautiful body. So if you want to have a better body, ask yourself, What do I need to do to have a beautiful brain?

Appendix B and an extended version of the test is online at www.amenclinics.com/cybcyb. These questionnaires are the next best thing to getting a brain scan and they have helped hundreds of thousands of people better target treatment for themselves. Of course, you should always talk to your own health care practitioner before embarking on a treatment program.

PRINCIPLE #9

One prescription does not work for everyone—we are all unique and you need to understand how your own personal brain functions.

Why would a doctor NEVER give a patient the diagnosis of chest pain? Because it is a symptom. It is too broad, and it has far too many causes to be considered a diagnosis or a single entity. What can cause chest pain? Many problems that range from the top of your head all the way to your pelvis, such as grief, panic attacks, hyperthyroidism, pneumonia, lung cancer, toxic fumes, a heart attack, abnormal heart rhythm, heart infection, rib injuries, indigestion, gastric reflux esophagitis, gallbladder stones, liver disease, kidney disease, and pancreatic cancer. Chest pain has many different possible causes and many possible treatments.

In the same way, what can cause obesity? Again, many different problems, such as a poor diet, no exercise, low thyroid, pituitary tumors, certain forms of depression, and some medications. Obesity can be caused by low activity in the brain, causing people to eat impulsively, or by overall increased activity in the brain, causing people to be anxious overeaters. Obesity can be caused by increased anterior cingulate hyperactivity (the compulsive sort of obesity) or by increased deep limbic activity (the emotional kind of overeating) or a combination of these plus still other problems. There are many different types of obesity.

How does chest pain relate to obesity, skin problems, low energy, or depression? All of these problems are just symptoms, not causes. As such, many physicians and patients view these common problems as single or simple disorders. Since they view these disorders in a simplistic way, they often have the idea that one treatment fits everyone with a certain disorder. From a brain imaging perspective this attitude just does not make sense, as there is not one type of obesity, stress response, anxiety, or depression. Understanding your individual variability is critical to getting the right help, whether it is to help your mood, your focus, your weight, or your overall health.

PRINCIPLE #10

Yes, you can change your brain and body!

This is one of the most exciting breakthroughs in medicine. By targeting specific interventions and lifestyle changes, you can improve your brain and your body. Working to enhance your brain can be the answer if you've been struggling with diets your entire life, have never been able to stick with a fitness routine, have been trying to quit smoking for years, or want to improve your overall health.

> **ACTION STEP**
>
> To get the body you want, you need to believe in your ability to change your brain.

Think of Becca, the impulsive, obese woman I mentioned in the introduction to this book. With low activity in her PFC, she wasn't capable of controlling her impulsive eating. It was only when treatment helped heal her brain that she was finally able to stick with a brain-healthy diet that allowed her to shed eighty pounds.

In my practice, I have seen this same pattern many times. When I boost someone's PFC, they become more thoughtful, more reliable, more consistent, and better able to follow through with a health plan. The same thing happens when we optimize other areas of the brain. When we calm someone's ACG, they become less worried, less negative, and happier, and they get better sleep, which helps them get a body they love. Stabilizing the temporal lobes improves memory under stress, which helps people remember what they need to do to reach their goals. Calming the basal ganglia makes people more relaxed and happier and results in fewer headaches and digestive problems. Boosting the cerebellum helps people learn better, makes them more apt to stick with a brain-healthy program, and improves athletic performance—yes, it can even improve your batting average or free-throw percentage.

The Brain-Body Solution

Brain Robbers	Brain Enhancers
Ignoring the health of your brain	Brain envy
Brain injuries	Brain protection
Alcohol or drug abuse	Multiple vitamins
Excessive caffeine	Fish oil
Smoking	Deep breathing
Excessive stress	Relaxation practice
Negative thinking	Gratitude
Poor diet	Healthy diet
Lack of sleep, poor sleep	Healthful, restful sleep
Lack of exercise	Exercise
Environmental toxins	Clean environment
Excessive TV	New learning
Excessive video games, cell phones, text messaging, computer time	Meditation
Dehydration	Hydration
Unbalanced hormones	Balanced hormones
Untreated mental disorders	Mental health

PART TWO

CHANGE YOUR BRAIN, CHANGE YOUR WEIGHT

2

THE CRAVING SOLUTION

Use Your Brain to Increase Your Willpower and Calm the Urges That Prevent You from Achieving Your Goals

From craving is born grief, from craving is born fear.
For one freed from craving, there's no grief—so how fear?

—Buddha

I had been good all day. I had a protein-fruit shake for breakfast; a spinach salad with turkey, blueberries, and walnuts for lunch; and sweet red bell pepper and apple slices with a little almond butter in the afternoon. All seemed right with my relationship with food, until I went to the Los Angeles Lakers basketball game. I know how to eat when I am away from home. But this night my brother bought a huge caramel apple with peanuts. I find that I now have total focus, not on the game, but on the sticky, gooey, sweet apple.

Our grandfather was a candy maker and some of my best memories are standing on a stool at the stove with him when I was a little boy making and then, of course, eating candy. Sweets have always been an emotional food for me. I am named after my grandfather, and he was my best friend growing up. Yet, I know how tired and foggy a sugar load makes me feel twenty to thirty minutes later.

Nonetheless, I am still totally focused on my brother's caramel apple. I try not to look at it, but the urge to look, sort of like when you are next to a very pretty woman, nudges me in that direction. The memories of the sweet taste try to hijack my brain. Dopamine, the pleasure and motivation brain chemical, pushes on an area in my brain called the nucleus accumbens, in the basal ganglia, which drives me toward asking for a piece, or heck, just getting up and buying an apple of my own. My prefrontal cortex, the brain's brake, fights back. Eating well earlier that day has given me a good blood sugar level, which helps to protect me against my urges. "I'll be back," I tell my brother, and I take a brief walk to reset my brain, let him finish the apple, and get my mind back on the game.

I come from a family of not only candy makers but also amazing cooks and overweight people. My brother, whom I adore, is at least one hundred pounds overweight. My grandfather, also overweight, had a heart attack in his sixties. If I was not focused on taking care of my brain, eating well, and exercise, I would, for sure, be overweight too. I am grateful for my neuroscience background, because it shows me how to maintain control over my urges.

In this chapter, I will share with you what I have learned on how to have the willpower to control your cravings to stay on track toward your goals of having a healthy brain and a vibrant body.

THE CIRCUITRY OF CONTROL

Understanding the brain circuits of willpower and self-control is an important step in gaining mastery of your brain and body. There are centers in the brain responsible for focus, judgment, and impulse control (the prefrontal cortex, in the front third of the brain). There is also a pleasure and motivation center, called the nucleus accumbens, which is part of the basal ganglia, large structures deep in the brain. The nucleus accumbens provides the passion and motivation that is one of the main drivers of behavior. Additionally, the brain has emotional memory centers that trigger behavior.

According to my friend, addiction specialist Mark Laaser, Ph.D., "the arousal template" in the emotional memory centers underlies many behaviors that get out of control. It is important to understand where you were and how old you were when you experienced your first pleasurable or arousing experience, such as standing at the stove making fudge with my grandfather when I was four years old. This intense, emotionally pleasurable experience often lays the neural tracks for later addictions, even if the experience happened as early as age two or three. The first experience gets locked into the brain, and when you get older, you seek to repeat the experience because it was the way you had the initial arousal or pleasurable experience, like the first time you tasted fudge, had sex, fell in love, or used cocaine. Understanding the triggers for emotional eating, smoking, or drinking can be very helpful to breaking addictions.

Four neurotransmitters are also important to mention here.

1. Dopamine is often thought of as the pleasure, motivation, and drive chemical in the brain. Cocaine and stimulants like Ritalin boost dopamine in the brain. Dopamine is often associated with "saliency," or the relative importance of something. At the moment I saw the caramel apple, it became much more salient or important in my mind.

2. Serotonin is thought of as the happy, antiworry, flexibility chemical. Most of the current antidepressants work on this neurotransmitter. When serotonin levels are low, people tend to suffer with anxiety, depression, and obsessive thinking.

3. GABA is an inhibitory neurotransmitter that calms or helps to relax the brain.

4. Endorphins are the brain's own natural pleasure and painkilling chemicals.

The relative strength and weakness of each of these brain areas and each of these neurotransmitters goes a long way in determining how much control we have over ourselves and how well we are able to stick to our plans, even around caramel apples with peanuts at the Lakers game. They all work together symphonically to give us beautiful control over our lives. When they are out of balance, the noise can be very irritating.

BRAIN AREAS INVOLVED WITH CRAVING AND WILLPOWER
- Prefrontal cortex (PFC)—focus, judgment, and impulse control
- Basal ganglia (nucleus accumbens)—pleasure and motivation center
- Deep limbic (emotional memory centers)—triggers of behavior

BRAIN CHEMICALS INVOLVED WITH CRAVING AND WILLPOWER
- Dopamine—motivation, saliency, drive, stimulant
- Serotonin—happiness, antiworrying, calming
- GABA—inhibitory, calming, relaxing
- Endorphins—pleasure and painkilling properties

In a healthy brain, there is good judgment and emotional control by a competent prefrontal cortex (PFC), but also plenty of emotion and drive from the deep limbic system to stay on track and get things done. Figure 2.1 shows a healthy self-control circuit. Healthy dopamine levels can drive passion, especially in the context of good activity in the PFC, which acts as the reins or the brake so you do not get out of control. Low levels of dopamine are associated with certain problems that rob us of motivation, such as Parkinson's disease, some forms of depression, and ADD. Addictions occur when the drive circuits hijack the brain and take over control.

When these chemicals and brain areas are in balance, we can be focused and goal oriented and have control over our cravings; we can walk away from caramel apples, chocolate cake, the bag of chips, French fries, and the myriad of other unhealthy choices. When these chemicals and brain areas are troubled (Figure 2.2), we often get off track and can do serious damage to ourselves.

For example, having low activity in the PFC from a head injury, poor sleep, persistent drug or alcohol use, or inheriting ADD, makes it more likely you

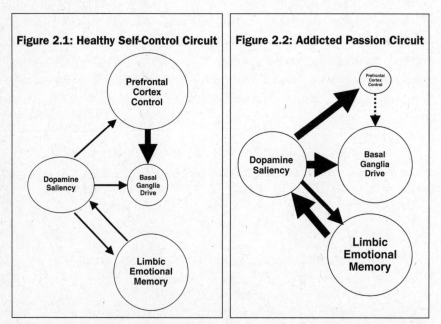

In the healthy self-control circuit, the prefrontal cortex (PFC) is strong and there is good balance between the chemical dopamine and the basal ganglia (BG) and limbic or emotional circuits in the brain. In the addicted circuit, the PFC is weak, so it has little control over unbridled passions that drive behaviors. Addiction actually changes the brain in a negative way, making it harder to apply the brakes to harmful behaviors. In the nonaddicted brain, the PFC is constantly assessing the value of incoming information and the appropriateness of the planned response, applying the brakes or inhibitory control as needed. In the addicted brain, this control circuit becomes impaired through drug abuse, ADD, sleep deprivation, or a brain injury, losing much of its inhibitory power over the circuits that drive response to stimuli deemed salient.

will have impulse-control problems and poor self-supervision. Even though the goal would be to stop drinking, hold the cigarettes, or maintain a healthy weight, you do not have the willpower (or the PFC power) to say no on a regular basis.

I once treated a forty-two-year-old woman who failed six alcohol treatment programs. Her impulse control was virtually zero. She could not be given a prescription for any medication because she would take them all at once. When I asked her initially if she had ever had a brain injury, she said no. But when I pushed her, she remembered that she had been kicked in the head by a horse when she was ten years old. Her brain SPECT scan showed severe PFC damage (Image 2.1). She had virtually no supervisor in her head. Comedian Dudley Moore once said that, "The best car safety device is a rearview mirror with a cop in it." The PFC acts like the cop in your head, and when it shows this level of damage, most people are in serious trouble. If I did not address the damaged PFC, she would never be well. Giving her a medication to enhance PFC function was very helpful to her.

If you have suffered an emotional trauma or you are under a lot of stress, the feel-good chemicals, such as serotonin and GABA, may be depleted and your emotional or limbic brain may become excessively active, making you feel sad. This makes you eat or drink in an attempt to calm your limbic brain.

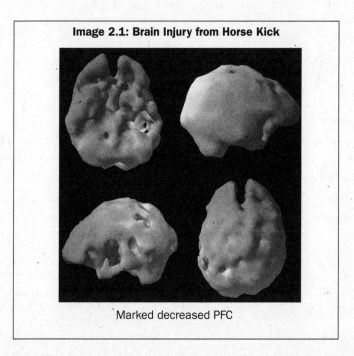

Image 2.1: Brain Injury from Horse Kick

Marked decreased PFC

MIT researchers demonstrated that simple carbohydrates, such as cookies or candy, boost serotonin levels. Many people unknowingly use these substances as a way to medicate their underlying negative feelings. But as with cocaine, over time these substances lose their effectiveness, and people engage in the corresponding behaviors not so much for the high or good feelings as for the attempt to prevent the terrible feelings of withdrawal.

Likewise, if you have engaged in excessive amounts of pleasure or used cocaine or too many excessively pleasurable foods, your brain may have been exposed to too much dopamine. Over time, it becomes numb to it, and it takes more and more to get the same pleasurable response. Keeping these brain chemicals and systems in balance is critical to maintaining focus and control over your cravings.

Anything that decreases activity to the brain, especially to the PFC, robs you of good judgment and self-control. Head injuries are obvious. Protect your brain. Poor sleep has been associated with overall decreased brain activity. Strive to get at least seven hours a night (see Chapter 10, "The Sleep Solution").

REGAINING CONTROL—BALANCE YOUR BRAIN SYSTEMS

1. Boost Your Prefrontal Cortex

To gain control over willpower and cravings, it is critical to strengthen your PFC. To do so:

- Treat any PFC problems that may exist, such as ADD, toxic exposure, or brain trauma. (See Chapter 15, "The Brain Health Solution.")
- Get good sleep—at least seven hours, more is better—to maintain adequate PFC blood flow.
- Maintain a healthy blood sugar level by eating frequent smaller meals. In a 2007 article by Matthew Gailliot and Roy Baumeister, the authors outline the critical nature of blood sugar levels and self-control. They write that self-control failures are more likely to occur when blood sugar is low. Low blood sugar levels can make you feel hungry, irritable, or anxious—all of which make you more likely to make poor choices. Many everyday behaviors can cause dips in blood sugar levels, including drinking alcohol, skipping meals, and consuming sugary snacks or beverages, which causes an initial spike in blood sugar then a crash about thirty minutes later.

Keeping glucose levels even throughout the day improves self-control. Several studies have examined the relationship between glucose and smoking cessation, and the majority of these studies have found that healthy glucose levels increase the likelihood of successfully quitting smoking. Coping with stress requires self-control because it requires that people make a concerted effort to control their attention, thoughts, and emotions. People with healthy blood sugar levels are therefore also able to manage stress more effectively than others. Maintaining your blood sugar levels with complex carbohydrates, lean protein, and healthy fat will significantly cut down on your cravings.

- Exercise to boost blood flow to the brain. Table tennis is a great choice. One study from Japan showed that ten minutes of table tennis boosted activity in the PFC.
- Practice meditation—numerous studies have found that it boosts activity and blood flow to the PFC.
- Create focused, written goals. The PFC is involved in planning and forethought. It needs clear direction. I have my patients do an exercise called the One-Page Miracle (OPM) because it makes such a dramatic difference in the lives of those who practice it. Here are the steps: On a piece of paper, write down the specific goals you have for your life, including your health, relationships, work, and money. There's a reason why your OPM includes more than just your physical goals. As you will learn throughout this book, your relationships, career, and financial situation—and the stress they can cause—all affect your body and your willpower.

Take your time with this exercise. Keep the paper with you so you can jot down ideas and goals as they come to you. After you complete your initial draft, place it somewhere where you are sure to see it every day, such as on the refrigerator, on your bathroom mirror, or on your desk at work. This way, on a daily basis, you will be focusing on what's important to you. When you are focused on what you want, it makes it much easier to match your behavior to make it happen. Ask yourself every day, Is my behavior today getting me what I want? Your mind is powerful and it makes happen what it sees. Focus and meditate on what you want. You will find that your willpower goes up dramatically. Here is an example.

TAMARA'S ONE-PAGE MIRACLE
What Do I Want for My Life?

RELATIONSHIPS—to be connected to those I love
> **Spouse/Significant other:** to maintain a close, kind, caring, loving partnership with my husband. I want him to know how much I care about him.
> **Family:** to be a firm, kind, positive, predictable presence in my children's lives. I want to help them develop into happy, responsible people. To continue to keep close contact with my parents, to provide support and love.
> **Friends:** to take time to maintain and nurture my relationships with my siblings

WORK—to be my best at work, while maintaining a balanced life. Specifically, for my work activities to focus on taking care of my current projects, doing activities targeted at obtaining new clients, and giving back to the community by doing some charity work each month. I will focus on my goals at work and not get distracted by things not directly related to my goals.

MONEY—to be responsible and thoughtful and help our resources grow
> **Short-term:** to be thoughtful of how our money is spent, to ensure it is directly related to our family's and my needs and goals
> **Long-term:** to save 10 percent of everything I earn. I pay myself and my family before other things. I'll put this money away each month in a pension plan for retirement.

HEALTH—to be the healthiest person I can be
> **Weight:** to lose thirty pounds so my body mass index (BMI) will be in the normal range
> **Fitness:** to exercise for at least thirty minutes three days a week and to start taking martial arts lessons. I promise no head injuries here.
> **Nutrition:** to eat breakfast every day so I don't get really hungry until lunchtime. To prepare a sack lunch at least three days a week so I'm not tempted to go to the fast-food restaurant across from work. To eliminate diet sodas and reduce the amount of sugar I eat. To take a multivitamin and fish oil every day.
> **Physical health:** to lower my blood pressure and cholesterol levels
> **Emotional health:** to meditate for ten minutes every day to help me calm stress

MY ONE-PAGE MIRACLE
What Do I Want for My Life?

RELATIONSHIPS
    Spouse/Significant Other   _____

                                   _____

    Family   _____

                                     _____

    Friends   _____

                                     _____

WORK   _____

                                     _____

                                     _____

MONEY
    Short-term   _____
    Long-term   _____

HEALTH
    Weight   _____

                                     _____

    Fitness   _____

                                     _____

    Nutrition   _____

                                     _____

    Physical health   _____

                                     _____

    Emotional health   _____

                                     _____

Along the same lines, having a clearly written set of rules also helps to boost the PFC.

For example, one of my rules is to stay away from mayonnaise. I like it, but not enough to make it worth the calories. Here is an example of some helpful rules.

- I treat my body with respect.
- I read my One-Page Miracle daily.
- I look for ways to optimize my nutrition.
- I eat breakfast every day.
- I eat frequently enough during the day so that I do not get hungry or a low blood sugar level.
- I get seven to eight hours of sleep at night whenever possible.
- I exercise three or four times a week.
- I do not poison my body with toxins such as nicotine or my mind with persistent negative thoughts.
- If I break a rule, I will not dwell on it and give up on the rest of the rules. I will be kind and forgiving.

No more than twelve rules. I once had a patient with obsessive-compulsive disorder who made up 108 rules.

Willpower is like a muscle. The more you use it, the stronger it gets. This is why good parenting is essential to helping children develop self-control. If we gave in to our six-year-old every time she wanted something, we would raise a spoiled, demanding child. By saying no, I teach her to be able to say no to herself. To develop willpower, you need to do the same thing for yourself. Practice saying no to the things that are not good for you, and over time, you will find it easier to do.

Long-term potentiation (LTP) is a very important concept. When nerve cell connections become strengthened, they are said to be potentiated. Whenever we learn something new, our brains make new connections. At first the connections are weak, which is why we do not remember new things unless we practice them over time. Practicing a behavior, such as saying no to the caramel apple, actually strengthens the willpower circuits in the brain. LTP occurs when nerve cell circuits are strengthened, practiced, and behaviors become almost automatic. Whenever

ACTION STEP
To improve your willpower, you have to practice it.

you give in to the caramel apple, it weakens willpower and makes it more likely you will not have any. You have to practice willpower, and your brain will make it easier for you.

2. Balance the Pleasure Centers and Calm Anxiety

As mentioned, the basal ganglia are large structures deep in the brain. They are involved with pleasure and motivation. When the basal ganglia are healthy, we feel happy and motivated. When they work too hard, we can be anxious or overly driven. When they are low in activity, we may feel low or unmotivated. Here are some ways to balance your pleasure centers.

- Be careful with too much technology. In Dr. Archibald Hart's book *Thrilled to Death*, he suggests that the evolution of technology in our society is wearing out our brain's pleasure centers. I believe it is having a very negative effect on our relationships and our bodies. With the onslaught of video games, text messaging, cell phones, Facebook, and Twitter, as well as online dating, pornography, and gambling, our pleasure centers are being worn out. Pretty soon, we will not be able to feel anything at all. As I mentioned above, our pleasure centers deep within the brain operate on a chemical called dopamine, which is the same chemical that cocaine stimulates and one of the main chemicals of new love. Whenever a little bit of dopamine is released, we feel pleasure. If dopamine is released too often or too strongly, we become desensitized to it and it takes more and more excitement to get the same response. More and more, I see people coming into our offices complaining about their partner or children being addicted to new technology.

Christina and Harold were having big problems in their relationship. Christina wanted more time with Harold, but he spent hours hooked on his video games. He became angry when she asked him to stop playing so much, and when he told her to stop nagging him, she moved out. Subsequently Harold became depressed and came to see us. This couple played out the same pattern I

> **ACTION STEP**
>
> Work to keep your pleasure centers healthy. Be careful with the high-excitement activities, limit video games, and stop ALWAYS being on your computer.

have seen with many other types of addictions—she didn't want to leave, but she didn't know what else to do.

As a society, we have unleashed massive amounts of technology on the population with virtually no study on what it all does to developing brains or to our families. We need to be more careful. Stop it. In a study sponsored by Hewlett-Packard, people who were addicted to their cell phones or their computers lost ten IQ points over a year. Find natural sources of pleasure, such as nature, a great conversation, and long, loving eye contact.

- Use relaxation techniques to help balance and calm this part of the brain.
- Engage in meaningful activities that give you motivation without putting you in overdrive.
- Use supplements to calm anxiety and balance the pleasure centers. These include vitamin B_6, magnesium, and N-acetyl-cysteine (NAC). See Appendix C, "The Supplement Solution," for more information.

3. Calm Your Brain's Emotional Centers and Eliminate Your Triggers

Emotional stresses and depression decrease willpower. If you have unresolved emotional issues, it is essential to understand and work through them, otherwise they will hijack your brain. Here are six tips to help get your emotions under control.

- Talk about what bothers you to someone close or a therapist. Talking about issues can help get them out of your head. If there has been past trauma, one of the psychotherapies I often recommend is called EMDR (eye movement desensitization and reprocessing). It is fast and very powerful. You can learn more about it at www.emdria.org.
- When you are upset, journal rather than eat, drink, or light up. Studies show that writing down your bothersome thoughts and feelings can have a healing effect.
- Write down five things you are grateful for every day. Our research suggests that focusing on gratitude helps to calm the deep limbic or emotional areas of the brain and enhances the judgment centers.
- Exercise. It not only boosts PFC activity, it also calms the limbic brain by boosting serotonin, the feel-good chemical.
- Correct the ANTs, or automatic negative thoughts (see Chapter 13, "The ANT Solution"). You do not have to believe every thought

that goes through your head. Whenever you feel sad, mad, or nervous, write down the thoughts that are bothering you and talk back to them.

- Try the supplement SAMe to help calm this area of the brain and boost the PFC. See Appendix C, "The Supplement Solution," for more information.

REGAINING CONTROL—BALANCE YOUR BRAIN CHEMISTRY

Beyond brain-system balancing, it is also important to balance the chemicals that drive behavior.

1. Dopamine

Dopamine is the chemical of motivation, saliency, drive, and stimulation. It is the chemical that both cocaine and Ritalin stimulate in the brain. Low levels are associated with low motivation, low energy, poor concentration, impulse-control problems, some forms of depression, Parkinson's disease, and ADD. You can boost dopamine levels by:

- Doing intense physical exercise
- Eating a protein-rich meal
- Working at a job or organization that is exciting or deeply meaningful
- Being wary of excitement-seeking behaviors, which may wear out your pleasure centers, deplete dopamine, and make you feel numb or unable to feel pleasure
- Taking natural supplements, such as L-tyrosine or SAMe. See Appendix C, "The Supplement Solution," for more information.

2. Serotonin

Serotonin is the chemical of feeling peaceful, happy, and flexible. When it is low, people suffer with some forms of depression, along with anxiety, obsessive thinking (such as about the caramel apple), or compulsive behaviors. You boost serotonin by

- Engaging in physical exercise, which allows the serotonin precursor L-tryptophan, a relatively small molecule, greater access to the brain.
- Practicing willpower. Giving in to obsessive behaviors solidifies them in the brain and establishes nerve tracks to make them more

automatic. Practicing willpower actually does the opposite and has been found to change the brain, much like serotonin medications, such as Prozac.

- Taking supplements, such as 5-hydroxytryptophan (5-HTP), L-tryptophan, inositol, or St. John's wort. Good scientific evidence supports 5-HTP's usefulness for helping people lose weight. Inositol is a natural chemical found in the brain that is reported to help neurons use serotonin more efficiently. St. John's wort comes from the flowers of the Saint-John's-wort plant and seems to increase serotonin availability in the brain. See Appendix C, "The Supplement Solution," for more information.

3. GABA

GABA, or gamma-aminobutyric acid, is an amino acid that helps to regulate brain excitability and calms overfiring in the brain. GABA and GABA enhancers, such as the anticonvulsant gabapentin and L-theanine (found in green tea), function to inhibit the excessive firing of neurons, which results in a feeling of calm and more self-control. Low levels of GABA have been found in many psychiatric disorders, including anxiety and some forms of depression. Rather than overeat or drink or use drugs to calm your anxiety, natural ways to boost GABA may help. I often recommend GABA supplements.

- Glycine is also an inhibitory neurotransmitter, which means it calms brain activity. It is an important protein in the brain, and recent studies have demonstrated its effectiveness in the treatment of obsessive-compulsive disorder and in reducing pain.
- L-theanine, one of the components of green tea, has also been shown to boost GABA, while at the same time helping with concentration and mental alertness.

4. Endorphins

Endorphins are chemicals linked to feeling pleasure and eliminating pain. They are the body's own natural morphine or heroinlike substances. These substances are heavily involved in addiction and the loss of control. Natural ways to boost endorphins include the following:

- Exercise, which is why some people feel a runner's high when they exercise intensely

- Acupuncture, which has been found to be effective for a number of pain syndromes. Its positive painkilling effect can be blocked by using endorphin-blocking drugs, such as naltrexone.
- Hypnosis, which has been shown to be helpful in pain syndromes

The craving solution involves balancing the brain areas and chemistry of pleasure and control. It involves using your PFC as the master controller and making sure there is a bridle on the pleasure and emotional centers to help them guide you to where you want to go.

The Craving Solution

Willpower Robbers	Willpower Boosters
Any brain problems	Brain health
Brain trauma	Focusing on brain protection
Poor sleep	Adequate sleep (at least seven hours)
Low blood sugar	Frequent small meals with at least some protein to maintain healthy blood sugar
Poor diet	Enriched diet
Alcohol	Freedom from alcohol
ADHD	Clearly focused, written goals (see One-Page Miracle, page 44)
Some forms of depression	Journaling when sad or anxious
Anxiety	Meditation for relaxation and to boost the PFC
Negative thinking	Killing the ANTs (automatic negative thoughts)
Focusing on problems and fears	Gratitude practice
Bad habits, giving in	Practicing willpower
Too much pleasure	Being careful with too much pleasure or too much technology
Artificial forms of pleasure	Finding natural sources of pleasure
Negative or meaningless behaviors	Engaging in positive and meaningful activities

Willpower Robbers	**Willpower Boosters**
Social isolation	Social support
Being in denial about problems	Effectively treating any brain problems
Lack of exercise	Exercise
Denial of feelings	Understanding emotional triggers
	Decreasing cravings with B_6, magnesium, and NAC
	Boosting dopamine (L-tyrosine, DL-phenylalanine, SAMe)
	Boosting serotonin (5-HTP, L-tryptophan, inositol, St. John's wort)
	Boosting GABA (GABA, glycine, L-theanine)
	Boosting endorphins (exercise, acupuncture, hypnosis)

3

THE WEIGHT SOLUTION

USE YOUR BRAIN TO ACHIEVE
YOUR OPTIMAL WEIGHT

I am what I ate . . . and I'm frightened.

—BILL COSBY

Rebecca, forty-four, couldn't stop herself from eating, especially at night. She thought about food constantly throughout the day. The thoughts haunted her, even though she did not want to have them. Over eight years, she had gained nearly ten pounds per year and was now eighty pounds overweight despite trying many diets and going to multiple weight-loss clinics. She hated how she looked and was thoroughly disgusted with herself. The Atkins diet—very high protein and low carbohydrate—made her irritable and emotional. Diet pills made her anxious. She felt as though she needed a glass—or two or three—of alcohol at night to settle her worries, but the extra calories were certainly not helping her weight problem. She came to our clinics because she was starting to have marital problems, in part because her husband was upset about her weight, and also because she had trouble letting go of hurts, held grudges, and worried incessantly.

Rick, thirty-seven, was growing larger by the year. At five feet eight inches tall, he was over 250 pounds. As a highly successful salesman for a large West Coast liquor company, he was always on the run and attended many fancy dinners and sporting events. His wife was starting to complain about his weight, which made him angry. Why doesn't she just love me the way I am? he thought, even though she married him when he was nearly seventy-five pounds lighter a decade earlier. Growing up, Rick had problems with focus and impulsivity. He barely finished his first year of college when he found a job in the liquor industry that he loved. Rick brought his son to our clinic for school-related problems, much like the problems Rick had experienced in school. After he saw how much better his son was on treatment, Rick decided to get an evaluation as well.

Cherrie, fifty-two, had been bulimic as a teenager, and the hidden truth for her was that she still had bouts of bingeing and purging, especially during times of stress. Cherrie was chronically thirty pounds overweight and hated how she looked. She would not undress in front of her husband and found that she often picked on him as a way to not have to have sex or be seen naked. Her own thoughts were extremely negative, and she vacillated between being obsessive about her work and housekeeping to being overwhelmed and disorganized. Cherrie grew up in an alcoholic home and had trouble talking about her feelings and trusting others.

She had tried a number of diet programs without success, until the fen-phen craze of the 1990s. On fen-phen, a combination of medications that increased the neurotransmitters serotonin (fenfluramine) and dopamine (phentermine), she did amazingly well, losing the unwanted pounds and feeling more emotionally stable than at any other time in her life. When the fen-phen was pulled from the market because fenfluramine was associated with a deadly illness called pulmonary hypertension, Cherrie relapsed and went back to her emotional roller coaster and lack of success at losing and keeping off weight. Cherrie came to see us on the advice of her sister, whom we were seeing for issues of depression.

Jerry, sixty-two, was baffled by his weight problem. As a child, he was fit, athletic, energetic, and loved being outside in the sun. He was raised in Southern California and made the most of the beach, surfing, and volleyball. In his thirties, still in great shape, he got a new job in the Northwest as a supervisor at Boeing. He loved his job, the new responsibility, and the income, but over time he noticed that particularly in the winter, his mood and energy would lag, and he started to gain weight despite trying to work out. Over time, he retained more of the weight he gained in the winter than what he could manage to lose in the summer. His weight gain and loss was like a yo-yo that was losing steam. He also complained of many more aches and pains. He came to our Northwest clinic to get a handle on his moods and weight.

Connie, twenty-eight, seemed to be constantly eating. She munched on the way to work, at work, on the way home, and late into the night. She found that when she tried to go without eating for a few hours, she felt anxious and nervous. She often felt a sense of dread and was often waiting for something bad to happen. She frequently complained of an irritable bowel, sore muscles, and headaches. Marijuana helped to calm her down in college, but it also gave her the munchies, so she used it only sporadically. Her weight continued to creep up; when she reached 165 pounds on her five-foot-two-inch frame, she knew something needed to be done. She came to our clinic because her family had complained about her level of anxiety and irritability.

Camille, sixty-four, could not keep on any weight. Two years before seeing us, she had gone through a difficult divorce, and the year before, her mother died. Camille had lost twenty-five pounds during that time and now none of her clothes fit. She had felt as if her whole system was in hyperdrive. She had trouble sleeping, her thoughts seemed to race, she had diarrhea, and both her heart rate and blood pressure were up. She came to our clinics to help calm her mind and body and put back on some weight.

ONE SIZE DOES *NOT* FIT EVERYONE

Rebecca, Rick, Cherrie, Jerry, Connie, and Camille all struggled with their weight. Yet they all had very different clinical presentations and brain patterns.

Rebecca was a compulsive overeater. She couldn't stop thinking about food. Her brain SPECT study showed too much activity in the front part of her brain (in an area called the anterior cingulate gyrus), likely due to low levels of the neurotransmitter serotonin. On a rational weight-loss program plus a regimen of 5-HTP to boost serotonin levels in her brain, she lost weight, felt much happier, was more relaxed, and got along better with her husband.

Rick was an impulsive overeater. He also had trouble controlling his behavior. His brain SPECT scan showed too little activity in his prefrontal cortex, likely due to low dopamine levels, so he had trouble supervising his own behavior. Like his son, he was also diagnosed with ADD. On treatment to boost his dopamine levels, he felt more focused and in better control of his impulses. Over the first year, he lost thirty-five pounds and was getting along better with his wife and child.

Cherrie was an impulsive-compulsive overeater. Cherrie had features of both impulsivity (the bulimia) and compulsivity (manifested by the repetitive negative thoughts and rigid behavior). Her brain SPECT scan showed areas in her prefrontal cortex that were both overactive and underactive, likely due to low serotonin and dopamine levels. In my research, I discovered that this pattern is common in children and grandchildren of alcoholics. On treatment to raise both serotonin and dopamine levels, she felt much more emotionally balanced and consistently lost weight.

Jerry was a SAD or emotional overeater. He struggled with his mood and weight, but only after he moved to a place where he got little sunlight. He suffered from seasonal affective disorder (SAD), which has been associated with low vitamin D levels, and his brain SPECT study showed increased activity in his emotional or limbic brain and decreased activity in his PFC. On a combination of vitamin D, bright light therapy, and SAMe, he did much better, experienced fewer pain symptoms, and returned to his premove weight over a two-year period.

Connie was an anxious overeater. She medicated her underlying anxiety with food. Her brain SPECT study showed increased activity in her basal ganglia, an area often associated with anxiety. By calming her anxiety with relaxation techniques and a combination of B_6, magnesium, and GABA, she stopped the constant grazing, felt more relaxed and more in control of her emotions and behavior. She lost twenty pounds over the next year and noticed a boost in her energy.

Camille was on adrenaline overload. This was causing her to waste away. The chronic intense stress from her divorce and the recent loss of her mother reset her brain and body to an overactive state. Her brain SPECT study showed overall increased activity in the deep centers of her brain, a pattern on SPECT we call the diamond pattern because of the hyperactivity of the different structures we see. On treatments to calm her brain—including a form of psychotherapy called EMDR for people who have been emotionally traumatized, plus phosphatidylserine, B_6, magnesium, and GABA—she was able to sleep, quiet her mind, and come back to a normal weight.

WHY MOST WEIGHT-MANAGEMENT APPROACHES DO NOT WORK

Weight-loss pills, clinics, books, programs, and cookbooks are everywhere you look. Why are there so many different approaches to weight loss and weight management? Why do they generally have such poor results? Why are people constantly searching for the next idea and the next fix? The problem with the whole notion of weight management is that one treatment, one program, or one method is advertised to work for everyone. Based on our brain imaging work with tens of thousands of patients, the premise for most weight-management programs that promote a single path or prescription is ridiculous. First, you need to know about your own individual brain and then target the interventions in a way that fits your own specific needs.

Looking at the descriptions below and taking the brief questionnaire in Appendix B, plus the extended online version at www.amenclinics.com/cybcyb, you will get an idea about how your own brain works and what specific needs you may have. Then, based on your answers, you will be better able to target the treatment interventions. Of course, you should do this in consultation with your own health-care provider.

SUMMARY OF THE AMEN CLINICS:
SIX TYPES OF WEIGHT-MANAGEMENT ISSUES

Type 1: The Compulsive Overeater

People with this type have trouble shifting their attention and tend to get stuck on thoughts of food or compulsive eating behaviors. They may also get stuck on anxious or depressing thoughts. The basic mechanism of this type is that they tend to get stuck or locked into one course of action. They tend to have trouble seeing options and want to have things their way. They struggle with cognitive inflexibility. This type is also associated with worry, holding grudges, and having problems with oppositional or argumentative behavior. Nighttime-eating syndrome, where people tend to gorge at night and not be hungry early in the day, usually fits this pattern.

The most common brain SPECT finding in this type is increased anterior cingulate gyrus activity, which is most commonly caused by low brain serotonin levels. High-protein diets, diet pills, and stimulants, such as Ritalin, usually make this type worse. Interventions to boost serotonin in the brain are generally the most helpful. From a supplement standpoint (see Appendix C), 5-HTP, L-tryptophan, St. John's wort, and the B vitamin inositol are helpful, as are the serotonin-enhancing medications, such as Prozac, Zoloft, and Lexapro. In fact, 5-HTP has good scientific evidence that it helps with weight loss, and in my experience, I have found that it works best for this type.

ACTION STEP

Behavioral interventions that boost serotonin to help compulsive overeaters:

- Exercise to allow more of the serotonin precursor, L-tryptophan, to get into the brain.
- If you get a negative or food-oriented thought in your head more than three times, get up and go do something to distract yourself.
- Make a list of ten things you can do instead of eating so you can distract yourself.
- People with this type always do better with choices, rather than edicts. Do not tell them where you are going to eat or what they are going to eat; give them choices.
- Avoid automatically opposing others or saying no, even to yourself.
- If you have trouble sleeping, try a glass of warm milk with a teaspoon of vanilla and a few drops of stevia.

Type 2: The Impulsive Overeater

People with this type struggle with impulsivity and trouble controlling their behavior, even though nearly every day they intend to eat well. "I am going to start my diet tomorrow" is their common mantra. This type results from too little activity in the brain's PFC. The PFC acts as the brain's supervisor. It helps with executive functions, such as attention span, forethought, impulse control, organization, motivation, and planning. When the PFC is underactive, people complain of being inattentive, distracted, bored, off task, and impulsive. This type is often seen in conjunction with ADD, which is associated with long-standing issues of short attention span, distractibility, disorganization, restlessness, and impulsivity.

Research published in the July 2008 issue of *Pediatrics* found that children and adolescents with ADD who do not currently take medications are at 1.5 times the risk of being overweight than non-ADD children. These individuals are more likely to be impulsive overeaters. On the other hand, those taking medication for ADD had 1.6 times more risk of being underweight compared to children without ADD, which is a side effect of their medication, which decreases appetite.

Impulsive overeaters may also be the result of some form of toxic exposure, a near-drowning accident, a brain injury to the front part of the brain, or a brain infection, such as chronic fatigue syndrome. The most common brain SPECT finding in this type is decreased activity in the PFC, which is most commonly associated with low brain dopamine levels. High-carbohydrate diets and serotonin-enhancing medications, such as Prozac, Zoloft, or Lexapro, or supplements, such as 5-HTP, usually make this type worse. Interventions to boost dopamine in the brain are generally the most helpful. From a supplement standpoint, green tea and rhodiola are helpful, as are stimulant medications, such as phentermine, Adderall, and Ritalin, which are commonly used to treat ADD.

ACTION STEP
Behavioral interventions that boost dopamine to help impulsive overeaters:

- Exercise, which helps increase blood flow and dopamine in the brain—especially doing an exercise you love.
- Clear focus—make a list of weight and health goals displayed where you can see it every day.
- Outside supervision—someone you trust checking in with you on a regular basis to help you stay focused.
- Avoid impulsively saying yes to offers for more food or drink and practice saying, "No, thank you, I'm full."

Type 3: The Impulsive-Compulsive Overeater

People with this type have a combination of both impulsive and compulsive features. The brain SPECT scans tend to show low activity in the PFC (associated with impulsivity, likely due to low dopamine levels) and high activity in the anterior cingulate gyrus (associated with compulsivity and low serotonin levels). This pattern is common in the children or grandchildren of alcoholics. People with this mixed type tend to have done very well emotionally and behaviorally on the fen-phen combination, which raised both dopamine and serotonin in the brain.

Using serotonin or dopamine interventions by themselves usually makes the problem worse. For example, using a serotonin medication or supplement helps to calm the compulsions but makes the impulsivity worse. Using a dopamine medication or supplement helps to lessen the impulsivity but

---

ACTION STEP
Behavioral interventions that boost both serotonin and dopamine to help impulsive-compulsive overeaters:

- Exercise.
- Set goals.
- Avoid automatically opposing others or saying no, even to yourself.
- Avoid impulsively saying yes.
- Have options.
- Distract yourself if you get a thought stuck in your head.

---

increases the compulsive behaviors. Treatments to raise dopamine and serotonin together, with either a combination of supplements, such as green tea and 5-HTP, or medications, such as Prozac and Ritalin, have worked the best in my experience.

Type 4: The SAD or Emotional Overeater

People with this type often eat to medicate underlying feelings of boredom, loneliness, or depression. Their symptoms can range from winter blues to mild chronic sadness (termed dysthymia) to more serious depressions. Other symptoms may include a loss of interest in usually pleasurable activities; decreased libido; periods of crying; feelings of guilt, helplessness, hopelessness, or worthlessness; sleep and appetite changes; low energy levels; suicidal thoughts; and low self-esteem. The SPECT findings that correlate with this type are markedly increased activity in the deep limbic areas of the brain and decreased PFC activity.

When this type occurs in the winter, it is usually in more northern climates, where there is often a deficiency in sunlight and vitamin D levels. Low vitamin D levels have been associated with depression, memory problems, obesity, heart disease, and immune suppression. In recent years, there is an increase in vitamin D deficiencies even in southern and western states in the summer. There are two reasons for this: People are wearing sunscreen more than ever, so they are not being exposed to the sun even when they are outside, and they are spending more and more time indoors on their computers or watching TV. Some researchers believe nearly half of the U.S. population suffers from a vitamin D deficiency. I screen all of my patients for it by ordering a 25-hydroxy vitamin D level. To treat SAD or emotional overeaters, check vitamin D levels and correct them when low by taking a vitamin D supplement. Bright light therapy may be helpful to correct vitamin D problems, help with mood states, and help people lose weight.

There is evidence that bright light therapy might also enhance the effectiveness of physical activity for weight loss. In studies, it significantly reduced the binge-eating episodes in people with bulimia and is an effective treatment for SAD. Research studies have also shown it to be more effective than Prozac for these patients. Using bright light therapy in the workplace was effective in improving mood, energy, alertness, and productivity.

ACTION STEP
Behavioral interventions that boost mood to help SAD or emotional overeaters:
- Exercise to increase blood flow and multiple neurotransmitters in the brain.
- Kill the ANTs (automatic negative thoughts) that steal your happiness.
- Write down five things you are grateful for every day (this has been shown to increase your level of happiness in just three weeks).
- Volunteer to help others, which helps to get you outside of yourself and less focused on your own internal problems.
- Surround yourself with great smells, such as lavender.
- Try melatonin to help you sleep.
- Work to improve your relationships.

Also, make sure to check your DHEA blood levels. DHEA is a master hormone that has been found to be low in many people with depression and obesity. Supplementing with DHEA has good scientific evidence that it is helpful for weight loss in certain patients. Another helpful treatment for emotional overeaters is the natural supplement SAMe, in dosages of 400 to 1,600 mg. Be careful with SAMe if you have ever experienced a manic episode, and take it early in the day as it has energizing properties and may interfere with sleep. I like the medication Wellbutrin for this type, which has been shown to have weight-reducing properties.

Type 5: The Anxious Overeater
People with this type tend to use food to medicate underlying feelings of anxiety, tension, nervousness, and fear. They tend to feel uncomfortable in their

own skin. They may be plagued by feelings of panic, fear, and self-doubt, and suffer physical symptoms of anxiety as well, such as muscle tension, nail biting, headaches, abdominal pain, heart palpitations, shortness of breath, and sore muscles. It is as if they have an overload of tension and emotion. People with this type tend to predict the worst and look to the future with fear. They may be excessively shy, easily startled, and freeze in emotionally charged situations. The SPECT finding in this type is increased activity in the basal ganglia, which is commonly caused by low levels of the calming neurotransmitter GABA.

Interventions to boost GABA, by using B_6, magnesium, and GABA, are generally the most helpful. From a medication standpoint, the anticonvulsant Topamax has strong evidence that it is helpful for weight loss, and in my experience, it is especially helpful for this type. Relaxation therapies can also be helpful to calm this part of the brain.

ACTION STEP
Behavioral interventions that boost GABA and calm the brain to help anxious overeaters:

- Exercise.
- Try relaxation exercises, such as:
  - meditation
  - prayer
  - hypnosis
  - deep diaphragmatic breathing exercises
  - hand-warming techniques
- Kill the anxious ANTs.
- For sleep, try self-hypnosis, kava kava, or valerian root.

Type 6: The Adrenaline-Overload Anorexic

For most people, excess stress leads to weight gain. But some people have trouble keeping a healthy weight on their bodies when they're under a lot of stress. The stress causes them to go into an emotional overload state, and they start to waste away. Typically, these people's thoughts often go too fast, they tend to have trouble sleeping, they may experience diarrhea, and they often complain of memory problems. Their brain SPECT studies show overall increased activity, especially in the deep centers of their brains, similar to what I see with post-traumatic stress syndrome.

Treatments to calm the brain are generally the most helpful, including EMDR—eye movement desensitization and reprocessing (see www.emdria.org for more information)—hypnosis, and cognitive therapy. The supplements phosphatidylserine (PS), B$_6$, magnesium, and GABA are also helpful to calm the stress. There are not any current medications I use to help people gain weight. Any medications I prescribe depend on what other factors may be contributing to the current stress.

ACTION STEP
Behavioral interventions—the same as those recommended for anxious overeaters—that boost GABA and calm the brain to help adrenaline overload anorexics:

- Exercise.
- Try relaxation exercises, such as:
  - meditation
  - prayer
  - hypnosis
  - deep diaphragmatic breathing
  - hand-warming techniques
- Kill the anxious ANTs.
- For sleep, try self-hypnosis, kava kava, or valerian root.

Knowing your brain type is essential to the Weight Solution and getting the right help for yourself. For any weight solution to be effective, it must be centered on your particular brain, your particular problems, and your particular needs. Any program that gives you a one-size-fits-all approach is destined to fail.

Do You Have More Than One Type?

Having more than one type is common, and it just means that you may need a combination of interventions. Type 3 Impulsive-Compulsive Overeaters is actually a combination of Type 1 Compulsive Overeater and Type 2 Impulsive Overeater. It is common to have Type 1 mixed with Type 4 SAD or emotional overeater or with Type 5 Anxious Overeater. In those cases, we may mix 5-HTP for Type 1 with SAMe for Type 4 or GABA with Type 5. Again, it is always smart to discuss these options with your health-care provider. If he or she does not know much about natural treatments, consult a naturopath or a physician trained in integrative medicine or natural treatments.

WEIGHT CONTINUES TO BE A RISING PROBLEM

Our poor eating habits are making us one of the fattest nations on the planet. More than half of American women have a waistline greater than thirty-five inches, while half of their male counterparts measure in at more than forty inches around the belly. Obesity is becoming an epidemic with a devastating impact on our health and our brains. Research from 2005 and 2006 indicates that fully one-third of adult men and more than 35 percent of adult women in the United States are obese. About six million people are considered to have morbid obesity, which is defined as being at least 100 pounds overweight. Obesity is determined by a person's body mass index (BMI), which is a ratio of their weight and height.

Body Mass Index (BMI) Categories

- Underweight: <18.5
- Normal weight: 18.5–24.9
- Overweight: 25–29.9
- Obese: 30 or higher
- Morbid obesity: 40 or higher

Sources: National Institutes of Health and American Society for Metabolic & Bariatric Surgery

Here are the steps to calculate your BMI: weight in pounds × 703/height in inches^2

1. Multiply your weight in pounds times 703.
2. Multiply your height (in inches) times your height (in inches).
3. Divide the number in step 1 by the number in step 2 to get your BMI.

For example: If you weigh 148 pounds and you are five feet six inches tall, the calculation would look like this:

1. 148 pounds x 703 = 104,044
2. 66 x 66 = 4,356
3. 104,044/4,356 = 23.9 BMI (normal)

Or, if you weigh 260 pounds and you are five feet six inches tall, the calculation would look like this:

1. 260 pounds x 703 = 182,780
2. 66 x 66 = 4,356
3. 182,780/4,356 = 42.0 BMI (morbidly obese)

Morbid obesity is associated with more than thirty medical conditions and diseases, including type 2 diabetes, heart disease, and high blood pressure, as well as brain-related conditions, such as stroke, chronic headaches, sleep apnea, and Alzheimer's disease. These diseases can devastate a person's life. Diabetes is a disease that occurs when blood sugar levels in the body aren't right. The high blood sugar level causes small blood vessels in the body to become fragile and break, which can lead to terrible consequences. I have a friend who is diabetic, and due to the disease, he has lost his sight and has had to have both of his legs amputated. If you have a disease such as diabetes or heart disease, it is even more important for you to eat right in order to prevent or delay progression of the disease. Obesity is also associated with significantly longer hospital stays for comparable conditions. Ultimately, obesity puts you at increased risk for death. A review of several long-term studies on obesity and longevity found that the risk of death rises as weight increases above normal weights.

People who are obese or overweight also have smaller brains than lean people, according to new research in the journal *Human Brain Mapping*. Scientists used brain scans to determine the amount of brain tissue in ninety-four people over the age of seventy. They found that obese individuals had 8 percent less brain tissue and their brains looked sixteen years older than the brains of people at normal weights. Overweight people had 4 percent less brain tissue and their brains appeared eight years older.

The loss of tissue occurred in several important areas of the brain. In obese people, losses affected the frontal lobes, anterior cingulate gyrus, hippocampus, temporal lobes, and basal ganglia. In the overweight crowd, brain loss occurred in the basal ganglia, corona radiata (white matter that speeds communication between different areas of the brain), and parietal lobe. Overall, the loss of brain tissue puts overweight and obese people at increased risk for Alzheimer's disease, dementia, and other brain disorders.

As if we needed more proof that gaining weight is bad for our health, researchers at the University of Pittsburgh used brain imaging to examine the effects of increases in BMI on forty-eight otherwise healthy postmenopausal women. They found that women whose BMI went up following menopause were more likely to have a reduction in gray matter.

What is even worse is that our kids are becoming overweight or obese at an alarming rate. Studies show that a whopping 34 percent of children and teens are either currently overweight or at risk of becoming overweight, and more than 16 percent of kids ages two to nineteen are obese. Among younger children, obesity is skyrocketing. This is putting our children at greater risk for a variety of diseases and conditions that negatively affect brain function.

If you are overweight or love someone who is overweight, it is important to think of this as a life-threatening problem. Mind-set here is critical. Some anxiety, or brain alarm, is often necessary for people to take the actions needed to be healthy. I think it is also important to treat obesity like a chronic disease, because it is. And we need to think about being on healthy diets for life, not just for a few months to fit into a wedding dress or a suit for a special occasion.

When it comes to the brain, size matters. A smaller brain means reduced brain function, which can affect every aspect of your life—your relationships, your career, and your mood.

FAT IS MORE THAN JUST FAT

I remember the first day of my anatomy dissection lab in medical school like it was yesterday. Some of my fellow students had weak stomachs and had to get the mop. Even before the vomit, there was a smell in the room unlike anything most of us had ever experienced. Some of the students were nervous. I was excited and fascinated. Anatomy and neuroanatomy were my favorite subjects. Irma was the woman who donated her cadaver so that my colleagues and I could become skilled physicians. Irma and I spent many, many hours together. I remember when I cut through her skin how amazed I was to see the bright yellow, greasy layer of fat below. I had no idea at the time that fat was anything more than, well, fat. Since that day in the fall of 1978, fat has taken on a whole new meaning. The fat on your body is not just an energy-storage reservoir; it is a living, biologically active, toxin-storing, hormone-producing factory, and more fat is definitely not better.

Fat produces the hormone leptin, which usually turns off your appetite. Unfortunately, when people are overweight, the brain becomes sensitized to leptin, and it no longer has a positive effect on curbing hunger cravings. Fat cells also produce the hormone adiponectin, which also helps to turn off appetite and increases fat burning. As fat stores increase, adiponectin levels drop, and the process of burning fat as fuel actually becomes less efficient. In addition, fat cells pump out immune-system chemicals called cytokines, which increase the risk of cardiovascular disease, insulin resistance, and high blood sugar, diabetes, and low-level chronic inflammation.

Inflammation is at the heart of many chronic illnesses. The level of fat on your body, especially abdominal fat, is also directly linked with higher total cholesterol and LDL (bad) cholesterol and lower HDL (good) cholesterol. Together, insulin resistance, high blood sugar, excess abdominal fat, unfavorable cholesterol and triglyceride levels, and high blood pressure constitute the metabolic syndrome, a major risk factor for heart disease, stroke, depression, and Alzheimer's disease.

In recent years, it has been found that fat stores toxic materials, so that the more fat on your body, the more toxins you have. The more animal fat you eat, the more toxins you have as well. Also, fat tends to increase the amount of estrogen in your body, especially if you are male. Fat cells store estrogen. They contain an enzyme that converts several other steroid hormones to estrogen. Having increased estrogen makes it difficult to lose fat. Estrogen binds with a receptor on the surface of fat cells, which promotes the growth and division of fat cells, especially in your butt and thighs.

THIRTEEN THINGS ALL OF US SHOULD DO TO MAINTAIN A HEALTHY WEIGHT

1. Know your type(s).
2. Get a complete physical and focus on having healthy vitamin D, DHEA, and thyroid levels.
3. Know your BMI and caloric need numbers.
4. Know the approximate number of calories you eat a day by keeping a food journal and calorie log and work on getting "high-quality calories in versus high-quality energy out."
5. Exercise four or five times a week, starting with walking fast and light strength training.
6. Optimize your hormone levels.
7. Get great sleep.
8. Use simple stress-management techniques.
9. Stop believing every negative thought that goes through your brain.
10. Use hypnosis to help keep you slim.
11. Take supplements to keep your brain healthy.

12. Using the advice in this book, keep your brain young and active in order to lose ten pounds.
13. Take control of your weight and do not let other people make you fat.

1. Know your type(s). From the more than 55,000 scans we have performed at the Amen Clinics, it is clear that not everyone with the same problem, such as obesity or depression, has the same brain pattern. The descriptions above and the questionnaire in Appendix B or at www.amenclinics.com/cybcyb will help you know your type or types.

2. Get a complete physical. Not the five-minute type, but a real physical where you spend time talking to your doctor about your health. Medical problems, such as being on certain medications or having a low or suboptimal thyroid, vitamin D, DHEA, or testosterone levels, or being depressed or anxious, can seriously sabotage any attempt to lose, maintain, or be at your ideal weight.

3. Know your BMI and daily caloric need numbers. This is critical. The basic principle of weight loss or weight gain is about energy balance. The BMI formula is given above. The Harris Benedict Formula is commonly used to help people understand the approximate number of calories a day they need to maintain their current weight. This is a key number for you to understand, because it will serve as a guide to help you lose or gain weight.

To find out your basic calorie needs without any exercise, your resting basal metabolic rate (BMR), fill out the following equation on yourself:

Women: 655 + (4.35 x weight in pounds) + (4.7 x height in inches) − (4.7 x age in years)
Men: 66 + (6.23 x weight in pounds) + (12.7 x height in inches) − (6.8 x age in years)
Take that number and multiply it by the appropriate number below.
1.2—if you are sedentary (little or no exercise)
1.375—if you are lightly active (light exercise/sports 1 to 3 days/week)
1.55—if you are moderately active (moderate exercise/sports 3 to 5 days/week)
1.75—if you are very active (hard exercise/sports 6 or 7 days a week)
1.9—if you are extra active (very hard exercise/sports and a physical job or strength training twice a day)

The total is the number of calories a day you need to maintain your current weight. Put this number where you can see it. This number helps to give you control over your health.

4. Know the approximate number of calories you eat a day by keeping a food journal and calorie log and work on getting "high-quality calories in versus high-quality energy out." People lie to themselves constantly about their food intake. They underestimate the number of calories they eat and subsequently, through ignorance or denial, ruin their brains and their bodies. I am not suggesting you count every calorie

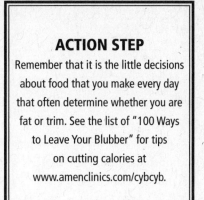

ACTION STEP

Remember that it is the little decisions about food that you make every day that often determine whether you are fat or trim. See the list of "100 Ways to Leave Your Blubber" for tips on cutting calories at www.amenclinics.com/cybcyb.

for the rest of your life, but I am suggesting that you use your brain to become educated about the calories and nutrition you put in your body, and then take control over them.

New York State recently passed a law making restaurants put the calories of their offerings on the menu. I love it! Why? It allows people to be informed consumers, to use their thoughtful brains rather than just impulsively ordering something because it looks good when their blood sugar and willpower are low. For example, when you look at the calories and fat in a Caesar salad, you realize it is not a healthy choice. Or, take one Cinnabon; it has 730 calories. My daily caloric intake needed to maintain my current weight is about 2,100 calories. If I have one Cinnabon a day, it fills more than 33 percent of my caloric needs with virtually no nutrition. Just knowing this fact will make me reach for a banana.

Likewise, knowing the calorie content of what you eat can help you make small adjustments that will make a big difference. Take having a Venti Peppermint White Chocolate Mocha at Starbucks. If you have them make it with whole milk and whipped cream, it is 700 calories! If you get a tall size of the same drink with nonfat milk and no whipped cream, it is only 320 calories, less than half.

To really know your calorie intake without cheating, keep a food journal where you write down absolutely everything you put in your mouth. Get a small weight scale and measure your portions of food. I can promise you that your idea of a serving will almost certainly vary substantially from what the food manufacturer puts on the label. Some of you may be thinking this is too much work. Yet I promise you it is worth the effort.

In our high school course Making a Good Brain Great, we have a lesson on nutrition. We teach the students that people gain weight when they eat more calories than they burn.

> Calories in versus calories out.
> Calories in = what you eat.
> Calories out = level of exercise.

The average male teen burns about 2,500 calories a day, while the average female teen burns about 2,000 calories a day. If you eat more calories than you burn, you gain weight. If you eat fewer calories than you burn, you lose weight. Calories are key.

> 1 pound (lb) = 3,500 calories (cals)
> 1 lb weight gain = eat 3,500 cals more than burn
> 1 lb weight loss = eat 3,500 cals less than burn
> For example, if you eat 500 extra cals a day (about one cheeseburger), you will
>   gain a pound a week

You need to know approximately how many calories you eat on a regular basis, otherwise they can seriously get away from you.

You cannot change what you do not measure.

In one of the laboratory exercises for the high school course, we have students write down the foods they typically order from their favorite fast-food restaurants and then have them go online to www.chowbaby.com to find the nutritional value of those meals. Most students are shocked by what they are putting in their bodies. When my son-in-law Jesse did this exercise (he helped me develop the course and did his master's thesis showing that it is highly effective in helping teens develop pro-social attitudes), he found out that for lunch alone he was eating almost 100 percent of his daily allotted calories. This knowledge encouraged him to make some simple adjustments that have helped him stay within his allotted calories and maintain a healthier weight.

You typically hear doctors talk about "calories in" versus "calories out." To be brain healthy, we must significantly upgrade this concept and think of "high-quality calories in" versus "high-quality energy out." For example, having 300 calories from Red Vines licorice or 730 calories from one Cinnabon is not the same as 500 calories from a piece of wild Alaskan Copper River Salmon, grilled veggies, and a sweet potato. I consider Red Vines and Cinnabon antinutrition, while the wild salmon, veggies, and a sweet potato are nutrition powerhouses. Likewise, "calories out" can come through taking supplements, such as caffeine or ephedra, to rev your metabolism and increase your stress hormones and anxiety and insomnia, or they can come from coordination exercises that burn calories and boost brain function. Aim for "high-quality calories in" versus "high-quality energy out"!

5. Exercise four or five times a week. One of the best exercises is walking fast. Walk like you are late, with periodic one-minute bursts of high-intensity walking or running. Some studies have shown that exercise can be as effective as antidepressant medications. The usual side effects of exercise are more energy and a healthier body. See Chapter 5, "The Exercise Solution," for more information. Coordination exercises, such as dance or table tennis, are also great for your brain and body.

6. Optimize your hormone levels. Much more information on this topic is found in Chapter 7, "The Hormone Solution." For now, let's look at three essential weight-management hormones: insulin, leptin, and ghrelin.

Insulin is produced by the pancreas and is considered a storage hormone. It gets stimulated primarily in response to a rise in blood sugar. Its function is to take nutrients from the bloodstream and store them in the body's cells. Insulin

---

ACTION STEP
Four tips to keep your insulin levels balanced:

- Have frequent small meals throughout the day rather than a few large meals. Larger meals tend to cause a greater insulin response.
- Control your carbohydrate intake. The more carbohydrates in a meal, the greater the insulin response.
- Emphasize more low-density carbohydrates and fewer high-density ones. The low-density carbohydrates, such as broccoli, cauliflower, green beans, and carrots, have more fiber and fewer carbohydrates than high-density carbohydrates, such as bread, pasta, rice, and cereals.
- Glucose-balancing agents—such as chromium, alpha-lipoic acid, cinnamon, and ginseng—may help. Chromium is a micronutrient (meaning that the human body doesn't need very much of it) that enhances the action of insulin and is involved in the metabolism of carbohydrates, fat, and protein. Alpha-lipoic acid is an antioxidant that may lower blood glucose levels.

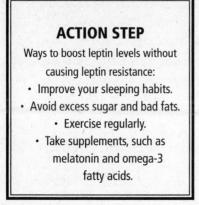

ACTION STEP

Ways to boost leptin levels without causing leptin resistance:
- Improve your sleeping habits.
- Avoid excess sugar and bad fats.
- Exercise regularly.
- Take supplements, such as melatonin and omega-3 fatty acids.

increases the uptake of glucose into the liver and muscles for storage as a substance called glycogen, and it also helps store excess glucose in fat cells. Since insulin is a storage hormone and not a mobilizing hormone, it also stops the body from mobilizing and using fat as a fuel source. Too much insulin stops fat burning. To maintain a healthy weight and burn fat adequately, it is important to keep insulin properly balanced.

Leptin is a hormone produced by fat cells that tells your body it is full. The more fat cells you have on your body, the more leptin you tend to have. Leptin works on the brain's hypothalamus to reduce your appetite when fat stores are high. When fat stores are low, such as after dieting, leptin levels are diminished, which causes a spike in appetite and sabotages weight loss. Leptin has been described as an antistarvation hormone because low levels lead to increased hunger. In the past, leptin was described as an antiobesity hormone, but researchers have since discovered that obese people, who produce large amounts of leptin, are often resistant to its effect in a similar way that some people are resistant to insulin. Leptin resistance may also result from overeating, as the hypothalamus becomes desensitized to its effects so you never know when you are full. Poor sleep also decreases leptin levels, which is interesting because many overweight people suffer from sleep apnea, a condition where people snore loudly, stop breathing frequently during sleep, and are chronically tired during the day. The lack of oxygen from sleep apnea is likely involved in lowering leptin levels. Poor sleep also impairs melatonin production, which can also lower leptin levels.

ACTION STEP

To stimulate the secretion of PYY3–36 in your stomach and help keep hunger at bay, eat with the acronym CRON (calorie restricted but optimally nutritious) in mind. For example, eating a 500-calorie spinach-and-salmon salad will keep you feeling full much longer than a 700-calorie cinnamon roll.

Ghrelin is a hormone secreted by the stomach that tells your brain you are hungry. I think of ghrelin as gremlins that force you to eat. In one study, when people were given ghrelin injections and then offered a buffet meal, they ate 30 percent more than they normally would! One of the main reasons it is thought that people tend to put weight back on after a diet is that ghrelin levels increase during dieting. This results in uncontrolled hunger and subsequent overeating. Naturally reducing ghrelin, keeping the gremlins away, is essential to maintaining a healthy weight. The substance peptide YY3–36 or PYY3–36, which is also produced in the stomach, blunts the effects of ghrelin. PYY3–36 is increased by having frequent small meals.

> **ACTION STEP**
> Pay attention to Chapter 13, "The ANT Solution," to clean up the ANTs that are stealing your happiness and increasing your waistline.

7. Get great sleep. For all of the brain types, being sleep deprived ultimately will make you fat and less intelligent. See Chapter 10 for more information.

8. Use simple stress-management techniques. Chronic, unrelenting stress upsets everything in your body, from your weight to your immune system to your memory. See Chapter 11 for more information.

9. Stop believing every negative thought that goes through your brain. People with weight issues typically are infested with a lot of ANTs. See Chapter 13 for more information. For many, these negative thinking patterns are one of the primary sources of worry, stress, depression, and anxiety, which often contribute to overeating or erratic eating.

A former professional football player who came to see us as part of a brain imaging study I am conducting on retired NFL athletes was six feet two inches and struggled at a weight of 365 pounds. When I asked him about it, he said, "I have no control over food." I asked, "Is that really true?" He said, "No, it isn't really true." I told him, "By saying or thinking that thought, I have no control over food, you just gave yourself permission to have no control over food and eat whatever you want."

In the same way, I was recently at dinner with a friend who was morbidly obese and ordered a large plate of nachos smothered in cheese. His wife was trying to get him on a healthy food plan, but he said, "I don't like any of that rabbit food." I responded by asking him what he meant. He said, "You know, all those vegetables and fruits." I told him that his way of thinking was giving himself permission to eat anything he wanted, and was going to kill him. "I don't like paying taxes," I said, "but I do it because I know there are consequences if I don't." Pay attention to your thoughts. They can help keep you on track toward your goals or completely give you permission to fail.

10. Use hypnosis to help keep you slim. When I was an intern at the Walter Reed Army Medical Center in Washington, D.C., one of my favorite teachers was the noted psychologist Harold Wain. He was the president of the American Society for Clinical Hypnosis and the chief of our Consultation-Liaison Service, the group of psychologists and psychiatrists who helped patients on medical wards who had psychiatric issues. Harold was a wonderful teacher. When he would use hypnosis for weight loss, he would help patients take their time to savor their food and drink. To patients in a trance he could describe drinking a cup of coffee in such a seductive way that it made them think drinking was as pleasurable as sex. He pointed out that people typically inhale their food and take little time to actually enjoy it. By using a simple, descriptive hypnotic technique, he could get people to slow down, feel full faster, and really start to enjoy the energy they put into their bodies.

I have personally been using hypnosis in my practice with patients for thirty years. To use it effectively for weight loss, it needs to be used in combination with a responsible weight-management program. There is also significant scientific evidence that suggests that hypnosis can be a powerful aid to weight loss. In one scientific review comparing a series of weight-loss studies with and without hypnosis, it was found that adding hypnosis significantly improved weight loss. The average post-treatment weight loss was 6.0 pounds without hypnosis and 11.83 pounds with hypnosis, nearly double. In a further follow-up period, the mean weight loss was 6.03 pounds without hypnosis and 14.88 pounds with hypnosis. The benefits of hypnosis increased over time.

Hypnosis can help people learn positive eating behaviors and create healthy long-term patterns of food intake. Some common hypnotic suggestions I give to patients include "feel full faster . . . eat more slowly . . . savor and enjoy each bite of your food . . . visualize yourself at your ideal weight and body . . . see the behaviors you need to do to get the body you want."

In addition, hypnosis has been found to be helpful to decrease stress, anxiety, insomnia, pain, and negative thinking patterns, all conditions that increase the potential for weight gain. Brain imaging studies have also shown that hypnosis boosts overall blood flow to the brain, which, as you will see below, helps to keep the brain young and may help you burn more calories. On our website (www.amenclinics.com), you can find a series of hypnosis CDs and downloads that I have created for you.

11. Take supplements to keep your brain healthy. Taking nutritional supplements can make a big difference in your efforts to reach your ideal weight. To all of my patients, I recommend taking a daily multiple vitamin/mineral supplement. Studies have reported that they help prevent chronic illness. In addition, people with weight-management issues often are not eating healthy diets and have vitamin and nutrient deficiencies.

I also recommend fish oil. Increased blood levels of omega-3 fatty acids from fish or fish oil have been recently linked to a lower incidence of obesity. Research results reported in the *British Journal of Nutrition* indicate that overweight and obese people have blood levels of omega-3 fatty acids that are lower than those of people with a healthy weight.

A considerable number of studies already support the benefits of the omega-3 fatty acids for heart, skin, eye, joint, brain, and mood health. In this particular study, researchers recruited 124 people of varying weights: 21 were classified as having a healthy weight, according to their body mass index (BMI); 40 were classed as overweight; and 63 were obese. People who consumed omega-3 supplements were excluded from the study. Blood samples were taken after the subjects fasted for at least ten hours. Researchers reported an inverse relationship between total omega-3 blood levels with BMI, the subjects' waist size, and their hip circumference. The researchers suggested that a diet rich in omega-3 fatty acids or omega-3 supplementation may play an important role in preventing weight gain and improving weight loss when used in combination with a structured weight-loss program.

Results from animal studies suggested that omega-3s may increase the production of heat by burning energy (thermogenesis). Another study suggested a role of omega-3s in boosting the feeling of fullness after a meal, and may help regulate the levels of hunger hormones like ghrelin and leptin, which impact appetite.

In addition, I recommend a craving supplement containing chromium picolinate, N-acetyl-cysteine, L-glutamine, and vitamin D and DHEA if levels of these are low. (See more about these supplements in Appendix C, "The Supplement Solution," and on our website: www.amenclinics.com.) Then, depending on your brain type, choose the supplements, if needed or desired, that best fit your brain. See the table at the end of this chapter.

I only consider recommending medication or surgery for weight loss if nothing else is working. People who have mild to moderate weight issues are often able to get a handle on the problem through natural means, but sometimes medications—especially those targeted to your type—or even surgery may be needed to save your life. The medications for each type are listed in the Summary Table of the Six Types of Weight-Management Issues at the end of this chapter. Obesity is a life-threatening problem, and sometimes lifesaving means are necessary. My friend Anthony Davis, a College Football Hall of Fame running back from USC, had bariatric surgery with great success.

There are several new weight-loss treatments currently being studied. For example, scientists are working on developing drug treatments that target abdominal fat. Another breakthrough technique involves brain surgery to treat obesity. Called deep brain stimulation, it delivers electricity to specific areas of the brain and has proved successful in eliminating or reducing tremors and tics in people with epilepsy, Parkinson's disease, and other neurological conditions. It has also been found to be useful in resistant depression and obsessive-compulsive disorder.

12. Using the advice in this book, keep your brain young and active in order to lose ten pounds. The brain uses 20 to 30 percent of the calories you consume each day. It is the major energy consumer in your body. Based on tens of thousands of brain scans that we have performed at the Amen Clinics, we have seen that the brain becomes dramatically less active as we age. In Image 3.1, you can see that the activity of the PFC peaks around age ten and then becomes less and less active. This happens in part because nerve cells are being wrapped with the white fatty substance myelin, which helps them work more efficiently, and brain connections that are not being used are pruned away. But this also happens because later in life there is overall decreased blood flow to the brain, which contributes to aging. This finding has also been reported by other researchers and may be one of the reasons why people need fewer calories with age.

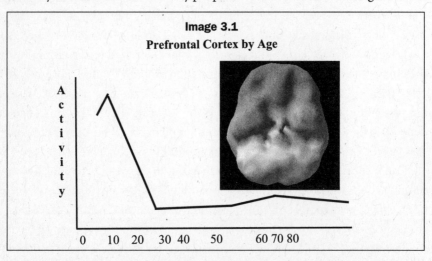

Image 3.1
Prefrontal Cortex by Age

This graph shows increased activity in the prefrontal cortex early in life, but dramatic decreased activity after age ten over the life span.

One way to lose ten pounds is to keep your brain young, healthy, and always challenged. By encouraging a youthful activity pattern and continually learning new things, you will keep your brain active, which will help you better manage your weight. So, learning a language or a musical instrument, playing bridge, or learning a new dance step all contribute to keeping your brain young.

13. Take control of your weight and do not let other people make you fat. My heritage is Lebanese. Like many cultures, Lebanese gatherings are often centered around and focused on food—usually tasty, high-calorie foods such as baklava, butter cookies, and rice fried in butter topped with tomatoes, green beans, and lamb. Too often, well-meaning, sweet people sabotage your efforts to maintain a healthy weight. "Eat this . . . try that . . . this is so amazing, you need to try just a bite . . . you are too skinny, eat more . . . here, have more or we will have to throw it away." Your own lack of focus, anxiety, and desire to please others allows these people to contribute to your early demise.

I see these interactions nearly everywhere I go. We were in Subway for lunch on a recent vacation and the store had run out of the little toys that come with the children's meal for our five-year-old. The clerk asked me if he could replace it with a cookie. I said, "No. Let's do an apple."

I was once at a store with a friend who asked me if I wanted an ice cream cone. I told her, "No."

She said, "Are you sure?"

"As sure as I can be," I replied.

When she came back, she had an ice cream cone for me.

"What part of *no* did you not understand?"

"The ice cream was on sale. I would get two cones for five dollars," she said innocently.

"Toss it or give it to the poor," I replied with a smile. "I get to have control over what goes into my body."

She didn't believe I would turn it down, but never disrespected my wishes again when it came to food.

Other people, at home, at parties, or in restaurants, often sabotage our efforts at health. Most of the times the behavior is innocent. Some of the time, it is because they feel uncomfortable being overweight and they would like you to join them. It is critical, if you want to be healthy, for you to be in control. Here are five ways to deal with people who, unknowingly or not, try to make you fat:

1. Be focused on your health goals. Before you go to a restaurant, party, or family gathering, know the approximate number of calories you want to spend on yourself.
2. Practice saying no, nicely at first: "No, thank you, I am full."
3. If the other person persists, add a little more detail: "No, thank you, I am on a special program, and it is really working for me."
4. If the other person is still persistent, pause, look them in the eye, and smile. Say something like, "Why do you want me to eat more than I want to?" That usually gets their attention. I was recently at the house of a friend who was very persistent. She asked me six times if I wanted something to eat. When I finally smiled and said, "Why do you want me to eat more than I want to?" she replied, "I am sorry, I just wanted to help." She then realized she was not being helpful, but irritating, and stopped.
5. Be persistent. We train other people how to treat us. When we just give in to their offers for food—so that they can feel helpful and important, or so we do not feel anxious—we train them to invade our health. When we are firm and kind, most people get the message and respect our wishes. Additionally, it may give you an opportunity to tell them about the exciting new information you are learning in this book.

IS FAT CONTAGIOUS?

A study published in the *New England Journal of Medicine* shows that one of the strongest associations in the spread of obesity is whom you spend time with. It is not a new virus that has been discovered, but the social and behavioral influence of your friends. The study was conducted using information gathered from more than twelve thousand people who had participated in a multigenerational heart study collected from 1971 to 2003. The study showed that if a subject had a friend who became obese, he had a 57 percent higher chance of becoming obese himself. That went up to a 171 percent higher chance if both friends identified each other as very close friends. Friendship was apparently the strongest correlation, and it didn't matter how far away geographically the friends were. Distance did not have a notable influence on the results. Sibling influence was also ranked high, with a 40 percent greater chance of becoming obese if another sibling was obese.

The study highlights the social network effect on health issues and makes an important point: Our health is heavily influenced by many factors, not the least of which are the role models around us. Whom you spend time with matters to the health of your brain and your body. This powerful influence works both ways, it seems, as the study's authors also stated that the same network effect showed up between friends who were *losing* weight. Health-conscious friends improve their health and their friends' health as well. By taking the information in this book seriously, you can influence your whole network of friends and family.

If you lead the way to better health in your circle of friends, your friends may also benefit. The author of the study said, "People are connected, and so their health is connected."

SUMMARY TABLE OF THE SIX TYPES OF WEIGHT-MANAGEMENT ISSUES

Type	Symptoms	Brain Findings/ Neurotransmitter Issue	Supplements	Medications
1: Compulsive Overeaters	Overfocused on food, worrying, have trouble letting go of hurts	Increased AC (anterior cingulate)/ low serotonin	5-HTP, St. John's wort, inositol	SSRIs, such as Prozac, Zoloft, or Lexapro
2: Impulsive Overeaters	Impulsive, bored, easily distracted	Low PFC (prefrontal cortex)/low dopamine	Green tea, rhodiola, ashwagandha	Phentermine, or stimulants such as Adderall or Ritalin
3: Impulsive-Compulsive Overeaters	Combination of types 1 and 2	High AC plus low PFC/low serotonin and dopamine	5-HTP plus green tea and rhodiola	SSRI plus phentermine or stimulant
4: SAD or Emotional Overeaters	Sad or depressed mood, gets the winter blues, has carbohydrate cravings, loses interest, sleeps a lot, has low energy	High limbic activity/low PFC; check vitamin D and DHEA levels	SAMe, vitamin D or DHEA if needed	Wellbutrin
5: Anxious Overeaters	Is anxious, tense, nervous; predicts the worst; eats to calm	High basal ganglia/low GABA levels	GABA, B_6, magnesium	Topamax
6: Adrenaline-Overload Anorexics	High stress, system overload, can't sleep, diarrhea, fast thoughts	Overall increased activity in emotional brain/ low-GABA, high-stress hormones	GABA, B_6, magnesium, and phosphatidylserine (PS)	Depends on other needs

The Weight Solution

Weight Boosters	Weight Trimmers
Thoughtless eating	Restricted and optimally nutritious calories
Low vitamin D level	Adequate vitamin D
Compulsive eating	Thought-stopping techniques
SAD eating	Finding healthier ways to be happy
Anxious eating	Deep relaxation
Adrenaline overload	Dealing with emotional issues
Only one diet tried	Tailoring the plan to your type
Low thyroid	Optimal thyroid
Ignorance/lying to self on calories consumed	Knowledge and honesty
Low blood sugar, which leads to impulsivity	Consistent blood sugar
Insomnia or low sleep	Adequate sleep, at least seven hours/night
Negative thinking, i.e., "I have no control"	Honest, optimistic thinking, i.e., "I do have control"
Sluggish brain	Active brain
Lack of exercise	Physical activity at least four or five times a week
Being unaware of calorie content	Counting calories
Hormonal imbalances	Balanced hormones
Chronic stress	Stress-management techniques

See www.amenclinics.com/cybcyb for "100 Ways to Leave Your Blubber."

4

THE NUTRITION SOLUTION

Feed Your Brain to Look
and Feel Younger

> Let food be your medicine and medicine be your food.
> —Hippocrates

s I was writing this book, I saw a feature on ESPN about Los Angeles Lakers forward Lamar Odom, who has a terrible sweet tooth, consuming up to eighty dollars' worth of candy a week. As a Lakers season ticket holder, I have suffered through years of Odom's erratic on-court performances. I decided to write a piece for my blog, which was picked up by the *Los Angeles Times*, which subsequently caused a firestorm of controversy during the 2009 NBA Finals. Here is an excerpt of the piece.

THE LAKERS' LAMAR ODOM, SWEET TOOTH, AND ERRATIC PLAY

I have been a huge Los Angeles Lakers fan since I was a child. I am really excited about my team being in the NBA Finals for the second year in a row. What I'm not as excited about is a piece I recently watched on ESPN about Lakers star Lamar Odom and his massive addiction . . . to candy. In it, you can see the 6-foot, 10-inch forward gobbling up massive quantities of the sugary treats.

Odom has been a giant source of frustration for Lakers fans. He is unbelievably talented, but often acts like a space cadet during games. Once, he was taking the ball out on the sidelines, when he walked onto the court before he threw the ball in, causing a turnover. During the Lakers last home game against the Denver Nuggets, Kobe Bryant threw him a pass, but the ball hit him on the shoulder because he had spaced out and was not paying attention. On talk shows, Odom is constantly criticized because no one knows if he will play well or not. He can play great, and be worth his fourteen-million-dollar-a-year salary or he can act like he is "missing in action."

Odom freely confesses that he just can't help himself when it comes to the sweet stuff and always keeps a stash on hand of Gummi Bears, Honey Buns, Lifesavers, Hershey's Cookies 'n' Crème white chocolate bars, Snickers bars, cookies, and more. He eats the sugary snacks morning, noon and night, and even says he sometimes wakes up in the middle of the night, chows down on some treats, then falls back asleep.

This is bad news for the Lakers. I've been telling my patients for decades that sugar acts like a drug in the brain. It causes blood sugar levels to spike and then crash, leaving you feeling tired, irritable, foggy, and stupid. Eating too much sugar impairs cognitive function, which may explain why Odom doesn't always make the smartest decisions on the court.

Excessive sugar consumption also promotes inflammation, which can make your joints ache and delay healing from injuries, which is definitely a bad thing for a professional athlete. It is also linked to headaches, mood swings and weight gain. Weight gain isn't a problem now for Odom, but it is for the average person who isn't playing full-court basketball for hours each day.

As a fan and a physician, it concerns me that our professional sports organizations and players are not more concerned about brain health, which includes nutrition. My advice to Odom and to all sugar addicts is to get your sugar consumption under control. You will feel so much better and your brain will function better, too.

After my piece ran, I was interviewed by ESPN radio, and reporters played part of my interview for Odom. Like most addicts, he denied it was a problem and said he had eaten candy for breakfast during games five, six, and seven of the last round of the playoffs against the Denver Nuggets, and he had played well in those games. The problem with the comment, however, was that there was no game seven. The Lakers won it in six games. Lakers coach Phil Jackson was also asked about my comments; he said he knows candy makes kids more troubled and that when you have kids, "Halloween is the worst night of the year." If Odom wants to be a world-class athlete who performs consistently, he needs to eat a brain-healthy diet. If you want your best physical body, you do, too.

In this chapter, I will provide you with the ingredients you need to eat right for your body, your brain, and your brain type. Here, you will discover five truths about the foods you eat, and you will learn eleven rules for brain-healthy nutrition.

FIVE TRUTHS ABOUT THE FOODS YOU EAT

1. You are what you eat.

You literally are what you eat. Throughout your lifetime, your body is continually making and renewing its cells, even brain cells. Your skin cells make themselves new every thirty days! Food fuels cell growth and regeneration. What you consume on a daily basis directly affects the health of your brain and body, and proper nutrition is the key. I often say if you have a fast-food diet, you will have a fast-food brain and an overweight body. To be your best self, get optimal nutrition from the food you put in your mouth.

2. Food is a drug.

You have probably noticed how the foods you eat affect your mood and energy level. Or maybe you have noticed that every time your child snacks on candy or cookies, he or she starts bouncing off the walls. Or that when your boss guzzles coffee, she gets impatient and demanding. That is because food is a drug.

Food can make you feel worse. If you chow down on three doughnuts for breakfast, about half an hour later, you are going to feel foggy, spacey, and stupid.

Food can make you sleepy. Have you ever noticed that after wolfing down a huge lunch, you feel like you need a nap?

Food can make you feel great. Eating the right foods gives you good energy that lasts all day long and helps you focus better.

3. Diet influences everything in your life.

Food does a lot more than just alleviate hunger pangs. It affects every aspect of your physical health and well-being.

Your overall health Eat a poor diet, and your health will suffer. Nosh on nutrient-rich foods throughout the day, and you will have a stronger immune system.

Your ability to think quickly and clearly Brain-friendly foods rev up mental sharpness to help you stay focused on your goals.

Your energy level Whether you are feeling peppy or pooped out depends on the foods you consume.

Your physical and athletic performance Good foods get you pumped up for physical activity, while bad foods zap your stamina.

Your weight Your eating habits directly affect the size of your body.

Your appearance People who have healthy diets tend to look healthier.

4. We're getting the wrong messages about food.

As a society, we're bombarded with bad messages about food. TV commercials, billboards, and radio ads are constantly encouraging us to adopt bad eating habits. Restaurants and fast-food joints train employees to "upsell" as a way to increase sales and, subsequently, expand our waistlines. Here are some of the sneaky tactics food sellers use to try to get you to eat and drink more.

> Do you want to supersize that for only thirty-nine cents?
> Do you want fries with your meal?
> Do you want bread first? (This makes you hungrier so you eat more!)
> Do you want an appetizer?
> Do you want another drink?
> Do you want a larger drink? It is a better deal!
> Do you want dessert? It comes with the meal!
> Free refills—you have to keep drinking to get your money's worth!
> Happy hour—you can drink more for less!
> All-you-can-eat buffet—you have to keep eating to get the most for your money!

Parents, grandparents, and teachers are sometimes just as guilty of sending out the wrong messages about food. We sometimes tell children, "If you behave, you can have a treat when we get home." Sure, this strategy might get Johnny to sit still in class or in church or to be quiet while you are trying to have a phone conversation, but there's a problem with this. Using poor nutrition as a reward for good behavior teaches children to reward themselves later in life with foods that are not good for them.

5. Who has the worst diets?

Teens and young adults often have the worst diets. Parents feel like they have little influence over their adolescent children, so they just give up and let them eat whatever they want whenever they want. The habits young people develop during this time can be hard to break later on, and they can have a major impact on their brain development. Because the brain is still undergoing intense development up until the age of twenty-five, the foods that teens eat can either enhance or impede their development. If young people want to have the best brain possible, they need the best diet possible.

On the other end of the life spectrum, older people often have poor nutrition habits, too. For example, when an elderly husband or wife dies, the surviving spouse may not be as motivated to eat right while dining alone. A spouse who cooked healthful meals throughout the marriage may not want to go to all that trouble to cook for one. He or she may shift to prepackaged meals or quick bites of whatever's handy. This is a trend that needs to be reversed.

Eleven Rules for Brain-Body–Healthy Nutrition

1. Drink plenty of water, some green tea, and not too many calories.
2. Watch your calories.
3. Increase good fats and decrease bad fats.
4. Increase good carbs and decrease bad carbs.
5. Dump artificial sweeteners and replace them with small amounts of natural sweeteners.
6. Limit caffeine intake.
7. Eat great brain foods.
8. Reduce salt intake and increase potassium intake.
9. Plan snacks.
10. Take a daily multivitamin/mineral supplement and fish oil.
11. Recognize when you or someone you care about has hidden food allergies.

1. Drink plenty of water, some green tea, and not too many calories.

Considering that your body consists of 70 percent water, and your brain is 80 percent water, proper hydration is the first rule of good nutrition. Even slight dehydration increases the body's stress hormones. When this happens, you get irritable and you don't think as well. Over time, increased levels of stress hormones are associated with memory problems and obesity. (See Chapter 11, "The Stress Solution," for more on stress hormones and how they affect your body.) Dehydration also makes your skin look older and more wrinkled.

I once did a SPECT scan of a famous bodybuilder. His scan looked like he was a drug addict, but he vehemently denied that. Then I learned that he significantly dehydrates himself before photo shoots to look leaner for the camera, and he was doing a shoot the day after we did his scan. When he was adequately hydrated the following week, his brain looked much better (see Images 4.1 and 4.2).

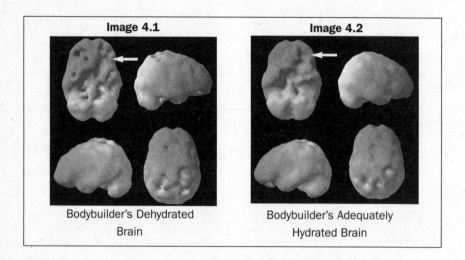

Bodybuilder's Dehydrated Brain

Bodybuilder's Adequately Hydrated Brain

To stay adequately hydrated, drink plenty of water every day. Based on weight, everyone's need is different. One rule of thumb is to drink half your weight in ounces every day. So, if you are 150 pounds, you should drink 75 ounces a day. Be aware that not all liquids are created equal. It is best to drink liquids that are free of artificial sweeteners, sugar, much caffeine, and alcohol. I also encourage my patients to drink unsweetened green tea two or three times a day. Researchers from China found that when people drank two to three cups of green tea per day, their DNA actually looked younger than that of those who did not. Interestingly, the DNA of people who took multiple vitamins also looked younger. Likewise, be careful of drinking too many of your calories. Research suggests that people forget about the calories they drink and are more likely to gain weight. My favorite drink is water mixed with lemon juice and a little bit of the natural sweetener stevia.

2. Watch your calories.

The bottom-line message about calories is that the fewer you eat, the longer you will live, according to many research studies. In a new twenty-year study on primates, researchers from the University of Wisconsin–Madison found that a nutritious but calorie-reduced diet blunts aging and significantly delays the onset of age-related disorders such as cancer, diabetes, cardiovascular disease, and brain deterioration. During the two decades of the study, half of the animals that were permitted to eat freely have survived, while 80 percent of the rhesus monkeys given the same foods, but with 30 percent fewer calories, are still alive. In terms of overall health of the monkeys, the authors note, the restricted diet leads to longer life span and improved quality of life in old age. "There is a major effect of caloric restriction in increasing survival if you look at deaths due to the diseases of aging." The incidence of cancerous tumors and cardiovascular disease in animals on a restricted diet was less than half that seen in animals permitted to eat freely. Amazingly, while diabetes is common in monkeys that can eat all the food they want, it has yet to be observed in any animal on a restricted diet. "So far," the researchers report, "we've seen the complete prevention of diabetes." In addition, the brain health of animals on a restricted diet was also better. In particular, the regions of the brain responsible for motor control and executive functions, such as working memory and problem solving, seem to be better preserved in animals that consume fewer calories.

Reducing calorie consumption overall helps you control weight and decreases the risk for heart disease, cancer, and stroke from obesity (a major risk factor for all these illnesses). Even better, restricting calories triggers certain mechanisms in the body to increase the production of nerve-growth factors, which are beneficial to the brain.

To get the most out of your food, think CRON (calorie restriction with optimal nutrition). That means making sure that every calorie you consume counts.

Counting calories is also one of the keys to lasting weight loss. Many diet programs today have discarded the traditional concept of calorie reduction. Instead, they insist that you need to eat a specific ratio of protein, carbohydrates, and fats in order to lose weight. Not so, according to a recent study in the *New England Journal of Medicine* conducted at the Harvard School of Public Health and Brigham and Women's Hospital. This study found that calorie reduction— regardless of the percentage of fats, carbohydrates, or proteins in a diet—is what leads to weight loss. For this study, the researchers enlisted 811 overweight individuals and assigned them to one of the following four diets:

1. 20 percent fat, 15 percent protein, 65 percent carbohydrates
2. 20 percent fat, 25 percent protein, 55 percent carbohydrates
3. 40 percent fat, 15 percent protein, 45 percent carbohydrates
4. 40 percent fat, 25 percent protein, 35 percent carbohydrates

At the conclusion of the two-year study, all four groups had achieved a similar weight loss of an average of nearly nine pounds. Regardless of the amount of fat, carbohydrates, or protein in their particular diet, the participants reported experiencing similar feelings of hunger and satiety. This study reinforces the concept that calorie restriction is essential if you want to lose extra pounds.

A lot of my patients ask me if it is possible to eat fast food while watching their calorie intake. The answer is yes. Many fast-food restaurants are adding healthier, low-calorie fare to their menu options. To help you make better choices at fast-food restaurants, here's a chart of calorie-busters to avoid and lighter options that get the green light.

ACTION STEP

	JUST SAY NO!	ORDER THIS INSTEAD!
Jack in the Box:	sirloin cheeseburger onion rings mango smoothie	chicken fajita pita fruit cup water
Total:	**2,020 calories**	**396 calories**
McDonald's:	Double Quarter Pounder (w/cheese) large fries large Coke	Chipotle BBQ Snack Wrap (grilled) Caesar salad (w/ low-fat balsamic dressing) small fruit 'n' yogurt parfait water
Total:	**1,550 calories**	**550 calories**
Wendy's:	Baconator hamburger large fries large strawberry shake	large chili baked potato water
Total:	**1,900 calories**	**550 calories**

Decreasing calories doesn't mean sacrificing flavor. Cook with brain-healthy herbs and spices to enhance the flavor of your food and boost your brain. You can find more information about the following and other brain-healthy spices at www.amenclinics.com/cybcyb.

- Turmeric, found in curry, contains a chemical that has been shown to decrease the plaques in the brain thought to be responsible for Alzheimer's disease.
- A number of studies have found that saffron extract is helpful in treating mild to moderate depression.
- Sage has A-level—the highest level possible—scientific evidence for memory enhancement.
- Cinnamon has been shown to enhance memory and focus and may aid in the prevention of Alzheimer's disease. Plus, cinnamon helps regulate blood sugar levels.

Restricting calories does not mean starving yourself. Crash diets and diets that severely limit the number of calories you consume aren't doing your brain or your body any favors. Extremely low calorie intake is associated with a lack of nutrients, which can deprive your brain and body of the fuel they need for optimal performance. Similarly, yo-yo dieting, in which you habitually lose and then regain weight, has been linked to certain health risks, including high cholesterol and high blood pressure. Adopting a brain-healthy eating plan for life is a more sensible way to shed pounds for good.

3. Increase good fats and decrease bad fats.

Fat has gotten a bad rap. Many myths and misconceptions surrounding dietary fat have led many of us to fear that eating any kind of fat is bad for our health and will make us fat. This isn't true. In fact, we all need some fat in our diets.

Our brains need fat, too. Did you know that 60 percent of the solid weight of your brain is fat? So if somebody ever calls you a fathead, say "Thank you." The hundred billion nerve cells in your brain need essential fatty acids to function. Myelin, the fatty protective covering that wraps around the nerve cells, keeps those neurons working at optimum levels. Any loss of myelin due to diseases, such as amyotrophic lateral sclerosis (ALS), commonly known as Lou Gehrig's disease, and multiple sclerosis (MS), compromises the nervous system. Of course, having too much of the wrong fat in your system leads to high "bad" cholesterol, which can kill you with heart disease and stroke. But did you know that really low cholesterol levels can kill you as well? Low cholesterol levels have been associated with depression and violence, and sometimes even homicide and suicide.

There are three main categories of fat—bad fat (saturated fats), really bad fat (trans fats), and good fat (unsaturated fats). Saturated fats contribute to hardening of the arteries and plaque formation. Plaque is the sticky, gooey stuff that accumulates on the inside of your blood vessels and can potentially block blood from flowing freely to the heart and brain. Saturated fats are found in red meat (like prime rib), eggs (especially in the yolks), and dairy foods (like butter and whole milk).

Diets high in saturated fats have long been associated with long-term health risks, such as heart disease. A 2009 animal study from British researchers has found that high-fat diets also cause more immediate problems. After eating a fatty diet for just ten days, rats showed short-term memory loss and less energy to exercise—in other words, they became more stupid and lazy. The researchers compared the performance of the rats on a high-fat diet (55 percent of calories as fat) with rats on a low-fat diet (7.5 percent of calories as fat). In the rats with the high-fat diet, their muscles worked less efficiently, which lowered their energy levels, caused their hearts to work harder during exercise, and caused their hearts to increase in size. The rats eating high-fat foods also took longer to make their way through a maze and made more mistakes than the rats eating low-fat foods. This is one of the first studies to show that it doesn't take long for a high-fat diet to make your brain and body more sluggish.

Scientific evidence also shows that consuming high-fat foods actually alters brain chemistry in ways that compel you to overeat. One animal study that appeared in the *Journal of Clinical Investigation* found that eating high-fat foods, such as milk shakes or burgers, caused the brain to release messages to the body telling it to ignore the feelings of fullness that typically make you stop eating. In this particular study, the brain switched off the fullness signal for up to three days and led to overeating. A similar trial found that high-fat, high-sugar diets alter brain receptors in an area of the brain that regulates food intake. Overconsumption of fat-laden, sugar-filled foods increased the levels of opioid receptors, which are linked to feelings of pleasure and euphoria. The researchers suggest that this could be a factor in binge-eating disorders.

The worst fats on the planet are referred to as Frankenfats. These man-made fats have been chemically altered by adding hydrogen and are more harmful than natural fats. On food labels, you will find these fats listed in the ingredients as "partially hydrogenated" oils and amounts listed as "trans fats."

The food industry uses these Frankenfats because they help foods—such as margarine, cakes, crackers, cookies, potato chips, and bread—have a longer shelf life and better flavor stability. Since 2006, the FDA has required manufacturers to list trans fats on nutrition labels, and many manufacturers have reduced or eliminated their use of these killer fats.

Unsaturated fats are good for your health and can actually lower cholesterol. There are two basic types of good fats: monounsaturated fats and polyunsaturated fats. Foods high in monounsaturated fats include avocados, olive oil, canola oil, peanut oil, and nuts (such as almonds, cashews, and pistachios). Foods high in polyunsaturated fats include safflower oil, corn oil, and some fish.

The polyunsaturated fats found in salmon and mackerel and the monounsaturated fats found in canola oil and soybean oil are high in essential fatty acids (EFAs), called omega-3 fatty acids. They are called *essential* fatty acids because our body needs them. When we don't have enough of these EFAs in our system, it can cause problems. For example, research has found that omega-3 fatty acid levels tend to be low in people with ADD, depression, and Alzheimer's disease; low in those who have trouble thinking; and low in those who attempt suicide.

Studies show that a diet rich in omega-3 fatty acids may help promote emotional balance and positive mood, two things that can reduce a tendency to overeat. In a Danish study that compared the diets of more than five thousand healthy older people, findings showed people who ate more fish in their diet were able to maintain their memory longer. Researchers in Holland found that consuming fish decreased the risk for dementia and stroke. And according to a French study, older adults who ate fish just once a week significantly lowered the risk of developing brain problems such as dementia.

Even though your body needs EFAs, it can't produce them itself, so you must get them through the foods you eat. Getting adequate amounts of omega-3 fatty acids from your diet isn't easy. EFAs tend to be scarce in many of the processed foods and fast-food meals we eat on a regular basis. I recommend that people eat one or two servings of fish per week, particularly fish such as salmon, which is high in omega-3 fatty acids. Be aware that even if you eat fish a few times a week, you may not be getting enough omega-3 fatty acids. That is because much of the salmon served in restaurants and sold in supermarkets is farm-raised and contains less of the important EFAs than salmon caught in the wild. For the highest amounts of omega-3 fatty acids, opt for wild salmon rather than farm raised. Because it can be so difficult to get all the EFAs you need from your diet, I recommend taking a daily fish oil supplement. Adults should take 2,000 to 4,000 mg of high-quality fish oil a day (500 to 2,000 mg a day for children). Amen Clinics, Inc., has its own brand, which we took years to develop. Knowing your good fats from your bad fats can get a little confusing, so use the following chart as a reminder.

Good Fats	versus	Bad Fats
Anchovies		Bacon
Avocados		Butter
Canola oil		Cheese (regular fat)
Flaxseed oil		Cream sauces
Lean meats (chicken/turkey)		Doughnuts
Low-fat cheeses		Fried foods
Nuts (walnut are the best)		Ice cream
Olive oil		Lamb chops
Peanut oil		Margarine
Salmon		Potato chips (fried)
Sardines		Processed foods
Soybeans		Steak
Tuna		Whole milk

4. Increase good carbs and decrease bad carbs.

Some of the latest diet trends are giving carbohydrates a bad name. But carbs are a necessary part of a healthy diet, as they provide the fuel your body needs to perform physical activity. The amount of carbs you need in your diet depends on your brain type. As we saw in the last chapter, Type 1 Compulsive Overeaters tend to feel better when they have more carbohydrates in their diets, while Type 2 Impulsive Overeaters typically do better with more protein.

No matter which type you are, it is important to understand that some carbs are better than others. There are two basic types of carbs: complex and simple. Complex carbs, which include fruits, vegetables, beans, legumes, and whole grains, get a thumbs-up. These foods take longer to digest and are loaded with vitamins, minerals, and fiber that promote good brain and body health. The carbs to avoid are the simple carbs, such as table sugar, pastries, candy, sodas, fruit juices, doughnuts, white bread, pasta, and white rice. Simple carbs are digested quickly, provide little or no nutritional value, and may promote disease and weight gain.

Reduce your sugar intake.

Curbing your intake of sugary foods is an important step to better health. Sugar spikes your blood sugar level then sends it crashing down about thirty minutes later, leaving you feeling lackluster and dim-witted. As we saw in the story of Lamar Odom at the beginning of the chapter, there is no doubt that sugar can be addictive. Sugar's empty calories can also lead to obesity and excess inflammation, which increases the risk of developing type 2 diabetes, heart disease, and stroke. Not only that, sugar also promotes seizure activity. In a number of studies from Johns Hopkins University, when neurologists took children completely off simple carbohydrates, it dramatically cut down on seizure activity, in some studies by more than half.

Sugar affects some people more than others. Jenny, twenty-six, is a prime example. She had been dealing with anxiety, depression, and fatigue for many years. She constantly craved sweets and would often experience headaches, mood swings, and dizziness throughout the day. When Jenny stopped eating treats made with refined sugar and gave up caffeine and alcohol, her symptoms disappeared.

Sugar consumption has been on the rise for decades and Americans currently consume an average of 22.2 teaspoons (almost half a cup) a day (355 calories a day) of added sugars. The number one source of added sugars in the American diet are soft drinks and other sugar-laden beverages. Recognizing the deleterious role excess sugar intake plays in our health, the American Heart Association issued a statement in 2009 recommending that Americans limit their intake of added sugars to no more than 100 calories per day for women and 150 calories per day for men.

If you want to cut down on your sugar intake, start by cutting out the sodas and limiting the cookies, candy, and ice cream you eat. I realize that it may not be easy. As noted earlier, according to Dr. David Kessler's *The End of Overeating: Taking Control of the Insatiable American Appetite,* the high-fat, high-sugar combos found in many mouthwatering snacks light up the brain's dopamine pathway similar to the same way drugs and alcohol do. He suggests that some people can actually get hooked on chocolate chip cookies the way other people get addicted to cocaine. Kessler and his team of researchers have seen this theory at work in animals, too. In one study, they found that rats will work increasingly hard for a high-fat, high-sugar milk shake, and that they will consume greater quantities of it if more sugar is added.

Because sugar is a common ingredient in thousands of processed foods—

NAMES FOR SUGAR USED ON FOOD LABELS

Sugar
Invert sugar
Lactose
Maltodextrin
Honey
Maltose
Glucose
Malt syrup
Galactose
Molasses
Fruit juice concentrate
Sorbitol
Fruit juice
Turbinado sugar
Fructose
Agave
Dextrose
Dehydrated cane juice
Corn syrup (or high-fructose corn syrup)
Cane juice crystals, extract
Cane sugar
Sucanat
Barley malt

even foods that don't taste sweet—start checking food labels. Spaghetti sauce, salad dressing, ketchup, peanut butter, and crackers often contain some form of sugar. If food labels simply said "sugar," it would be easy to figure out what to cut out of your diet, but they don't. On food labels, sugar may be listed using any of a wide variety of names (see the box to the left). This list is only the beginning— Manufacturers use many more names, so you have to be on your toes. When you start looking for these names on labels, you will soon realize just how many foods contain sugar. You will also notice that a food might not have sugar listed as one of the top few ingredients, but it might have three, four, or more different types of sugar included.

When you add up all of them, it comes to a huge amount of sugar. I went to the store the other day looking for a healthful snack and picked up one of those so-called health bars. The packaging screamed "health," but the list of ingredients told another story.

LIST OF INGREDIENTS OF A SO-CALLED HEALTH BAR

- granola
  whole-grain rolled oats
  sugar (SUGAR!)
  rice flour
  whole-grain rolled wheat

  whole wheat flour
  molasses (SUGAR!)
  sodium bicarbonate
  soy lecithin

partially hydrogenated soybean
and cottonseed oils with TBHQ
(tert-Butylhydroquinone)
and citric acid sunflower oil with
natural (trans fat) tocopherol

- corn syrup (SUGAR!)
- crisp rice

    whole-grain rolled oats

    rice

    sugar (SUGAR!)

- sugar (SUGAR!)
- corn syrup solids (SUGAR!)
- glycerin
- high fructose corn syrup (SUGAR!)
- peanuts
- partially hydrogenated soybean and/or cottonseed oil
- sorbitol (SUGAR!)
- calcium carbonate
- fructose (SUGAR!)
- honey (SUGAR!)
- natural and artificial flavors
- salt
- molasses (SUGAR!)
- soy lecithin
- water
- BHT
- citric acid

caramel color (SUGAR!)
barley malt (SUGAR!)
salt
nonfat dry milk

salt
barley malt (SUGAR!)

Some form of sugar is listed an incredible fourteen times! When you inspect the food label, this "healthy" snack doesn't seem so healthy anymore.

In looking at the list of sugar names, you might be wondering about fruit juice and fruit juice concentrate. After all, isn't fruit one of those complex carbs that are so good for you? Let me clear this up. Yes, fruit is great for you, but fruit juice isn't so good. Orange juice, for example, consists of a small amount of vitamin C, a lot of sugar, and water. It doesn't contain any of

GLYCEMIC INDEX (GI)
High GI (70 and above)
Medium GI (56–69)
Low GI (55 and under)

GI RATINGS

Low-fat yogurt	14
Asparagus	15
Broccoli	15
Cherries	22
Kidney beans	27
Low-fat milk	33
Apples	38
Carrots	39
Spaghetti	41
Apple juice	41
Grapes	46
Oatmeal	49
Whole-grain bread	50
Yams	51
Orange juice	52
Sweet potato	54
Brown rice	55
Bananas	55
Popcorn	55
Potato chips	56
Cheese pizza	60
Ice cream	61
Pineapple	66
Watermelon	72
Cheerios	74
White bread	75
French fries	75
Doughnuts	76
Waffles	76
Rice cakes	77
Rice Krispies	82
Cornflakes	83
Baked potatoes	85
Dates	103
White rice	110

Sources: The Glucose Revolution, GlycemicIndex.com, NutritionData.com, SouthBeachDietPlan.com, and Diabetesnet.com.

the fiber you get from eating an orange. Orange juice is better than a Diet Coke, but it isn't as good as eating an orange.

Get to know the glycemic index.

To help you figure out how carbs affect your blood sugar, understand the glycemic index (GI). The GI rates carbs based on their effect on blood sugar levels. Low-glycemic carbs cause only small fluctuations in blood sugar levels, which helps you maintain energy throughout the day. High-glycemic carbs cause blood sugar levels to spike then crash. This roller-coaster effect gives you an initial boost of energy, but then leaves you feeling sluggish and slow. The key to good brain health is to make sure the majority of the carbs you consume are low-glycemic.

Eating low-glycemic carbs that contain a lot of fiber is even better for your brain. Dietary fiber promotes health and can lower cholesterol, which promotes good blood flow. Good sources of high-fiber foods include vegetables, fruits, whole grains, and beans and legumes. When choosing fruits and vegetables, it is best to go for non-starchy vegetables and low-sugar fruits—think broccoli rather than potatoes, and blueberries instead of pineapple. Check the GI Ratings box for tasty low-glycemic, high-fiber foods you should stock up on.

Hold the bread before meals.

Why do restaurants serve baskets of bread before each meal for free? Why not cheese? Why not almonds, or chunks of beef or chicken? The reason is that bread makes you hungrier and encourages you to eat more. Bread, especially white bread made from bleached and processed flour, spikes your blood sugar and boosts the natural feel-good neurotransmitter serotonin in the brain. Serotonin helps you feel happier and less anxious.

On brain SPECT scans, I have seen that serotonin interventions help to relax or lower function in the PFC. When I prescribe antidepressant medications or supplements that boost serotonin in the brain, my patients often say they feel better but that they are also less motivated. Anything that lowers PFC function makes you more impulsive and less worried about long-term consequences. The bread or simple carbohydrate to start a meal helps you feel better, but also more impulsive when the dessert tray comes by later on. Hold the bread, wait for your meal, and you will be happier with the end result.

5. Dump artificial sweeteners and replace them with small amounts of natural sweeteners.

I love sweet things. I wish it wasn't so, but growing up with a grandpa whom I adored who was a candy maker put me at a decided disadvantage. When I found it was essential to watch my weight, I was grateful for artificial sweeteners. No calories! How cool. Have as much as you want, I thought. Diet sodas became a regular companion for me and I drank a ton of them from age twenty-five to thirty-five. Then, at age thirty-five, right as we started our brain imaging work, I found that I had problems getting off the floor when I played with my young children, because my joints hurt. Being a writer, I became even more concerned when my fingers and hands started to hurt as well.

Initially, I just wrote it off to old age. At thirty-five? Then, as I became much more interested in learning about brain health, I discovered that there was a large body of information reporting that artificial sweeteners, like aspartame in diet sodas, may be associated with arthritis, gastrointestinal problems, headaches, memory problems, neurological problems, and a myriad of other maladies. I had a patient who told me her arthritis and headaches went away after she stopped aspartame. Another patient told me her confusion went away as she got rid of artificial sweeteners, and yet another patient told me that it was only after he stopped diet sodas that he was able to lose weight.

So I stopped aspartame, and within four weeks, my arthritis went away. Just to test, as diet sodas have been a big part of my life, I tested it again with a diet soda at lunch. Within twenty minutes, my fingers started to hurt. So I decided to eliminate aspartame from my diet. The other artificial sweetener choices at the time either tasted bitter to me or had been reported to be possibly associated with cancer.

Then sucralose (Splenda) came along, and I felt as though I was in sweet heaven again, plus it had no aftertaste, and I did not have arthritis with it. In fact, sucralose was reported to be six hundred times sweeter than sugar. Putting regular sugar in tea or lemonade was bland by comparison. Then, yet again, reports began to emerge that it was associated with health troubles, including decreasing the healthy bacteria in the intestinal tract.

Besides the reported health problems, one of the significant problems with artificial sweeteners is that they may increase sugar cravings. The empty calories prime the brain's appetite centers to expect something good, and when nothing comes, it wants more. Artificial sweeteners also desensitize your taste buds, and even naturally sweet things, such as a regular portion of sugar, are not enough to satisfy you.

Changing the sensitivity of your taste buds is clearly possible. If you were a diet soda drinker like me, remember how disgustingly sweet regular sodas tasted after you had not had them for a while? When you dump the artificial sweeteners, your taste buds will adapt back to normal within a few weeks.

My favorite natural sweetener, stevia, which has been reported to have anti-inflammatory and blood pressure–lowering properties, has not been associated with negative health effects. Xylitol and agave are other natural sweeteners. With any of them, use sparingly, and you will be better off in the long run.

Another terribly disturbing trend is the artificial sweeteners that are ending up in gum, candy, packaged foods, sauces, vitamins, medications, nutritional powders, nutritional bars, popcorn, toothpaste, and water. The sweeter it is, these companies know, the more hooked you are likely to become. Fight back and do not collude with the food companies in your own demise.

ACTION STEP

Read the labels of everything you eat! It is important to know what you are putting in your body.

6. Limit caffeine intake.

Most of us associate caffeine with coffee, but it can also be found in tea, dark sodas, chocolate, energy drinks, and pep pills. If your caffeine intake is limited to one or two normal-size cups of coffee or two or three cups of tea a day, it probably is not a problem. But any more than that can cause problems.

Caffeine restricts blood flow to the brain, and anything that compromises blood flow leads to premature aging.

Caffeine dehydrates the brain (remember, your brain is 80 percent water and needs adequate hydration), which makes it harder to think quickly.

Caffeine interferes with sleep, which is essential for good brain health, appetite control, and skin rejuvenation. Caffeine disrupts sleep patterns because it blocks adenosine, a chemical that tells us when it is time to hit the hay. When this chemical is blocked, we tend to sleep less, which leads to sleep deprivation. And when we aren't getting enough sleep, we feel like we absolutely must have that cup of joe in the morning in order to jump-start our day.

Caffeine can be addictive in high amounts. When you try to kick the habit, you are likely to experience withdrawal symptoms, including severe headaches, fatigue, and irritability.

Caffeine can accelerate heart rate and raise blood pressure. In some people, drinking too much caffeine leads to a temporary spike in blood pressure and a racing heart.

Caffeine can give you the jitters. Ingesting more caffeine than you normally do can leave you feeling jittery and nervous.

Caffeine increases muscle tension. Tight muscles have been linked to caffeine intake.

Caffeine can cause an upset stomach. Gastrointestinal troubles are common with excessive caffeine use.

Caffeine can elevate inflammatory markers. Two studies showed that 200 mg of caffeine (equivalent to two cups of coffee) raised homocysteine levels, a marker for inflammation and heart disease.

Caffeine can interfere with fertility. Pregnant women should be careful with caffeine because it has been associated with premature births, birth defects, inability to conceive, low birth weight, and miscarriage.

To be fair, there are also a number of studies suggesting that coffee can be helpful for you. It has been shown to decrease the plaques that cause Alzheimer's disease, lower the risk for Parkinson's disease, and lower the risk of colon cancer and diabetes. It may be other substances in the coffee, not just the caffeine, that are actually helpful, and decaffeinated varieties may give you

THE BEST ANTIOXIDANT FRUITS AND VEGETABLES

- Açaí berries
- Blueberries
- Blackberries
- Cranberries
- Strawberries
- Spinach
- Raspberries
- Brussels sprouts
- Plums
- Broccoli
- Beets
- Avocados
- Oranges
- Red grapes
- Red bell peppers
- Cherries
- Kiwis

Source: U.S. Department of Agriculture

the benefits without the troubles noted above. A Harvard University study found that those drinking decaf coffee also showed a reduced diabetes risk, though it was half as much as drinking caffeinated coffee. Another study, however, found that caffeine reduced insulin sensitivity and raised blood sugar—both bad news for you.

One question you should ask yourself whenever you read a scientific study promoting the benefits of certain medications, alcohol, or caffeine is, Who funded the research? One of the university departments that advocate for coffee use is funded, in part, by Kraft Foods, the makers of Maxwell House coffee.

7. Eat great brain foods.

You will be glad to know that there are plenty of delicious foods that are great for your brain regardless of your brain type. Foods that contain high amounts of antioxidants help your body and brain stay young. Several studies have found that eating foods rich in antioxidants, which include many fruits and vegetables, significantly reduces the risk of developing cognitive impairment. How do they work? Antioxidants neutralize the production of free radicals in the body. Free radicals are chemicals that play a major role in the deterioration of the brain with age. The body produces free radicals every time a cell converts oxygen into energy. When produced in normal amounts, free radicals help rid the body of harmful toxins, thus keeping it healthy. When produced in toxic amounts, free radicals damage the body's cellular machinery, resulting in cell death and tissue damage. This process is called oxidative stress. It is similar to the way metals rust, or oxidize, when exposed to moisture in the air. Antioxidants act like the body's rust busters.

Foods rich in antioxidants include a variety of fruits and vegetables. Blueberries are very high in antioxidants, which among neuroscientists has earned them the nickname "brain berries." In laboratory studies, rats that ate blueberries showed a better ability to learn new motor skills and gained protection against strokes. That is not all. In one study, rats that ate a diet rich in blueberries lost abdominal fat, lowered cholesterol, and improved glucose levels. Similar studies showed that rats that consumed strawberries and spinach also gained significant protection.

THE FIFTY BEST BRAIN FOODS

1. Almonds, raw
2. Almond milk, unsweetened
3. Apples
4. Asparagus
5. Avocados
6. Bananas
7. Beans, black, pinto, garbanzo
8. Bell peppers, yellow, green, red and orange
9. Beets
10. Blackberries
11. Blueberries
12. Broccoli
13. Brussels sprouts
14. Carrots
15. Cheese, low fat
16. Cherries
17. Chicken, skinless
18. Cranberries
19. Egg whites, DHA enriched
20. Grapefruit
21. Herring
22. Honeydew
23. Kiwi
24. Lemons
25. Lentils
26. Limes
27. Oats
28. Olives
29. Olive oil
30. Oranges
31. Peaches
32. Peas
33. Plums
34. Pomegranates
35. Raspberries
36. Red grapes
37. Soybeans
38. Spinach
39. Strawberries
40. Tea, green
41. Tofu
42. Tomatoes
43. Tuna
44. Turkey, skinless
45. Walnuts
46. Water
47. Whole wheat
48. Wild salmon
49. Yams and sweet potatoes
50. Yogurt, unsweetened

When it comes to antioxidants, I always say eat from the rainbow. By that, I mean eat fruits and vegetables of many different colors—eat blue foods (blueberries), eat red foods (pomegranates, strawberries, raspberries, cherries, red bell peppers, and tomatoes), eat yellow foods (squash, yellow bell peppers, small portions of bananas and peaches), orange foods (oranges, tangerines, and yams), green foods (spinach, broccoli, and peas), purple foods (plums), and so on. This will ensure that you are getting a wide variety of antioxidants to nourish and protect your brain.

Balance the foods you eat.

Your brain needs a balance of lean protein, such as skinless chicken or turkey, complex carbohydrates, and good fats. It is a good idea to include lean protein at each meal to balance blood sugar levels, especially if you are a Type 2 Impulsive Overeater. Adding lean protein to snacks and meals slows the fast absorption of simple carbs and helps prevent the brain fog that typically follows consumption of sugary snacks.

In 2000, I conducted a five-month study on the effects of a balanced diet on five college students who had all been diagnosed with ADD, including my own son. Each student followed the Zone diet by Dr. Barry Sears, which advocates eating a balance of lean protein, complex carbohydrates, and good fats. In addition, they all took high-dose purified fish oil. To track their progress, we did before-and-after SPECT scans. After five months of sticking with the dietary regimen, all of the students performed better in school and lost weight. Their brain scans showed positive changes as well, enhancing the concentration centers of the brain and calming overactive areas involved in mood control. It was clear to me that a healthy diet and fish oil helped balance brain function.

Use the form on this page to create

MY TOP 20 BRAIN FOODS

1. _____
2. _____
3. _____
4. _____
5. _____
6. _____
7. _____
8. _____
9. _____
10. _____
11. _____
12. _____
13. _____
14. _____
15. _____
16. _____
17. _____
18. _____
19. _____
20. _____

your own list of your top twenty brain-healthy foods and include them in your diet each week. The simple act of writing down your favorite brain foods will help you be more mindful of what you are eating.

8. Reduce salt intake and increase your potassium intake.

A lot of people erroneously blame salt for making them fat. Salt in and of itself does not cause weight gain, but it does cause your body to temporarily retain water, which can make it harder to zip up your jeans. Part of the problem with salt is that it is commonly found in large quantities in high-calorie processed foods at the grocery store, fast-food fare, and restaurant meals. So eating a diet that is high in high-salt foods is likely to make you gain weight over time.

Take note that salt is not the same as sodium. Sodium accounts for about 40 percent of table salt. It is found naturally in many foods and in the human body. Sodium and potassium are electrolytes that are involved in a variety of bodily functions. For optimal function, these electrolytes need to be balanced. When they are out of balance, with much higher sodium levels and lower potassium levels, as in most Americans, they can lead to weight gain, hypertension, insulin resistance, and a depressed immune system.

A low-salt diet, such as the DASH (Dietary Approaches to Stop Hypertension) diet, has been proven to lower hypertension in just fourteen days, according to numerous studies. It has also been shown to reduce the risk of stroke and heart disease. One study found that participants who reduced salt intake lowered their risk of dying from heart disease ten to fifteen years later by 25 percent. As a bonus, because the diet is based on eating an abundance of great brain foods—such as fruits and vegetables, whole grains, lean protein, and healthy fats—it can result in weight loss and enhanced brain function.

Just as important as cutting back on salt is increasing potassium intake. A recent study found that eating twice as much potassium as sodium can cut in half the risk of dying from heart disease. A 1997 study in the *Journal of the American Medical Association* that reviewed the results of thirty-three clinical trials found that individuals who took potassium supplements lowered their blood pressure. Foods high in potassium include bananas, spinach, honeydew melon, kiwi, lima beans, oranges, tomatoes, and all meats.

ACTION STEP

Dietary guidelines currently recommend getting at least 4,700 mg a day of potassium and no more than 2,300 mg a day of sodium (about one teaspoon of salt).

9. Plan snacks.

If anybody has ever told you to avoid snacking throughout the day, don't listen! Going too long without eating can wreak havoc on your brain function and make your blood sugar levels drop too low. Low blood sugar levels are associated with poor impulse control and irritability. It can also cause emotional stress. Phil is a fifty-six-year-old man who suffered from anxiety attacks. Every Wednesday night, Phil ate dinner in a restaurant, and every Wednesday before he left his home for the restaurant, he had an anxiety attack. It eventually was revealed that Phil normally ate dinner at 6 p.m., but on Wednesdays, the dinner didn't start until 8 p.m. Waiting the extra two hours for dinner was causing his blood sugar to drop. When Phil started eating a snack of an apple and a few almonds at 6 p.m. on Wednesdays, his anxiety attacks disappeared.

Eating approximately every three to four hours throughout the day can help balance your blood sugar. This isn't a license to gorge all day long. When snacking, opt for low-calorie foods and include a balance of protein, complex carbs, and good fats, if possible. Personally, I love to snack. Since I travel frequently, I've learned to pack brain-healthy snacks for the road. Otherwise, I am tempted to grab candy bars from the airport gift shop. One of my favorite low-calorie snacks is dried fruits, without any added sugar or preservatives, and fresh raw vegetables—I add a few nuts or some low-fat string cheese to balance out the carbohydrates in the fruits and vegetables with a little protein and fat. Be wary when buying dried fruits and vegetables, though; many brands add sugar, preservatives, or other ingredients, which renders them less than healthy. Read the food labels. Look for brands that don't add anything.

Here are a few more of my favorite midafternoon snacks:

Low-fat yogurt and nuts
Low-fat cottage cheese with fruit and a couple of almonds or macadamia nuts
1 ounce of string cheese and a half cup of grapes
Turkey and apple with a macadamia nut or three almonds
Deviled eggs with hummus (Slice the eggs in half, discard the yolks, and fill with
    1 tablespoon hummus; add paprika to taste.)

10. Take a daily multivitamin/mineral supplement and fish oil.

Ninety-one percent of Americans do not eat at least five servings of fruits and vegetables a day, the minimum required to get good nutrition. For years, I have been advocating that everybody take a daily multivitamin. The *Journal of the American Medical Association (JAMA)* agrees. For twenty-two years, the AMA recommended against taking a daily multivitamin, but eventually reversed its position. The AMA now recommends daily vitamins for everybody because they help prevent chronic illness. Many people argue that if you are eating a balanced diet, you don't need a supplement. That may be true, but how many of us are really eating a perfectly nutritious diet every day?

In addition to a daily multiple vitamin/mineral supplement, I almost always prescribe a fish oil supplement for my patients as well. Fish oil, a great source for omega-3 fatty acids, has been the focus of many research studies. The two most studied fish oils are eicosapentaenoic acid (EPA) and docosahexaenoic acid (DHA). DHA is a vital component of cell membranes, especially in the brain and retina. DHA is critical for normal brain development in fetuses and infants and for the maintenance of normal brain function throughout life. DHA appears to be a major factor in the fluidity and flexibility of brain cell membranes, and it could play a major role in how we think and feel. See Appendix C, "The Supplement Solution," for more detailed information.

11. Recognize when you or someone you care about has hidden food allergies.

Many people know that food allergies can cause hives, itching, eczema, nausea, diarrhea, and, in severe cases, shock or constriction of the airways, which can make it difficult to breathe and can be fatal. But can certain foods and food additives also cause emotional, behavioral, or learning problems? You bet. These types of reactions are called hidden food allergies, and they could be hampering your efforts for a better body.

My patient Mark had ADD and symptoms of anxiety and depression. He explained that whenever he ate foods with MSG, he became violent. To see why this was happening, we scanned his brain twice—once having avoided anything with MSG and once after he ate a Chinese dinner laced with MSG. The MSG scan showed a marked difference in activity in Mark's left temporal lobe, the area associated with temper control. I told Mark he could either stay away from MSG or take medication to prevent the problem. To my surprise, he opted for the medication. He explained that if he lost his temper one more time, his wife was going to divorce him, and "you never know what has MSG in it. Sometimes it is listed on the label as natural flavorings." If you have problems with your temper, you might want to hold the MSG.

Although Mark's case is extreme, sensitivity to food additives, such as

ACTION STEP

If you suspect a food allergy or
sensitivity, try an elimination diet.

MSG, artificial sweeteners, or food colorings, is probably more widespread than we realize. As far as food allergies go, the most common culprits are peanuts, milk, eggs, soy, fish, shellfish, tree nuts, and wheat. These eight foods account for 90 percent of all food-allergic reactions. Other foods commonly associated with allergies include corn, chocolate, tea, coffee, sugar, yeast, citrus fruits, pork, rye, beef, tomato, and barley.

Physical symptoms that might tip you off to a food allergy or sensitivity include dark circles under the eyes, puffy eyes, headaches or migraines, red ears, fatigue, joint pain, chronic sinus problems (congestion or runny nose), or gastrointestinal issues. Behavioral problems that can be caused by foods include aggression, sleep problems, lack of concentration, and changes in speech patterns (turning into a motormouth or slurring words).

When a food allergy or food sensitivity is suspected, a medical professional may recommend an elimination diet. An elimination diet removes all common problem foods for a period of one or more weeks. These diets aren't easy to follow because they're very restrictive. After the initial diet period, potential allergens are reintroduced one by one. Foods that cause abnormal behaviors or physical symptoms should be permanently eliminated from the diet. Working with a nutritionist may make a big difference.

Here's how an elimination diet worked for a thirty-seven-year-old woman who complained of fatigue, anxiety, and panic attacks. When she went on the elimination diet, all of these symptoms disappeared. After reintroducing foods to her diet, she discovered that sugar, corn, cheese, and grapefruit caused her symptoms to flare up. Now, as long as she avoids these foods, she remains symptom-free.

In a 2008 study from Holland, researchers found that putting children with ADD on a restricted elimination diet reduced their symptoms by more than 50 percent in 73 percent of them. This is basically the same effectiveness as prescription ADD medication without any of the side effects. Basically, during the study, the children could eat only rice, turkey, lamb, vegetables, fruits, margarine, vegetable oil, tea, pear juice, and water. But the results were stunning. In this study the researchers also found that the children's moods and oppositional behaviors were improved.

In 2003, a SPECT study was performed to determine if eliminating problem foods could affect brain function. The study tested cerebral blood flow in thirty people with celiac disease (an intolerance for wheat and wheat products). Half of them had been following a gluten-free diet for almost one year, while the other half had not eliminated gluten from their diet. Twenty-four healthy individuals were also tested as a control group. Researchers concluded that the celiac patients who followed a gluten-free diet were significantly less likely to experience decreased cerebral blood flow than those who continued to eat gluten. Only 7 percent of the patients who eliminated gluten from their diet experienced lower blood flow in at least one area of the brain, compared to 73 percent of those who continued to eat gluten showing reduced blood flow in at least one area of the brain. Once again, this shows that the foods you eat directly affect your brain.

In my practice, I've found that many adults and children with emotional, learning, or behavioral problems improve when they eliminate specific foods or food additives from their diets. In particular, I work with many children who have autism or Asperger's syndrome. When I put these kids on a diet free of gluten (wheat, barley, rye, oats, and any products made from these grains) and casein (milk protein and all dairy products), I've noticed that some of their behavioral problems diminish and their language tends to improve.

TREAT EATING DISORDERS EARLY

Eating disorders, such as anorexia nervosa, bulimia, and obesity, are very common. It is estimated that seven million women and one million men are affected by anorexia nervosa and bulimia. Obesity was discussed in the prior chapter. People with anorexia nervosa starve themselves, which causes extreme weight loss. Even though they may look emaciated, people with the disorder may still be convinced they are too fat. People who have bulimia engage in a vicious cycle of binge eating and purging, either self-inducing vomiting or using laxatives, diuretics, or enemas to eliminate what they've consumed. They may also exercise excessively in order to burn off the calories consumed in a binge. These conditions can have devastating consequences on health and brain function. Treating eating disorders early is key to recovery and a healthier life.

The Nutrition Solution

Antinutrition Boosters	Nutrition Boosters
Low blood sugar	Frequent small meals with at least some protein to maintain healthy blood sugar
Dehydration	Adequate hydration
Overeating	CRON (calorie restriction with optimal nutrition)
Trans fats	Monounsaturated fats
Saturated fats	Polyunsaturated fats
Simple carbs	Complex carbs
Sugar	Low-glycemic foods
Artificial sweeteners	Natural sweeteners
Excessive caffeine	Limited caffeine
Empty calories	Antioxidants
High-salt processed foods	Fruits and vegetables with potassium
Office vending machine products	Healthy snacks from home
Junk food	Multivitamins and fish oil
Food allergens	Elimination diet

See www.amenclinics.com/cybcyb for a list of ways to be a "brain-healthy" shopper at the supermarket. Also, find many brain-healthy recipes for breakfast, lunch, dinner, desserts, and snacks.

5

THE EXERCISE SOLUTION

Exercise Your Body to
Strengthen Your Brain

Those who think they have not time for bodily exercise will sooner or later
have to find time for illness.
— Edward Stanley, former prime minister
of the United Kingdom

Physical activity was a natural part of daily life for our ancestors. They
hunted animals for food, tended to their gardens, built their own homes,
and walked wherever they had to go. In our thoroughly modern world,
we drive to work, sit at a desk all day, drive home, and loaf around on the
couch. We've almost completely eliminated movement from our day-to-day
lives. This is bad news for our brains—not to mention our bellies, our butts,
and our backs.

If you want to have a healthy brain and body, you've got to get off your butt
and move! Physical activity is the single most important thing you can do to
enhance brain function and keep your body looking young. Whether you are
six years old or ninety-six years old, exercise acts like a fountain of youth. If
you can only follow one of the solutions in this book, make it this one.

THE MANY WAYS PHYSICAL EXERCISE
PUMPS UP YOUR BRAINPOWER

Physical exercise acts like a natural wonder drug for the brain. It improves
the heart's ability to pump blood throughout the body, which increases
blood flow to the brain. That supplies more oxygen, glucose, and nutrients
to the brain, which enhances overall brain function. The number of ways

that physical exercise benefits the brain is truly remarkable. Here are just some of the things exercise can do for your brain and body.

Exercise encourages the growth of new brain cells. Aerobic activity that gets the heart rate up for extended periods of time boosts brain-derived neurotrophic factor (BDNF), a chemical that plays a role in neurogenesis, or the growth of new brain cells. Think of BDNF as a sort of Miracle-Gro for your brain. When you exercise, your brain sprouts new cells. When your brain doesn't create as many new cells as it loses, aging occurs.

Research studies on laboratory rats show that exercise generates new brain cells in the temporal lobes (involved in memory) and the prefrontal cortex (involved in planning and judgment). These new cells survive for about four weeks, then die off unless they are stimulated. If you stimulate these new neurons through mental or social interaction, they connect to other neurons and enhance learning. This indicates that it is necessary to exercise consistently to encourage continual new cell growth in the brain. It also explains why people who work out at the gym and then go to the library are smarter than people who only work out at the gym.

Physical activity enhances cognitive ability at all ages. No matter how old you are, exercise increases your memory, your ability to think clearly, and your ability to plan. In Dr. John J. Ratey's book *Spark*, he details how a revolutionary physical education program at a school in Naperville, Illinois, has transformed the student body into some of the smartest kids in the nation. In 1999, eighth graders there took an international standards test called TIMSS (Trends in International Mathematics and Science Study), which focuses on math and science. For years, U.S. students have been lagging far behind pupils from other nations—including Japan, Korea, Singapore, and China—in these two subjects. The Naperville eighth graders defied that trend, ranking first in the world in science and sixth in math. Compare those results to U.S. students' national rankings of eighteenth in science and nineteenth in math.

What's so special about Naperville's PE program? It sidelines traditional sports in favor of high-intensity aerobic activity—a brief warm-up, a one-mile run, and a cool-down. The only rule: Students must keep their average heart rate above 185 for the mile-long run. The burst of activity is obviously paying off. I hope other schools from around the country take notice and start implementing similar PE programs. I highly recommend that you pick up a copy of *Spark* to learn more about the many ways this fitness program is benefiting the students.

There's a lot more evidence that exercise boosts brainpower. In 2005, the California Department of Education (CDE) released a study that compared the relationship between physical fitness and academic achievement. The study revealed that students in the fifth, seventh, and ninth grades with the highest fitness levels also scored highest on standardized reading and math tests. On the other end of the scale, the students in these grades who were the least physically fit had the lowest academic test scores.

In a 2005 issue of *Pediatrics*, a panel of thirteen researchers published the results of a large-scale review of 850 studies about the effects of exercise on the nation's youth. The panel concluded that for optimal academic performance, school-age children should participate daily in one hour or more of moderate to vigorous exercise that includes a variety of physical activities.

Another study, published in *Brain Research*, found that physically fit thirteen- and fourteen-year-olds showed significantly greater cognitive processing ability than their couch-potato peers. A host of other studies have found a laundry list of benefits tied to exercise. Physical activity boosts memory in young women aged eighteen to twenty-five, and it improves frontal lobe function in older adults. Getting your body moving also protects the short-term memory structures in the temporal lobes (hippocampus) from high-stress conditions. Stress causes the adrenal glands to produce excessive amounts of the hormone cortisol, which has been found to kill cells in the hippocampus and impair memory. In fact, people with Alzheimer's disease have higher cortisol levels than do normal aging people.

Exercise enhances your mood. People who exercise consistently report a general sense of well-being that people who lead a sedentary lifestyle do not experience. Getting your heart pumping allows more of the natural mood-enhancing amino acid L-tryptophan to enter the brain. L-tryptophan is the precursor to the neurotransmitter serotonin, which balances moods. It is a relatively small amino acid, and it often has to compete with larger amino acids to cross the blood channels into the brain. With exercise, the muscles of the body utilize the larger amino acids and decrease the competition for L-tryptophan to enter the brain, which makes you feel better.

Exercise helps alleviate depression. In any given year, almost fifteen million American adults and about 5 percent of children and adolescents

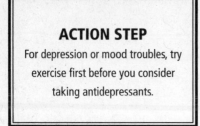

ACTION STEP

For depression or mood troubles, try exercise first before you consider taking antidepressants.

experience major depressive disorder. Millions of these adults and children turn to prescription medication for help, and antidepressants have become the most commonly prescribed drug in the nation, according to a study by the U.S. Centers for Disease Control and Prevention. What would you say if I told you that exercise can be as effective as prescription medicine in treating depression?

I teach a course for people who suffer from depression, and one of the main things we cover is the importance of exercise in warding off this condition. I encourage all of these patients to start exercising and especially to engage in aerobic activity that gets the heart pumping. The results are truly amazing. Over time, many of these patients who have been taking antidepressant medication for years feel so much better that they are able to wean off the medicine.

The antidepressant benefits of exercise have been documented in medical literature. One study compared the benefits of exercise to those of the prescription antidepressant drug Zoloft. After twelve weeks, exercise proved equally effective as Zoloft in curbing depression. After ten months, exercise surpassed the effects of the drug. Minimizing symptoms of depression isn't the only way physical exercise outshined Zoloft.

Like all prescription medications for depression, Zoloft is associated with negative side effects, such as sexual dysfunction and lack of libido. Plus, taking Zoloft may ruin your ability to qualify for health insurance. Finally, popping a prescription pill doesn't help you learn any new skills. On the contrary, exercise improves your fitness, your shape, and your health, which also boosts self-esteem. It doesn't affect your insurability, and it allows you to gain new skills. If anyone in your family has feelings of depression, exercise can help.

The power of exercise to combat depression is yet another reason why I think schools need to make physical education a requirement for all grades. If 5 percent of kids and adolescents suffer from depression, why not get them to try exercise as a way to reduce or eliminate their need for medication? Getting depressed kids to take part in PE could even prove to be a lifesaver. Consider this fascinating report from the Secret Service: National Threat Assessment Center on school shootings. The researchers examined thirty-seven school shootings involving forty-one perpetrators between the ages of eleven and twenty-one. Aside from the fact that all the shooters were male, what was the one and only characteristic they shared? A history of depression. More than half of the shooters reported having experienced feelings of depression. In fact, 75 percent of them had threatened to commit suicide or had actually tried to kill themselves before they carried out their attacks.

Exercise calms worries and anxiety. Anxiety disorders are very common in the United States, affecting approximately forty million adults and as many as one in ten young people. Millions more of us spend far too much time worrying about the little things in life. When worry or negative thoughts take over, exercise can provide a welcome distraction. Research shows that high-intensity activity can soothe anxiety and reduce the incidence of panic attacks. If, for example, you or your family members are stressing out about an upcoming test or dwelling on an argument you had, physical activity can help clear your mind.

Exercise helps prevent, delay, and lessen the effects of dementia and Alzheimer's disease. Canadian researchers conducted a large-scale, five-year study to determine the association between physical activity and the risk of cognitive impairment and dementia. From 1991/1992 to 1996/1997, they gathered information on 4,615 men and women sixty-five years or older. The researchers evaluated the participants at the study's debut and again at its conclusion five years later. The results showed that 3,894 participants remained without cognitive impairment, 436 were diagnosed as having cognitive impairment but no dementia (mild cognitive impairment), and 285 were diagnosed as having dementia. Physical activity was associated with lower risks of cognitive impairment, Alzheimer's disease, and dementia of any type. High levels of physical activity were associated with even further reduced risks. The researchers concluded that regular physical activity could represent an important and potent protective factor against cognitive decline and dementia in elderly people.

A number of other studies support these findings and show that physical exercise prevents or delays the cognitive decline associated with dementia and Alzheimer's disease. Research has shown that in people over sixty-five, mild to moderate exercise reduces the risk of cognitive impairment and dementia due to Alzheimer's disease by about 50 percent. A study conducted at Case Western Reserve University examined how much TV people watch each day, which

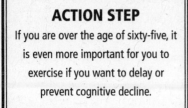

ACTION STEP

If you are over the age of sixty-five, it is even more important for you to exercise if you want to delay or prevent cognitive decline.

correlates inversely to their exercise level—the more TV people watch, the less they tend to exercise. People in the study who watched two or more hours of TV a day (couch potatoes) were twice as likely to develop Alzheimer's disease. In contrast, people over forty years of age who exercised at least thirty minutes per session two or more times a week reaped many protective benefits.

People already suffering from dementia or Alzheimer's disease may also see rewards from physical activity. Australian researchers found that memory-impaired older adults who followed a six-month exercise program experienced a decrease in cognitive decline over an eighteen-month follow-up period.

Exercise eases symptoms of ADD. The best natural treatment for ADD is physical exercise. In my experience, I have seen a direct correlation between the level of exercise a person gets and the severity of their symptoms. I have noticed that when my patients exercise on a regular basis, their ADD medication works better. In particular, I work with a lot of children and adolescents with ADD. In the spring, these patients will sometimes complain that their medications aren't working as effectively as before. When I hear this, I always ask them if they've changed their exercise routine. Often, they will tell me that they had been playing basketball, a highly aerobic sport, but the season ended, so they aren't doing any physical activity at the moment. When I get them to exercise again, their medication starts working better again. I could just as easily raise the dosage of their medication, but there are side effects associated with that. Exercising has no side effects and a wealth of benefits, so I prefer trying that route first.

If you want more proof that exercise is a great natural treatment for ADD, look at Olympic gold medalist Michael Phelps. Diagnosed with ADD at the age of nine, Phelps had trouble concentrating in class and struggled with his schoolwork. He started taking prescription stimulant medication for ADD to ease his symptoms. In the sixth grade, he told his mother he wanted to stop taking the medication. By then, he was spending hours a day swimming in the pool, and thanks to the intense aerobic activity, he managed to stay focused without medication.

Physical fitness sparks better behavior in adolescents. Researchers at the University of California, Irvine, studied 146 healthy adolescents to determine the effects of physical exercise on their lives. The results showed that teens who were more physically fit were less impulsive, felt happier, and were more likely to do good things with their lives than their less-fit peers.

People who exercise regularly sleep better. Regardless of your age, engaging in exercise on a routine basis normalizes melatonin production in the brain and improves sleeping habits. If you've ever watched your kids horse around in the backyard for hours and then collapse into bed at night, you know how true this is. In Chapter 10, you will learn why sleeping is critical for maintaining optimal brain function throughout your lifetime. Remember, although regular exercise is advised, it is best to avoid doing vigorous exercise too close to bedtime. Try to complete physical activity about four hours before going to bed.

Exercise helps women cope with hormonal changes. Evidence shows that regular exercise tends to minimize symptoms associated with PMS. It also helps women deal with the hormonal fluctuations that occur during pregnancy, perimenopause, and menopause.

EXERCISE IS KEY TO BETTER HEALTH, BETTER ENERGY, AND A BETTER MOOD

Exercise promotes better health and helps you live longer. Regular exercise increases the chemical nitric oxide, which tells the smooth muscles in your blood vessels to relax and open, allowing blood to flow more freely throughout your body. You probably never think of your blood vessels as having muscles, but they do. Every time you exercise, you give your blood vessels a workout too. With consistent exercise, your blood vessels become more robust. That helps keep blood pulsing to your heart, organs, and tissues. This boosts the health of vital organs and reduces the risk for high blood pressure, stroke, and heart disease—all of which have been linked to cognitive decline.

Physical activity also enhances insulin's ability to prevent high blood sugar levels, thereby reducing the risk of diabetes. In addition, exercise increases the production of glutathione, which is the major antioxidant in all cells. Pumping up the levels of glutathione protects muscles and other tissues from free radical damage and premature aging. Research has also shown that mild to

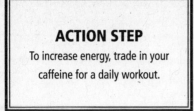

ACTION STEP

To increase energy, trade in your caffeine for a daily workout.

moderate exercise reduces your risk of developing osteoporosis, breast cancer, and colon cancer. For the elderly, physical activity improves muscle tone and endurance, which lowers the risk of falling.

When you make exercise a habit, it also pumps up your energy levels and keeps you from feeling lethargic. Instead of sprawling on the couch all day, you will have a good helping of get-up-and-go. That makes you more likely to go out and do the things you love to do, which burns even more calories and keeps you looking and feeling good.

ADD EXERCISE TO YOUR BEAUTY REGIMEN

What's good for the brain is good for the heart is good for the genitals is good for the skin. Exercise improves blood flow to every organ in your body, so it makes sense that it would benefit your skin, which is the largest organ. Thanks to increased circulation, greater amounts of oxygen and nutrients are delivered to your skin cells. This encourages cell renewal and the production of collagen, the supportive protein that helps keep your skin from sagging and wrinkling. It also helps skin battle back against the daily assaults from pollution and other environmental toxins. Some forms of exercise, such as yoga, help keep acne breakouts at bay. How? Yoga and other types of exercise reduce stress, which minimizes the production of stress hormones that are often associated with acne flare-ups.

Improved blood flow also gives your skin a rosy-looking glow. According to a team of researchers at the University of St. Andrews in Scotland, people perceive a rosier complexion as healthier and potentially more attractive. The study, featured in the journal *Psychological Science*, involved having college-age participants alter the color of faces in digital photos to make them appear healthier. The researchers found that the students almost invariably added redness to the faces to enhance the appearance. This is more evidence that exercising does more than just improve your shape—it makes you more attractive.

ACTION STEP

If you think you look too old and are considering a face-lift or laser treatment to rejuvenate your appearance, try exercise first in order to boost blood flow to your skin.

In an animal study conducted at the University of Illinois, researchers found that moderate regular exercise has another benefit for the skin: it speeds the wound-healing process. The researchers concluded that exercise speeded healing times by decreasing inflammation. For people such as diabetics who typically have poor wound healing, this study shows that exercise can be especially beneficial.

GET MOVING TO BURN FAT

To melt away fat, you need to burn more calories than you consume, and exercise can help. A quick review of the scientific literature on the effect of exercise on fat reveals thousands of studies showing that physical activity helps you lose weight. Engaging in aerobic exercise also increases your body's metabolism, which boosts your calorie-burning power. Metabolism is a complex process that converts the foods you eat into energy and also determines how quickly you burn that energy. Daily exercise and activity that builds muscle tissue help you burn more calories, which allows you to prevent weight gain or to shed a few pounds if that's your goal. When you exercise, your body looks and feels better, which makes you feel better about yourself. Other physical benefits include better coordination, agility, speed, and flexibility.

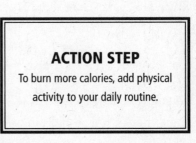

ACTION STEP

To burn more calories, add physical activity to your daily routine.

EXERCISING LEADS TO
MORE BRAIN- AND BODY-HEALTHY CHOICES

Did you know that when you are physically active, you are more likely to eat foods that are good for you, to get more sleep, and to take better care of your health in general? One study examined the effects of a twelve-week exercise program on sixty-two university students. At the end of three months, the students who engaged in physical activity reported eating a healthier diet, taking more responsibility for their own health, seeking out more social support, and managing stress better.

In a remarkable study that was published in a 2006 issue of *Pediatrics*,

ACTION STEP

If you want to quit smoking, stop drinking, calm stress, or eat a healthier diet, exercising can help you achieve these goals.

researchers found that compared to teens who watch a lot of TV, those who take part in a wide variety of physical activities are less likely to engage in risky behavior, such as drinking, smoking, drugs, violence, sex, and delinquency. This fascinating study also revealed that teens who participated in physical activities with their parents were the least likely to get into trouble with such behavior. These teens also tended to have higher self-esteem than both sedentary teens and active adolescents who didn't exercise or play sports with their parents. Conversely, the study showed that teens who spent a lot of time watching TV or playing video games tended to be at higher risk for engaging in all of these risky behaviors and had lower self-esteem.

This research reinforces what I've been advocating for years: Turn off the TV and the video games, and get active.

WHY COUCH POTATO SYNDROME
IS BAD FOR YOUR BRAIN AND BODY

Adopting a sedentary lifestyle is one of the worst things you can do for your brain, your overall health, and your body. Lack of physical exercise negatively affects blood flow in the body. When you don't get your blood pumping thanks to aerobic activities, the levels of nitric oxide drop. This causes the blood vessel walls to become distorted, which limits blood's ability to pulse freely. This puts you at increased risk for heart disease, high blood pressure, and stroke.

Without adequate blood flow, the blood vessels in the deep areas of the brain also become distorted, increasing the risk of tiny strokes. As the years go by, these tiny strokes accumulate and cause these deep brain areas to shut off and stop working. The deep brain areas control leg movement, coordinated body movement, and speed of thinking and behaving. These are some of the areas of the brain that are affected by Parkinson's disease, which explains why these strokes produce a clinical picture that closely resembles this disease. This explains why people over the age of forty who don't exercise aren't as mentally sharp as those who are physically active.

Being a couch potato also makes you more vulnerable to high blood pressure, which in turn increases the risk of developing other brain-related health problems. New research in the journal *Neurology* shows that people as young as forty-five with hypertension are more likely to experience problems with memory and thinking skills. In particular, middle-aged people with high diastolic blood pressure (the number on the bottom) are at greater risk than people with normal readings. For every 10-percent increase in the diastolic reading, the odds of an individual having cognitive problems jumped by about 7 percent. With nearly twenty thousand people involved in this study, it is the largest to investigate the link between hypertension and memory problems.

These findings support those of the Honolulu Study of Aging, which concluded that middle-aged people between the ages of forty and sixty who have untreated high blood pressure are at greater risk for developing dementia. For middle-aged people with a systolic blood pressure of 160 mmHg or higher, or a diastolic blood pressure of 90 mmHg or higher, the risk of dementia after age seventy was 3.8 to 4.8 times greater than for those whose hypertension was treated. The damage from inactivity can be devastating. Basically, when you shun exercise, you can say good-bye to all the brain, health, and body benefits you read about earlier in this chapter.

BEST KINDS OF EXERCISE

The best exercises combine aerobic activity to raise your heart rate and get your blood pumping, resistance to strengthen muscles, and coordination to activate your brain.

Cardiovascular exercise Aerobic exercise is one of the keys to brain health and plays a role in neurogenesis, or new cell growth. Ideally, aerobic exercise involves a brief warm-up period, twenty to forty-five minutes of sustained moderate to intense activity, and a cool-down. Some evidence suggests that higher-intensity activity—even for shorter periods of time—is also beneficial to the brain. Running, fast walking, swimming, rowing, and stair climbing are just some of the many aerobic exercise options available.

Your brain will benefit whether you get your heart pumping outdoors or in the gym. Animal studies show that running on a treadmill produced a significant enhancement in memory, similar to the cognitive improvements seen in outdoor aerobic activities. One of the best things about many aerobic activities is they don't require a lot of expensive equipment—you just throw on a pair of running shoes and go.

Resistance training For many years, experts have been touting the benefits of aerobic activity on the brain. According to a new study published in the *British Journal of Sports Medicine,* it appears that resistance training may also have protective powers for the brain. After a review of three exercise trials, researchers concluded that resistance training may prevent cognitive decline in older adults. Resistance training builds strength and tones muscles by working against any type of resistance, such as dumbbells, medicine balls, resistance tubing, or your own body weight. For example, you can use your own body weight to build strength by doing push-ups, pull-ups, or squats. Some resistance-training exercises—rowing, swimming, and stair climbing—double as aerobic activities, which makes them even more beneficial to your brain.

Coordination activities Exercise that requires coordination activates the cerebellum, which is located at the back of the brain and enhances thinking, cognitive flexibility, and processing speed. This means that participating in activities like dancing, tennis, and basketball, which require coordination, can make you smarter! And that's not all. Animal studies have shown that physical exercise that involves the planning and execution of complex movements actually changes the brain's structure.

Researchers from Brazil put this theory to the test when they compared the brains of competitive judo players and non-judo participants. Judo is a form of martial arts that relies on quick reactions and cunning to outsmart and outmaneuver an opponent. (I think judo is a wonderful activity as long as you don't engage in any sort of contact that could result in a brain injury.) Results of the study showed that the judo players had significantly higher gray matter tissue density than people who didn't practice judo. More gray matter translates into more brain cell bodies, which equals better brain function.

Combo exercises It is a good idea to engage in various types of exercises. Aerobic activity spawns new brain cells, which might make you think that if you want to boost your brainpower, you should limit your workouts to high-intensity aerobics. But it is coordination exercises that strengthen the connections between those new cells so your brain can recruit them for other purposes, such as thinking, learning, and remembering.

THE WORLD'S BEST BRAIN SPORTS

My favorite physical activity is table tennis, which also happens to be the world's best brain sport. It is highly aerobic and gets both the upper and lower body moving in every which way—twisting, bending down low, reaching up high, and shuffling from side to side. Plus, it gives your brain one heckuva workout. It is great for hand-eye coordination and reflexes (cerebellum and parietal lobes). You have to focus (prefrontal cortex) so you can track the ball through space (parietal lobes and occipital lobes), figure out spins (parietal lobes and occipital lobes), and plan shots and strategies (prefrontal cortex and cerebellum). Then you have to follow through and execute those tactics successfully (prefrontal cortex and cerebellum). All the while, you have to stay calm so you don't get too nervous on game point (basal ganglia). And you can't dwell on that point you blew a few minutes ago (anterior cingulate gyrus) or blow your top when you make a mistake (temporal lobes). It is like aerobic chess.

ACTION STEP

For better brain function, try a variety of activities that combine aerobic exercise and complex movements.

One of the things I love best about table tennis is that it involves very few brain injuries. In 1999, I played in the U.S. National Table Tennis Tournament with hundreds of other players, and there wasn't a single brain injury. A fascinating brain imaging study from Japan found that table tennis helps balance your brain. The researchers examined a group of people before and after playing table tennis for a period of ten minutes. The "after" images revealed increased activity in the prefrontal cortex, the thoughtful part of your brain, and the cerebellum.

Another reason why I'm such a fan of table tennis is that it is a sport the whole family can play. I was lucky enough to have a Ping-Pong table in my backyard when I was growing up, and I played a lot as a child with my siblings and my parents. My mother was a fierce competitor with lightning-fast reflexes, and she usually reigned as queen of the court. I always had such a great time playing that I never realized that I was "exercising," or improving my brain function. It was just fun.

Other great brain sports include dancing and tennis. Dancing is very aerobic and is especially good for your brain if you are learning new steps rather than just grooving to the music. That's why taking classes in ballroom, hip-hop, or jazz dancing where you have to memorize routines is ideal. Tennis, like table tennis, is a high-intensity activity that pumps up your brainpower. The main difference is that traditional tennis is slower so your reflexes don't get as much of a workout as they do with table tennis.

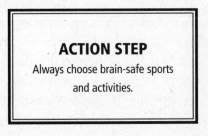

ACTION STEP

Always choose brain-safe sports and activities.

MOVE IT!
START AN EXERCISE PLAN NOW

There's no time like the present to get on the move to better brain-body health through exercise. If you are new to fitness, ease into it gradually. Trying to do too much too fast can lead to injuries and burnout. It is just like when you were a kid. You had to crawl before you walked, and you had to use training wheels before you could ride a two-wheeler bike.

Making exercise a habit takes time. A habit is a series of actions your brain executes—when you tell it to do so—relatively automatically and without effort. It takes numerous repetitions before your brain learns to perform a function automatically. The best chance of making exercise a habit is to schedule a specific time and place to exercise each day or at least on several specific days each week. This doesn't mean you have to do the same form of exercise each time. In fact, it is better to vary your routine. This prevents boredom and helps keep you motivated. After a few months of sticking to the routine, you will find that you no longer think about whether or not to work out; you just do it. By this time, exercise will have become a habit that will help keep your brain and body healthy for a lifetime.

ACTION STEP

Make it a rule to exercise. Don't give yourself the option of exercising or not. It should be a daily habit just like brushing your teeth.

FIND THE BEST PHYSICAL ACTIVITIES
FOR YOUR BRAIN

When it comes to exercise, one type doesn't fit all. Depending on your brain, you may gravitate toward exciting, stimulating, competitive, or even dangerous activities or you might be more inclined to seek out calming, soothing, or solitary activities. Whatever type of exercise suits you, make sure you get an aerobic workout at least three times a week for at least twenty minutes. For example, if you find that yoga helps you focus and calm stress, do it! Just remember that yoga doesn't usually get your heart rate up high enough for aerobic benefit. So, if you love yoga, alternate that with sessions of aerobic exercise.

See the following chart to find physical activities that are good for your brain type.

ACTION STEP

Try physical activities that can help heal your brain and keep your body looking great.

If you have:	**Try this type of exercise:**
PFC problems (ADD, short attention span, impulsiveness, poor planning)	LOTS of high-intensity aerobic activities, table tennis, meditation
Basal ganglia problems (anxiety, panic attacks, constant worry)	Yoga, aerobic activity
Deep limbic problems (depression, PMS)	Aerobic activity in social activities such as dancing
ACG problems (holding grudges, getting stuck on negative thoughts)	Intense aerobic exercise to boost serotonin
Temporal lobe problems (memory troubles)	Dancing or aerobics classes that involve music steps
Cerebellum problems (slow thinking)	Coordination exercises

Here are more brain-friendly activities from which to choose.

- Table tennis
- Tennis
- Dancing and dance classes
- Dance Dance Revolution (this is one video game that earns my seal of approval)
- Running
- Walking
- Golf (walk the course quickly; no carts, please!)
- Hiking
- Frisbee
- Swimming
- Basketball

- Volleyball
- Jumping rope
- Walking the dog
- Running/walking for charity
- Working out at the gym
- Aerobics classes
- Badminton
- Martial arts (no contact, and please don't break boards with your forehead!)

Remember that whichever activities you choose, the idea is to drive up your heart rate. Any of the activities on this list can provide aerobic benefits—if you put enough effort into them. Many people make the mistake of thinking that the sport they play as a hobby fulfills their exercise quota, but it depends on the sport and the intensity you put into it.

I once outlined a nutrition and exercise program as part of a treatment plan for an overweight patient. After several weeks on the plan, he complained to me that he wasn't losing any weight even though he was exercising more than ever. When I asked him what kind of exercise he was getting, he told me he was playing two whole rounds of golf a week. I had to break it to him that although walking a golf course is physical activity, it often doesn't count as aerobic activity because you have to stop all the time to hit the ball. He looked at me like I was nuts and said, "I don't walk the course. I get out of the cart, walk to hit the ball, then get back in the cart. That's a lot of activity, hopping in and out of that cart!"

Even though golf isn't the best aerobic exercise, it is a great recreational activity that gets your brain working. You can always fuel the intensity by walking the course very quickly and doing a few jumping jacks or push-ups while waiting your turn (as long as you don't distract the other players).

When choosing physical activities, always keep brain safety in mind. For example, martial arts provide a high-intensity workout involving coordination and discipline. That's great for the brain, but only if there isn't any contact involved. To protect your brain, avoid martial arts classes that include sparring with other participants or stupid stunts like breaking boards with your forehead.

Getting involved in brain-friendly sports is easy. If you want to try table tennis, the best brain sport in the world, get a table and start hosting friendly competitions at home, at the office, or at school. Or join one of the many table tennis clubs located throughout the nation. To find a local club, visit the United States of America Table Tennis (USATT) website (www.usatt.org). I often recommend getting a USATT coach to ramp up skill quickly. The game is faster, more fun, and more challenging if you play well. Plus, whenever you do something well, you want to do more of it.

You may notice that many common physical activities aren't included on the list above. Biking may be one of the most popular aerobic activities, but it also happens to be the number one cause for head injuries. I have seen far too many SPECT scans of brains that have been damaged by bike accidents. If you absolutely must ride a bike, wear a helmet that fits correctly. Helmets that don't fit provide little to no protection. Skateboarding is another activity that isn't advised. One of the worst brain scans I have ever seen is of a young skateboarder who wasn't wearing a helmet. He lost nearly all function in approximately one-fourth of his frontal lobe. His life will never be the same.

> **ACTION STEP**
>
> Organized sports, gym workouts, and recreational activities aren't the only ways to inject physical activity into your daily life. Try these simple tricks to add more exercise to your day:
> - Take the stairs instead of the escalator or elevator.
> - Walk to work or school.
> - Do the housework at a quick pace.
> - Use a jogging stroller or baby backpack and walk to the store instead of driving.
> - Rake leaves, pull weeds, and mow the lawn.

NO EXCUSES

I recommend exercise as part of a treatment plan to many of my patients, and I can tell you that I've heard every excuse in the book as to why they can't exercise.

"My back aches."
"My knees hurt."
"My feet hurt."
"I don't have the time."
"I'm too tired."

> **ACTION STEP**
>
> Stop using excuses to avoid exercise. In many cases, exercise will help eliminate or minimize the source of your excuse, such as pain or health conditions.

"I'm not very coordinated."
"I don't like to sweat."
"I have a health condition."
"I hate exercise."

Pain is one of the most common excuses I hear. Our scans have taught me that the use of chronic pain medications, such as Vicodin or OxyContin, is harmful to brain function. The brains of people who use these medications on a long-term basis look very similar to the brains of alcoholics. If you suffer from back pain, neck pain, or any other kind of pain, consider natural supplements that may ease your discomfort. Some of my patients have experienced pain relief from SAMe. In my practice, I have found that some patients get stuck on the pain. It is all they can think about. For these individuals, 5-HTP, which boosts serotonin, and fish oil may help get them unstuck.

The Exercise Solution

Exercise Robbers	Exercise Boosters
Fatigue	Adequate sleep (at least seven hours)
Chronic pain	Natural pain relief (SAMe, fish oil, 5-HTP, no artificial sweeteners)
Lack of time	Making exercise a priority
Lack of coordination	Practicing coordination activities
Lack of focus	Clearly focused, written goals
Bad habits, giving in	Practicing willpower
Depression	Any physical activity
Being in denial about problems	Effectively treating any brain problems

PART THREE

CHANGE YOUR BRAIN, BEAUTIFY AND STRENGTHEN YOUR BODY

6

THE SKIN SOLUTION

Brain Signals to Soothe

and Smooth Your Skin

The health of your skin is an outside reflection of the health of your brain.

On a rare, sunny, glorious, fall day in Seattle, my friend Cynthia, whom I had known for the past twelve years, greeted me at the front entrance of the lecture hall. Cynthia was the founder of ADD Resources, a support group for people and families affected by attention deficit disorder. I had spoken to her group many times. Cynthia, who has ADD herself, is famous for saying exactly what is on her mind. You always know what Cynthia is thinking. As I hugged her hello, she said, "I have to know what you are taking. Your skin is beautiful."

I blushed. "Fish oil and sleep," I said.

"That's it," she said.

"That is a big part of it," I replied. "Plus, I eat a brain-healthy diet, exercise, don't believe every stupid thought that comes into my head, and deal with the stress in my life without caffeine or alcohol."

The health of your skin is directly tied to the health of your brain. People, especially women, spend so much time and money working on their skin, when the first organ you want to take care of to have great-looking skin is your brain. The cosmetics counter, the dermatologist, the plastic surgeon— this is where you run when you want to reverse the aging process. But skin-care products, laser treatments, and the scalpel are often only temporary fixes. The real fix lies in your brain. It is your brain that tells your skin to produce more or less oil. It is your brain that supervises the production of supportive

ACTION STEP

Boost blood flow to rejuvenate
your skin.

collagen. And it is your brain at the command post of skin-cell regeneration. We all need to stop thinking about skin care from the outside in and start thinking about it from the inside out.

While writing this book, I went to my father's eightieth-birthday party. Two of my childhood friends were there. One was a longtime smoker. As we stood next to each other, I could see that his skin was deeply wrinkled. Smoking constricts blood flow to your brain and skin and prematurely ages both. As I wrote in the Introduction, my other friend had lost his wife to cancer a year earlier. The chronic stress had aged him what looked like twenty years. As he complained about his energy and memory, I worried that his brain would look aged as well.

I have often said that whatever is good for your heart is good for your brain, and whatever is bad for your heart is bad for your brain. It is all about healthy blood flow. Here we can definitely add that whatever is good for your heart is good for your brain is good for your skin, and whatever is bad for your heart is bad for your brain is bad for your skin. The same things that boost blood flow to the brain and enhance overall brain function will rejuvenate your skin and give it a healthy glow. By the same token, many things that harm the brain also damage your skin and make you look older.

THE BRAIN–SKIN CONNECTION

You might wonder what your brain has to do with your skin. After all, your skin is on the outside of your body, right? Isn't it more affected by our environment and the things we put on our faces—creams, lotions, makeup, aftershave, wrinkle removers—than by our brains? No. Scientific evidence points to a powerful brain-skin connection. Your skin and brain are completely connected to each other. It is not uncommon to hear:

"He is so mad that he is turning red."
"You can tell she is embarrassed because she is blushing."
"Whenever I get upset, I break out in hives."
"I am so excited I have goose bumps."
"He must be the nervous type, because his hands are cold."
"Whenever I get nervous, my hands start to sweat."

I remember the first time I was on television. It was on a small station in Connecticut about twenty years ago. I was so nervous that I unconsciously spent the whole interview rubbing my hands on my trousers trying to keep them dry. When I watched the video later, I was horrified.

> **ACTION STEP**
>
> Counteracting responses to stress helps you feel calm and relaxed, and makes your skin look healthier.

Scientists measure both hand temperature and skin sweat gland activity to understand the body's response to stress. Lie detector tests use these two measures as part of their battery to determine when people lie. As a biofeedback therapist, I have spent many hours teaching my patients to both warm and dry their hands as part of relaxation protocols. When we feel anxious or upset, our skin temperature immediately starts to become colder and we start to sweat.

UNRESOLVED EMOTIONS MAY COME OUT THROUGH YOUR SKIN

When I was a resident at the Walter Reed Army Medical Center in Washington, D.C., one of my first psychotherapy cases was a U.S. Army colonel named Bob who had a persistent rash over his whole body that was resistant to treatment. Bob was referred to our clinic because the rash had started shortly after his wife had died in a car accident two years earlier. He had no idea why he needed to see a shrink but was happy to cooperate if it could help. The rash was interfering with everything in his life. Plus, he noticed that whenever he became stressed, the rash would intensify.

One of the unique features of his story was that Bob never cried over the loss of his wife. He told me he had always had problems expressing his feelings, and he had four children at home who needed him now more than ever. After several sessions, I decided to use hypnosis with Bob to help him with what I believed to be unresolved grief. Bob was highly hypnotizable, which is often true of many intelligent people. During our first hypnotic session, Bob cried for the first time. The tears started silently, almost reluctantly, then the sobs came, which became more intense as the session progressed. The next four hypnosis sessions were filled with tears and the expression of grief over his lost love and best friend. He had been so

> **ACTION STEP**
>
> Don't bottle up your emotions or it might cause skin problems.

overwhelmed by having to take care of his children and his job that his unconscious mind did not allow him to grieve, fearful he would lose total control. In a safe place, he allowed himself to feel the pain. Over the next three months, his rash went away.

YOUR SKIN IS "THE BRAIN ON THE OUTSIDE"

Change your brain, change your skin. Numerous studies have shown that when you experience psychological stress, your brain responds by sending signals to your skin to react as if it is under physical attack. This can result in a rash, flushing, blushing, or an increase in the production of protective oils and a decrease in the skin's less-critical functions, such as hair growth. More oil and less hair growth typically equal more blemishes and thinning hair. If you are stressed out about your new job, a test, or a big date, your skin is more likely to break out.

More evidence of the brain-skin link comes from research out of Sweden, where researchers have found that it is possible to study the biological roots of mental health diseases like bipolar disorder and schizophrenia by looking at certain skin cells rather than having to take tissue samples of the brain. That's because certain skin cells function similarly to the brain cells that are believed to be involved in these disorders. In a sense, this study shows that your skin cells mirror your brain cells.

On the flip side of the brain-skin connection, your skin can change your brain. In 2008, Wake Forest University's Gil Yosipovitch and colleagues published findings from a very interesting study using brain scans to see how scratching affects the brain. The researchers studied what happened when thirteen healthy adults had their lower right leg gently scratched although the area didn't itch. Participants were scanned before, during, and after the scratching sessions using functional MRI imaging. The scans showed that scratching activated certain areas of the brain, including the prefrontal cortex, inferior parietal lobe, and cerebellum. At the same time, it deactivated the anterior and posterior cingulated cortices. These areas are associated with unpleasant emotions and memories. This means that the simple act of scratching your skin changes your brain and can make you feel better. You might also want to try this with your partner or children to soothe them when they are upset.

The brain-skin connection is so strong that some people have begun calling the skin "the brain on the outside." In fact, the skin has been found to produce many of the same neuropeptides—including melatonin, serotonin, and cortisol—used by the brain. It is clear that the health and appearance of your skin are a reflection of the health of your brain.

BAD BRAIN HABITS AND CONDITIONS THAT CAN CAUSE SKIN PROBLEMS AND PREMATURE AGING

When you look in the mirror, what do you see? If it is a face full of wrinkles, fine lines, or sagging, don't run to the plastic surgeon just yet. Take a look at these common brain causes of premature aging first. The same goes for those of you with blemishes and acne. Before you rush to the cosmetics counter for a bunch of pricy acne treatments, take a moment to think about what is going on inside your body and your brain and how your lifestyle and environment are affecting both your skin and brain. In many cases, by taking care of your brain, you will be able to improve the appearance of your skin.

Caffeine Too much caffeine from coffee, tea, chocolate, or some herbal preparations dehydrates your skin, which makes it look dry and wrinkled.

Alcohol Alcohol has a dehydrating effect on the body, sapping moisture from your skin and increasing wrinkles. It also dilates the blood vessels and capillaries in your skin. With excessive drinking, the blood vessels lose their tone and become permanently dilated, giving your face a flush that will not go away. Alcohol also depletes vitamin A, an important antioxidant involved in skin-cell regeneration. Alcohol abuse damages the liver and reduces its ability to remove toxins from the body, resulting in increased toxins in the body and skin that make you look older than you really are.

Smoking Nicotine reduces blood flow to the skin, robbing it of that healthy, rosy glow. It also destroys elasticity, which promotes wrinkles. The act of puffing on cigarettes also adds fine lines to the area above your upper lip. Smoking for ten or more years can give you "smoker's face." That's a term Dr. Douglas Model introduced in 1985 when he published a study in the *British Medical Journal* showing that he could identify long-term smokers by doing nothing more than looking at their facial features. The smoker's face made the people look older than their true age and included the following characteristics: lines above and below the lips, at the corners of the eyes, on the cheeks, or on the jaw; a gaunt appearance; a grayish tone; and a reddish complexion. More bad news: Smokers are three times as likely to develop a certain type of skin cancer called squamous cell carcinoma than nonsmokers, according to a study in the *Journal of Clinical Oncology*.

Poor diet The foods you eat fuel the regeneration of your skin cells, which make themselves new every thirty days. Your skin reflects the nutritional quality of your diet. If you eat a diet deficient in omega-3 fatty acids, you are more likely to look older than your age.

Too much sugar Eating too many sweets and high-glycemic foods can cause wrinkles. A study in the *British Journal of Dermatology* found that consuming sugar promotes a natural process called glycation, in which sugars attach themselves to proteins to form harmful molecules called advanced glycation end products (AGEs). AGEs damage your brain and also damage collagen and elastin, the protein fibers that help keep skin firm and supple. The more sugar you consume, the more damage to these proteins, and the more wrinkles on your face.

Yo-yo dieting and massive weight loss Every time you gain weight, your skin stretches to accommodate the increased girth. When you lose weight, your skin has to contract back to your new smaller shape. A lifetime of ups and downs in weight diminishes your skin's elasticity until it can no longer shrink to fit your size. Gaining a lot of weight—a hundreds pounds or more—can stretch your skin to the point of no return. After massive weight loss, you may be stuck with loose, hanging skin on your body and face.

Inadequate water intake When you don't drink enough water, your skin becomes dehydrated.

ACTION STEP

Avoid too much alcohol, too much caffeine, or too little water. They dehydrate the skin and make it look dull and wrinkled.

Lack of sleep Without adequate rest, your skin misses out on the ever-so-important rejuvenation process that occurs during sleep. The result? Premature aging of the skin, bags under the eyes, and an increase in wrinkles.

Lack of exercise Being a couch potato decreases blood flow to the skin and deprives you of the antiaging benefits of physical activity.

Stress Researchers have pinpointed a strong brain-stress-skin connection. In response to stress, your brain sends signals to your skin that can result in pimples and breakouts. Scientific evidence has found that psychological stress worsens the symptoms of several common skin diseases, such as psoriasis and eczema.

Unresolved emotional conflicts or post-traumatic stress disorder As in Colonel Bob's case above, unresolved grief or emotional conflicts cause chronic stress and may be reflected in your skin. If you emotionally repress or bury your problems, they may be reflected negatively through your skin. Get help when you need it.

Hormonal changes The hormonal fluctuations that occur during puberty, pregnancy, PMS, perimenopause, menopause, polycystic ovarian syndrome (high testosterone levels in some women), and andropause (low testosterone levels in men) may be at the root of breakouts and other undesirable changes in your skin. Dry skin is commonly associated with hypothyroidism when the thyroid gland is underactive.

Untreated or undertreated psychiatric conditions Skin picking and cutting are symptoms of certain types of mental disorders.

Dementia and memory problems With impaired cognitive function, you may not remember to take medications, to wear sunscreen, or to follow a skin-healthy beauty regimen.

Medications Some prescription and over-the-counter medications can affect your skin in a negative way. For example, birth control pills may either worsen or improve the appearance of acne and oily skin.

Sun exposure The damaging rays of the sun accelerate the effects of aging and cause age spots, wrinkles, sagging, and in some cases, skin cancer. Scientific studies show that due to our changing climate and ozone depletion, the risk for skin cancer is on the rise. Although most types of skin cancer are treatable, they may leave unsightly scars. Some sun exposure is important to get healthy levels of vitamin D. But balance is also important.

Pollution and environmental toxins Daily exposure to toxins can damage your brain and your complexion. A study published in the *International Journal of Cosmetic Science* found that exposure of the skin to troposphere ozone, the major oxidant in photochemical smog, reduced vitamin E by 70 percent. It also increased lipid hydroperoxides, which are a sign of oxidative damage in cell membranes.

Climate If you live in a dry, desert area, your skin may look as parched as you feel.

Twelve Brain Ways to Get Smoother, Younger-Looking Skin

1. Get more sleep for a better brain and skin that glows.

Skin cell regeneration, in which dead skin cells are replaced with fresh new cells, revs up while you sleep to rejuvenate your skin. Getting adequate sleep is a better antiaging treatment than anything you could find at the cosmetics counter. Sleep also repairs skin from daily pollution and toxins and helps prevent breakouts by regulating the body's hormones. For more on the importance of sleep, see Chapter 10, "The Sleep Solution."

2. De-stress for antiaging your brain and skin.

By reducing the stress in your life, you can take years off your appearance and delay the skin's aging process. With stress hormones under control, you are likely to experience fewer wrinkles and breakouts. For more information on how stress affects your skin, check out Chapter 11, "The Stress Solution."

3. Exercise to improve both brain and skin circulation.

Getting your heart pumping improves blood flow to your brain and skin. Improved cell regeneration, collagen production, and wound healing are some of the many benefits of enhanced circulation. Chapter 5, "The Exercise Solution," included more ways that exercise improves the skin.

4. Balance your hormones for better skin and brain function.

Acne, dry skin, oily skin, wrinkles, sagging—these can all be signs of hormonal imbalances in your body. For example, the hormone estrogen helps delay the aging process to keep your skin looking firm and supple. Estrogen is responsible for collagen crosslinking, in which collagen intertwines with other collagen to form a sort of mesh network that provides elasticity and smoothness and keeps the skin from sagging. It is similar to the way spandex works—you can stretch it out, and it will snap back to its original shape. Estrogen levels decrease with age, which causes you to lose the protection of crosslinking. This makes your skin more similar to a delicate wool sweater—if you stretch it out, it stays stretched out and doesn't spring back into shape. This is when gravity starts to take its toll on your face. By keeping your hormone levels in check, your skin will be softer, smoother, and clearer. See Chapter 7, "The Hormone Solution," for more on balancing your hormones.

5. Have more sex.

Having great sex—and a lot of it—can boost the levels of hormones, such as estrogen and DHEA, both of which promote smoother, tighter skin. According to fascinating research, making love on a regular basis is so good for your skin, it can make you look ten years younger. More on this intriguing research in Chapter 14, "The Passion Solution."

6. Limit caffeine and alcohol.

To keep your skin looking soft and supple, avoid any beverages that dehydrate it.

7. Quit smoking—now!

If you quit smoking, you can reverse some of the damage you've done to your skin.

8. Eat a brain-healthy diet.

A diet full of brain-friendly antioxidants gives you healthier skin and enhances the skin-cell regeneration process.

9. Maintain a healthy weight.

By stabilizing your weight, your skin is more likely to maintain its tone and elasticity.

10. Drink more water.

Drinking an adequate amount of water keeps your skin hydrated to prevent wrinkles and fine lines.

11. Balance your sun exposure.

Some sun is essential for healthy skin, to boost vitamin D levels in your body. Too much sun can cause premature aging and age spots. Try to get twenty minutes of good sun exposure during the day, after which you should protect yourself with sunscreen.

12. Treat mental disorders and memory problems.

When your brain works better, your skin will likely look better too. The chronic stress from having depression, anxiety, substance abuse, or attention deficit disorder robs your skin of its vitality and elasticity. Early treatment is essential.

SUPPLEMENTS TO ENHANCE YOUR BRAIN AND YOUR SKIN

See Appendix C, "The Supplement Solution," for more detailed information.

Vitamin D is an essential vitamin for both your brain and skin. I have written about it many times in this book in regards to brain health for mood and memory, but it is also important for your skin.

Fish oil is another supplement I have written extensively about for the brain, and it is often helpful for your skin.

Evening primrose oil contains an essential fatty acid called gamma-linolenic acid (GLA), which scientific evidence says can help with eczema and rashes.

DMAE, also known as deanol, is an analog of the B vitamin choline. DMAE is a precursor of the neurotransmitter of acetylcholine; it has strong effects on the central nervous system. DMAE is commonly used to increase the capacity of neurons in the brain and is also thought to have antiaging properties that diminish wrinkles and improve the appearance of the skin.

Phenylalanine is an amino acid that has been found to be helpful for depression and pain. There is also good scientific evidence that it may be helpful for vitiligo, a chronic relatively common skin disorder that causes white patches of skin. It occurs when the cells responsible for skin pigmentation die or become unable to function.

Alpha-lipoic acid (ALA) is made naturally in the body and may protect against cell damage in a variety of conditions. In a number of studies it has been found to be helpful for skin issues as well.

Grape seed extract comes from grape seeds that are waste products of the winery and grape juice industries. Extensive research suggests that grape seed extract is beneficial in many areas of health because of its antioxidant ability to bond with collagen, promoting youthful skin, elasticity, and flexibility.

The Skin Solution

Skin Damagers	Skin Enhancers
Too much caffeine	Limit caffeine
Alcohol	Freedom from alcohol
Smoking	No nicotine products
Poor diet	Brain-healthy diet
Too much sugar	Reduced sugar intake
Yo-yo dieting	Stable weight
Dehydration	Adequate water intake
Lack of sleep	Adequate sleep, at least seven hours
Lack of exercise	Physical activity at least four or five times a week
Chronic stress	Meditation, deep-breathing exercises
Post-traumatic stress disorder (PTSD)	Therapy
Hormonal imbalances	Balanced hormones
Thyroid conditions	Balanced thyroid levels
Psychiatric conditions	Treatment, such as therapy and medication
Memory problems	Brain-healthy habits or treatment, such as medication
Sun exposure	Sun exposure limited to twenty minutes, then wearing sunscreen
Aging	Supplementation with vitamin D, fish oil, evening primrose oil, DMAE, phenylalanine, alpha-lipoic acid, grape seed extract

7

THE HORMONE SOLUTION

BALANCE YOUR HORMONES TO
TURN BACK THE CLOCK

Your hormones play a critical role in the way you think, act, and look.

Did you know that hormones have a huge impact on brain function, for both men and women? When your hormones are balanced, you tend to feel happy and energetic. When your hormones are off, everything and everyone in your life suffers. For example, did you know that low thyroid hormone is associated with overall decreased brain activity, which makes you feel depressed, irritable, and have significant trouble thinking (Image 7.1)?

Likewise, low testosterone levels have been associated with low libido, depression, and memory problems and have been implicated in Alzheimer's disease. We are only beginning to talk about male menopause, but for many men it is a real issue that needs to be treated. Low testosterone levels may be a significant cause of midlife crises and divorce. As his testosterone levels go down, he feels more negative, blames his wife, who is having her own hormonal issues, and looks outside of the marriage to feel young again. Of course, the new love usually doesn't make him happy.

Low testosterone levels also affect women. I once had a female physician come up to me at a lecture and tell me that at age fifty-one she had no interest in sex, her marriage was in trouble, and her mother had just died from Alzheimer's disease. She had NO idea that low testosterone levels could be part of her problem. Later she e-mailed me that her testosterone levels were near zero and that taking testosterone made a huge difference for her sexuality, her memory, and her marriage.

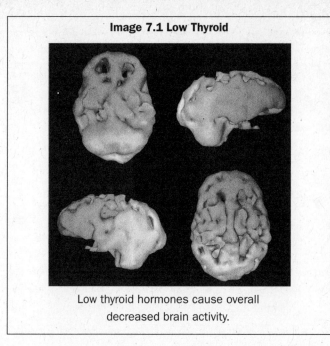

Image 7.1 Low Thyroid

Low thyroid hormones cause overall
decreased brain activity.

When testosterone levels are too high, men or women can be "too competitive," have commitment issues, be hypersexual, and struggle with acne or being too aggressive. A common condition in women associated with too much testosterone is called polycystic ovarian syndrome (PCOS). More on this in a bit.

Do you believe in PMS? I have five sisters and three daughters. I believe in PMS! But it wasn't until I met Becky that I finally had evidence that PMS was, in fact, a brain disorder. Becky came to my office after a brief stay in jail. In the week before her period, she often became moody, anxious, aggressive, and tended to drink too much. Shortly before she saw me, during the worst time of her cycle, she got into a fight with her husband, attacked him with a knife, and was arrested. When I met her, I decided to scan her during the worst time of her cycle, and then again two weeks later, during the best time. Becky's scans were radically different. During the difficult time of her cycle, her worry center was overactive, indicated by the arrow on Image 7.2, and her judgment center was low in activity, which may have been why she grabbed the knife. You can see the holes in the front of her brain. During the best time of her cycle, her brain looked much better (Image 7.3). Seeing her scans was so instructive, and on treatment she did much better. Hormone fluctuations can change your brain and literally rip apart your family.

Image 7.2
PMS Worst Time of Cycle

Image 7.3
PMS Best Time of Cycle

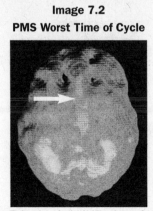 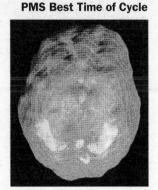

This view is looking down from the top, where gray is average activity and white is the top 15 percent of activity. The white area by the arrow indicates increased anterior cingulate activity and trouble shifting attention. The holes in the front part of the scan indicate lower prefrontal cortex activity and poor judgment.

Along the same lines, menopause is often associated with lower overall brain activity, which can lead to depression, anxiety, insomnia, and concentration and memory problems. Images 7.4 and 7.5 show a woman's SPECT scan both off and on her hormones.

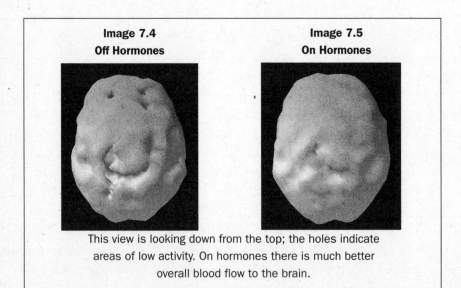

Image 7.4
Off Hormones

Image 7.5
On Hormones

This view is looking down from the top; the holes indicate areas of low activity. On hormones there is much better overall blood flow to the brain.

Again, these hormonal shifts can cause seismic problems in relationships. Carefully testing and treating hormonal issues for both men and women is critical to the health of the brain as well as to the health of relationships. Let me give you a very personal example of how issues with hormones can affect your relationships.

I am married to a neurosurgical ICU nurse. While Tana is both beautiful and smart, she was also used to being very assertive, working around neurosurgeons all day long. She often joked, "What is the difference between a neurosurgeon and God? . . . At least God knows he is not a neurosurgeon." Tana also has a black belt in tae kwon do and her approach to romance was more like the typical guy's—we'd be cuddling together and she'd say, "Okay, that's enough, I've got to go work out." She also loved masculine dogs and had a big dog named Mack.

One of our first fights was over what type of dog we should get together. I wanted a King Charles cavalier spaniel—they're cute, little, fluffy, smart, and sweet. She wanted none of it. She actually said that the little dogs were nothing more than chew toys for the bigger dogs. So we compromised on an English bulldog. Frasier was cute, but not the kind of cute I was looking for.

When Tana was about thirty-eight years old, she went off birth control pills and noticed that her face started breaking out and her menstrual cycles became very irregular. Despite her young age, she thought she must be going

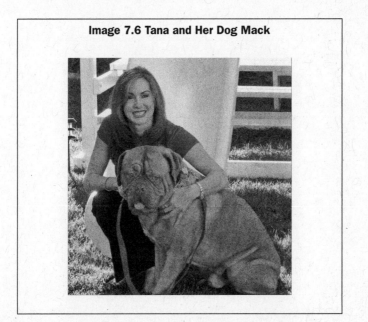

Image 7.6 Tana and Her Dog Mack

through perimenopause, a period of time that can last several years prior to menopause. To figure out what was going on, she went to see her doctor. To her astonishment, she was informed that her cholesterol and triglycerides were high and that she was prediabetic. What?! Tana is five feet six inches tall, weighs 118 pounds, has about 15 percent body fat, works out like a nut, and eats all the right foods. That's crazy, she thought, I'm the healthiest person I know.

As we were both concerned about her health, a friend of ours introduced us to Dr. Christine Paoletti, a gynecologist in Santa Monica. It took only about ten minutes for Dr. Paoletti to suspect that Tana had a condition called polycystic ovarian syndrome (PCOS), which causes a woman to have too much testosterone. It is also linked to irregular menstrual cycles, skin breakouts, high cholesterol, and insulin resistance. An ultrasound confirmed the diagnosis. Why didn't any other doctors catch it? Tana doesn't fit the typical physical profile of a woman with PCOS. Most women with PCOS are overweight and have excessive facial and body hair.

Dr. Paoletti treated Tana with glucophage, a medication used to balance insulin and reduce testosterone levels. The changes were dramatic. Within a few months, her cholesterol dropped fifty points, her insulin levels normalized, her skin cleared up, and her cycle became perfectly regular. Even more dramatic were the changes in her personality. All of a sudden, she wanted to cuddle more, was less intense, less anxious, and after about six months she had to have a pocket poodle and called her Tinkerbell.

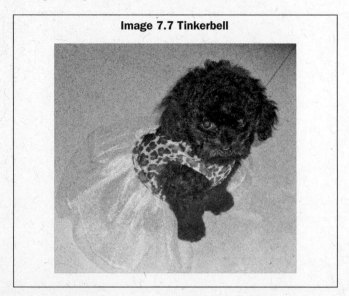

Image 7.7 Tinkerbell

Now, I like to say, change your hormones, change your brain, change your body, change your personality, change your relationships . . . and even the type of dog you have. It is clear that our hormones are heavily involved in making us who we are.

YOUR BRAIN, YOUR BODY, AND THE HORMONAL CASCADE

There are many myths and misconceptions about hormones. First, people usually think hormones are just a female issue. Wrong! Hormones are essential for health and vitality in both men and women. Second, most people—and even some doctors—think of our hormone-producing glands as the sole source of any hormonal problems. Wrong again! In reality, the brain controls all the hormones in your body. Think of your hormones as airplanes flying through the air and your brain as the air traffic controller. Your brain tells them how fast they can fly, when they can land, and where they can land. For example, if your thyroid gland is overproducing, it doesn't know it. Your brain filters your blood to check up on your thyroid levels, sees that there is too much, and asks the thyroid gland to lower production. The hormone-producing glands don't communicate with each other, only with the brain, which controls them all.

Third, most of us think of our hormones—estrogen, testosterone, thyroid, and others—as individual and unconnected systems. Wrong again! For example, when a woman approaches menopause, many doctors look only at the ovaries. And when thyroid levels are off, they only test and treat the thyroid gland. This approach is wrong, because our hormones all work together to maintain balance. Think of the hormonal system as a symphony, with the brain as the conductor. If all the players are playing the right notes at the right time, it is a wonderful concert. But if the conductor takes a break and a single player hits a sour note, it ruins the whole effect. Similarly, when one hormone system is out of balance, it causes imbalances with the other hormone systems.

When your hormones are in sync, a magnificent mind, a slimmer body, clearer skin, better energy, a happier outlook, and improved health are the rewards. Hormonal imbalances lead to cloudy thinking, make you fat, give you acne and wrinkles, sap your energy, sour your mood, and increase your risk for disease.

What exactly are hormones? They are little chemical messengers that travel through the bloodstream, allowing the brain and bodily organs to communi-

cate. You might be surprised to learn that hormones are derived from cholesterol. Cholesterol gets a bad rap in the media, but cholesterol isn't the enemy.
Yes, it is true that when cholesterol is too high, it is associated with heart disease. But when it is too low, it is associated with homicide, suicide, and severe
depression. Your brain and body need some cholesterol. Approximately 60
percent of the solid weight of the brain is fat, so you need healthy levels of
cholesterol for optimal function. From cholesterol, your body makes a chemical called pregnenolone, a mother hormone, from which all the other hormones are derived. This hormonal tree is referred to as the hormonal cascade
(Figure 7.1).

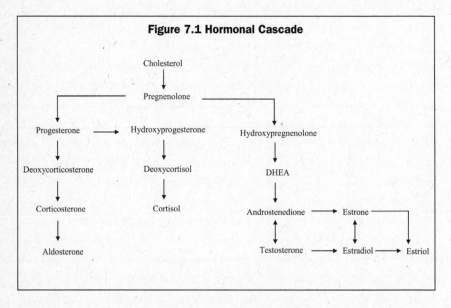

Figure 7.1 Hormonal Cascade

Like most people, you are probably most familiar with the body's reproductive hormones: estrogen, progesterone, and testosterone. But these are only
some of the many hormones that help keep your brain and body balanced. In
this chapter, you will discover how many other hormones play a vital role in
the health of your brain and how your body looks, feels, and functions.

BALANCE YOUR THYROID
FOR A BRIGHTER MIND, MORE ENERGY,
SLIMMER SHAPE, AND A BETTER MOOD

The small, butterfly-shaped thyroid gland located in the lower neck has
become big news ever since Oprah revealed that she was suffering from

hypothyroidism. Oprah isn't alone. Tens of millions of people worldwide are estimated to have thyroid problems. The thyroid is the hormone of metabolism, regulating how fast the processes in your body work. It is similar to a car's idle.

Low thyroid activity (hypothyroidism) When your thyroid is low, your body works more slowly or sluggishly. Your heart rate is usually slower, your bowels move slower, your digestion rate is slower, and your thinking is slower. On SPECT scans of people with hypothyroidism, we see decreased brain activity. Many studies on hypothyroidism have shown overall low function in the brain, which leads to depression, cognitive impairment, anxiousness, and a sense of being in a mental fog or feeling spacey. Some people have what's called subclinical hypothyroidism. These are patients whose thyroid levels are in the normal range but who have symptoms. When other hormonal systems within the body are out of balance, it can affect thyroid activity and alter it.

Common signs of hypothyroidism Fatigue, weight gain, dry skin, chronically low temperature below 98.6, fuzzy thinking, depression, and being cold when others feel fine.

High thyroid activity (hyperthyroidism) When the thyroid gland is producing too much thyroid, everything in your body works too fast. Your heart beats faster, your bowels move faster, your digestion works faster. It is like you've had too much caffeine and you feel jittery or edgy.

Common signs of hyperthyroidism Sleeplessness, anxiety, irritability, racing thoughts, and being hot when others feel fine.

Get it balanced A simple blood test is all you need to see if you have thyroid problems. Unfortunately, many doctors look only at the overall functioning of the thyroid, by a test called a TSH, or thyroid-stimulating hormone. Thyroid problems often go undiagnosed because TSH levels can be normal even when a problem exists. Ask your doctor to perform a test that looks at your T4 and free T3 levels, which are the actual levels of thyroid floating in your system. What does that mean? It is very simple. Nearly all the hormones in the body float around in the bloodstream attached to a protein. When they're attached to this protein, they aren't available for use. The hormones that are active, or available for use, are free-floating in the bloodstream rather

ACTION STEP

Be sure to have your physician test
your T4 and free T3 levels when
checking your thyroid levels.

than attached. So it is these free-floating levels that are very important to test.

If you are diagnosed with a thyroid imbalance, a number of medications can be prescribed. Typically, when medication is prescribed, it will have to be taken throughout your lifetime. Many supplements support the thyroid, including iodine and selenium.

BALANCE YOUR ADRENAL HORMONES TO CALM STRESS, REDUCE ABDOMINAL FAT, AND DECREASE YOUR RISK FOR DISEASE

The triangle-shaped adrenal glands, which sit on top of your kidneys, are critically important in helping your body deal with stress. The adrenals produce DHEA and cortisol, which is known as the stress hormone. Our adrenal glands have the ability to put us in "fight-or-flight" mode. For example, let's say you are hiking and you come across a bear. Your body produces adrenaline, which gives you the strength to either fight the bear (usually not a good idea) or run from the bear. DHEA has been called coping fuel and the "universal promoter of goodness." DHEA is one of the most abundant hormones in the body, second only to cholesterol. A lack or deficiency of DHEA impacts the person's ability to cope with stress, potentially leading to damaging effects and behavioral changes and ultimately leading to emotional burnout, early aging, and physical exhaustion. With age, DHEA declines.

Adrenal fatigue In today's hustle-and-bustle world, we are faced with stress on a daily basis. Rush-hour traffic, family issues, and work demands mean that we are stressed from the minute we wake up until we go to sleep. This puts our adrenal gland on overdrive so it is constantly producing cortisol. After months or even years of unrelenting stress, the adrenal glands can burn out. We call this adrenal fatigue or adrenal gland failure, and it means your body no longer has the capacity to deal with daily stress. You have trouble getting out of bed, struggle to function, and may even have trouble getting yourself to work. Adrenal fatigue makes you fat—especially in your abdomen, which not only looks bad but also increases your risk for cardiovascular disease. Chronic exposure to stress hormones also kills brain cells in the hippocampus, a major memory structure in the brain.

Part of the reason why adrenal fatigue is becoming so common is that so many of us are skimping on sleep. If you don't get seven to eight hours of sleep at night, your system automatically goes on stress overload. Then you do terrible things to try to make up for the lack of sleep. You drink coffee,

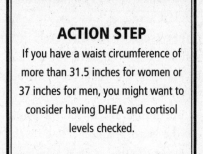

ACTION STEP

If you have a waist circumference of more than 31.5 inches for women or 37 inches for men, you might want to consider having DHEA and cortisol levels checked.

which is a stress inducer, to wake up. Then you drink wine in the evening to calm you down, but when the alcohol wears off, it puts your body into another stress response and wakes you up at two o'clock in the morning. It is a never-ending cycle of stress.

Common signs and symptoms of adrenal gland failure Abdominal fat, tiredness, low stress tolerance, craving sweets, difficulty concentrating, mental fog, low libido, and poor memory.

Overactive adrenal system When the adrenal system is working too hard, it is a very serious medical condition that can lead to a rare kind of tumor, which is usually noncancerous, called pheochromocytoma.

Common signs of overactive adrenals High blood pressure and high heart rate.

Get it balanced Diagnosing adrenal fatigue or overactive adrenals involves checking cortisol and DHEA-S levels with a blood test. Ways to combat adrenal fatigue include learning stress-management techniques, meditating, using self-hypnosis, and getting an ANTeater in your head to talk back to the automatic negative thoughts (ANTs). See Chapter 13 for more on ANTs (automatic negative thoughts) and ANTeaters. B vitamins—either in foods like green leafy vegetables or in supplements—support the adrenal system and help our bodies deal with stress. 5-HTP helps you sleep and boosts serotonin levels in the brain, which helps you calm stress and lose weight. Phosphatidylserine can also be helpful for adrenal fatigue. See Appendix C, "The Supplement Solution," for more information on these and the rest of the supplements mentioned in the chapter.

DHEA, if low, is an important supplement to counteract adrenal fatigue. DHEA serves as a precursor to male and female sex hormones (androgens and estrogens). DHEA levels in the body begin to decrease after age thirty, and are reported to be low in some people with anorexia, end-stage kidney disease, type 2 diabetes (non-insulin-dependent diabetes), AIDS, adrenal insufficiency, and in the critically ill. DHEA levels may also be depleted by a number of drugs, including insulin, steroids, opiates, and Danazol. According to the NaturalStandard.com website, there is good scientific evidence supporting the use of DHEA in the treatment of adrenal insufficiency, depression, systemic lupus erythematosus, and obesity. Dosages of 25 to 200 mg have been generally recommended. It is usually well tolerated. Acne and facial hair are common side effects, as it increases the body's testosterone levels. To avoid getting acne or facial hair, many doctors prescribe a metabolite of DHEA called 7-keto-DHEA. It is more expensive, but if acne and facial hair are an issue, it is worth it.

The main worry about DHEA for some professionals is that it will partly convert itself into sex hormones such as testosterone and estrogens. This seems to be an obvious advantage for the healthy person looking to combat age-associated hormonal decline. Unfortunately, this means advising people who are at risk for hormonally dependent cancers (prostate, breast, ovarian) against taking DHEA. For these, 7-keto-DHEA is a good solution.

BALANCE TESTOSTERONE
FOR BETTER SEXUAL FUNCTION AND A BETTER BRAIN

We typically think of testosterone as a sex hormone, but it does a lot more than just drive your libido. If you get a Y chromosome from your father, you get a spike of testosterone in the womb, which makes your brain more male. If you get an X chromosome from your dad, you don't get that spike of testosterone. This makes a huge difference in the kind of brain you have. Female brains have better language ability, are more interconnected, more communicative, more relationship driven, and less competitive. Male brains are wired for competing and dominating, but not as much for commitment.

Testosterone's effect on the brain goes far beyond typical male/female differences. Emerging scientific evidence is revealing that testosterone offers neuroprotection, helping prevent cognitive impairment, Alzheimer's disease, and depression. Researchers are also uncovering a relationship between low testosterone levels in men and chronic pain. Studies are currently under way to determine if balancing a man's testosterone levels can improve pain tolerance and reduce the perception of pain.

We tend to think of testosterone as a male hormone, but it is also vitally important for women. It is involved in her sex drive, her ability to build muscle, her outlook on life, and her memory.

Low testosterone in men For men, testosterone levels peak at age twenty-two and slowly decline thereafter. On average, men lose 10 percent of their testosterone every decade after age thirty, or about 1 to 3 percent each year. Recent research also indicates a link between low testosterone and Alzheimer's disease. As testosterone drops, there's less blood flow to the brain, which causes problems with sexual and cognitive function. It can also affect body weight, muscle mass, sex drive, mood, and energy. We call this male menopause or andropause. Some of my patients like to joke that it puts men on pause.

Common signs of low testosterone in men Declining libido, erectile dysfunction, depression, lack of energy, and memory problems.

Low testosterone in women Without enough testosterone, a woman's libido can go out the window. I treat a lot of women who are on the brink of divorce. In many cases, I find that their testosterone levels are off, or their husband's levels are low, and that is actually the source of their dissatisfaction with the marriage. So many times, I hear someone tell their spouse, "You are not the same person I married." And they aren't! That's because their hormone levels are nowhere near the same levels as when they got married. I think that before you file for divorce and throw away twenty or thirty years of a good marriage, you should both get your hormones checked.

Common signs of low testosterone in women Lack of libido, depression, and poor memory.

High testosterone in men Guys who produce too much of this hormone tend to fly off the handle for no reason. Men with the most testosterone are

> ### ACTION STEP
>
> There is a simple test I like to do. Hold up your hand and look at the ratio of your ring finger to your index finger. If your ring finger is longer, you got a lot of testosterone in the womb. Some say that the size of the ring finger also correlates to the size of a man's genitals.

also the least likely to get married and stay married. That may be why so many men tend to wait until they're older to tie the knot.

Common signs of high testosterone in men Aggression, moodiness, acne, and extreme competitiveness.

High testosterone in women Some women produce too much testosterone, which is often associated with PCOS—the same condition my wife has. PCOS can cause big changes in your body that affect your weight, skin, mood, and overall health.

Common signs of high testosterone and PCOS in women Obesity, irregular periods, acne, oily skin, excessive facial and body hair, aggression, high cholesterol, high blood pressure, diabetes.

Get it balanced For the best results from this blood test, make sure your doctor looks at two levels: your total testosterone and your free testosterone. New research shows *that spikes in blood sugar can lower a man's testosterone levels* by as much as 25 percent. So if you want an accurate reading on your test, you may want to skip having anything like doughnuts, candy, or Gatorade for at least a few hours before your blood test. For men with low testosterone, options include creams, gels, and injections. For women who need more of the hormone, creams are the most common treatment method. Treatment for women with high testosterone or PCOS is highly individualized and may include birth control pills, diabetes medications, fertility medications, and antiandrogens. DHEA is often helpful in raising testosterone levels.

BALANCE YOUR ESTROGEN
TO CONTROL YOUR WEIGHT AND MOODS
AND TO STRENGTHEN YOUR BONES, HEART, AND MEMORY

Estrogen is an amazing hormone that affects every organ system in the body—the bones, cardiovascular system, reproductive system, and the brain. Most people think of estrogen as a female hormone, but men need it too— only in much smaller doses. When women first start menstruating, estrogen levels begin rising and falling in a cyclic fashion. During a normal twenty-eight-day cycle, estrogen peaks and falls like a gentle rolling hill twice (see Figure 7.2).

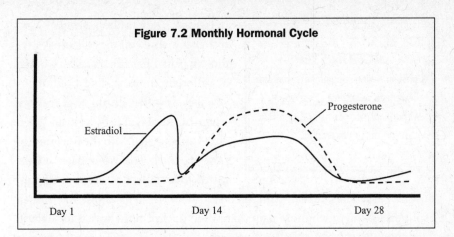

Figure 7.2 Monthly Hormonal Cycle

In their thirties and forties, when women enter perimenopause, the hormone system doesn't work as efficiently and changes start to take place in this pattern. Instead of gentle ups and downs, estrogen spikes and then crashes dramatically right before her period starts, which can cause severe PMS symptoms. This seesaw effect of going from estrogen dominance to estrogen withdrawal isn't fun and can make her feel like she is crazy, literally. An eye-opening study found that 40 percent of women being committed to mental institutions were admitted during the two days prior to the start of their period. By the time menopause hits, estrogen withdrawal is in full swing, which affects weight, cognitive function, and health.

Women have three kinds of estrogen: estrone, estradiol, and estriol. During the childbearing years, estradiol is the most abundant of the three. Like a fountain of youth, estradiol protects the brain, heart, and bones, provides antiaging protection for the skin, and helps prevent weight gain. Researchers at Yale University have found that estradiol suppresses appetite using the same pathways in the brain as leptin, one of the hormones involved in regulating the appetite. (See more on leptin later in this chapter.) The scientists concluded that impaired estrogen signaling, which may occur during menopause, may be the cause of menopausal weight gain and obesity. In perimenopause and menopause, estradiol begins to wane, and its protective qualities are lost.

Estrogen withdrawal When estrogen levels decline during the menstrual cycle, perimenopause, or menopause, women have more trouble with short-term memory and are more likely to have crying spells and depression. A woman may find herself wondering, Where did I park the car? or Why did I walk into this room? Low levels of estrogen can also make her more sensitive

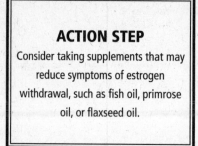

ACTION STEP

Consider taking supplements that may reduce symptoms of estrogen withdrawal, such as fish oil, primrose oil, or flaxseed oil.

to pain. A study in the *Journal of Neuroscience* focused on the effects of estradiol on pain. Researchers tested women at different times during their menstrual cycle—first during their period, when estradiol is at its lowest, and then after being treated with the hormone to raise its level. The women were subjected to a controlled amount of pain and were asked to rate their pain. When estradiol was at its lowest, the women reported feeling much more pain than when the hormone was at its highest. This shows that when estrogen levels are low, such as during menopause or during your period, women are likely to feel pain more acutely.

Common signs of estrogen withdrawal Fuzzy thinking, trouble focusing, and depression or bad moods.

Estrogen dominance High estrogen levels in conjunction with low levels of progesterone can cause heavier periods, cramping, and shorter cycles. In some women, this leads to a seemingly nonstop period.

Common signs of estrogen dominance Weight gain, retaining water, bossiness, aggressive behavior, and depression.

Get it balanced A simple blood test is used to determine levels of the three types of estrogen. Estrogen pills, birth control pills, creams, and vaginal inserts are just some of the options for estrogen replacement. Living a brain-healthy life by exercising and limiting caffeine, sugar, and alcohol can also help alleviate symptoms. Fish oil, primrose oil, and flaxseed oil may ease symptoms.

BALANCE YOUR PROGESTERONE
FOR BETTER MOODS, DEEPER SLEEP,
AND ENHANCED COGNITIVE FUNCTION

Say hello to the "feel good" hormone. Progesterone is like nature's Xanax—it calms you down, makes you feel peaceful, and helps you sleep. But while Xanax clouds your brain, progesterone sharpens your thinking. Progesterone is sometimes referred to as the pregnancy hormone because it promotes pregnancy. When you get pregnant, your progesterone levels shoot sky high, giving you a glow, great energy, and a flood of enthusiasm and love.

Like estrogen, progesterone follows a rolling-hill pattern during the second half of the menstrual cycle, rising and falling along with estrogen. By the time a woman hits her thirties, her body starts to produce progesterone less efficiently. In her late thirties and forties, those nice rolling hills of progesterone decrease to little more than bumps. Without the nice rise, she starts having progesterone-withdrawal symptoms. If estrogen is on a hill or a spike while progesterone is low, it really exacerbates the symptoms of estrogen dominance.

Low progesterone Without enough progesterone, you lose the brain's natural sleeping pill and antianxiety hormone. A deficiency of this hormone can also lead to addictions. Wendy, age forty-five, came to the Amen Clinics after her husband threatened to divorce her if she didn't stop drinking. She started to drink heavily around the age of forty because she had increasing issues with anxiety and insomnia. When I tested her, she had very low progesterone levels. Research shows that progesterone levels start to decrease eight years before a woman goes into menopause. Balancing her progesterone levels helped to calm her anxiety, improve her sleep, and end her addiction.

Common signs of low progesterone Trouble sleeping, headaches, migraines, anxiety, fuzzy thinking, poor memory, mood swings, and difficulty concentrating. Bossiness, aggressiveness, and water retention are intensified when coupled with high estrogen.

High progesterone It is rare to have high progesterone levels unless you are pregnant or your dosage of hormone replacement therapy is too high. Typically, it can make you feel like you are experiencing the first few weeks of pregnancy.

Common signs of high progesterone Morning sickness, extreme fatigue, and backaches.

Get it balanced Most doctors check progesterone levels using saliva, blood, or urine tests. For the best results, tests are usually done on day twenty-one of your menstrual cycle. Synthetic and bio-identical hormone replacement is available.

PREMENSTRUAL SYNDROME (PMS)

Lisa Nowak, the astronaut in the scandalous love triangle that made the news some time ago, put on a diaper and drove nine hundred miles to confront the girlfriend of her love interest. She was later accused of attempted kidnapping. During pretrial motions, I appeared on Fox News to talk about what could have caused a highly successful woman to do such a crazy thing. I was on a panel with five women. She had just filed an insanity plea—not guilty by reason of insanity—when the moderator asked me, "If you were the consulting psychiatrist for her defense team, what would you want to know?" I told him I would want to know where she was in her menstrual cycle when she committed the crime. All five women on the panel were aghast and one said, "Oh my God, I can't believe he just said that!" I explained that we've scanned many women at different times of their cycle, and that during the worst time of their cycles for women with PMS, their brains change. The way our society reacts to saying that a woman may fluctuate with her hormones is, in my mind, stupid because it is just so obvious.

PMS is real. From a hormonal perspective, the days prior to your period coincide with the days when your estrogen and progesterone levels hit rock bottom. Brain scans show that during the last two weeks of the cycle, the anterior cingulate gyrus starts to fire up. That's the part of your brain that helps you shift attention, be flexible, and go with the flow. This is due to a deficiency of serotonin, a natural antidepressant, feel-good chemical. We've seen that as estrogen levels fall, serotonin does too. Also, during the worst time of the cycle, the prefrontal cortex tends to go low, which is why women may struggle with focus and impulse control.

Common signs of PMS This crash causes emotional difficulties, intensifies feelings of depression, and can affect sleep. By now, you know that this can be a precursor to poor eating habits, which pack on unwanted pounds. It also robs your skin of the nighttime rejuvenation it needs. Other symptoms include bloating, breast tenderness, irritability, anger, worry, focusing on negative thoughts, poor concentration and impulsivity.

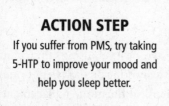

ACTION STEP

If you suffer from PMS, try taking 5-HTP to improve your mood and help you sleep better.

Get it balanced Replacing a small amount of progesterone during the sec-

ond half of your cycle may neutralize symptoms. Medications that boost serotonin, such as Prozac and Zoloft, have been shown to be helpful to calm the
anterior cingulate symptoms of worry, depression, and anxiety. In my practice, I've noticed that 5-HTP reduces symptoms of PMS.

PERIMENOPAUSE

Perimenopause is the ten to fifteen years leading up to menopause. It is the
time when your hormone fluctuations gradually start to change from your
regular cycle and you don't know where your hormones will be on any given
day. Most women don't think about perimenopause until estrogen levels have
fallen to a point where they get hit with hot flashes and night sweats, the most
common symptoms. But by the time you are having hot flashes, you've probably been going through perimenopause for up to ten years. And you may
already be saddled with the effects of estrogen dominance.

Common signs of perimenopause Hot flashes, night sweats, weight gain,
depression, anxiety, irritability, and poor memory.

Get it balanced It is a good idea to
get your hormone levels checked when
you are about thirty-five years old so
you have a baseline. Then get them
checked every two to three years. Synthetic or bio-identical hormone replacement therapy may be helpful in
the form of creams, pills, and vaginal
inserts. The best way to treat hot flashes

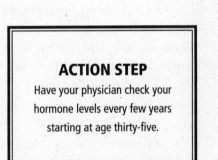

ACTION STEP
Have your physician check your
hormone levels every few years
starting at age thirty-five.

is with a combination of estradiol and estriol. Natural treatments include supplements, such as B vitamins, fish oil, primrose oil, and flaxseed oil. Plus,
adopt brain-healthy habits. Get plenty of exercise, adequate sleep, drink lots
of water, eat whole foods, and meditate.

MENOPAUSE

Menopause is a woman's last period, after which she is said to be postmenopausal. Menopause can also be surgically induced if your ovaries are
removed during a hysterectomy. If you are postmenopausal, you may continue

to experience many of the same side effects associated with perimenopause. By this time, estrogen and progesterone have usually fallen to such low levels that it also makes you more vulnerable to conditions such as heart disease, stroke, and Alzheimer's disease.

Common signs of menopause Menopause is often associated with lower overall brain activity, which can lead to depression, anxiety, insomnia, weight gain, and concentration and memory problems. Hot flashes and night sweats may continue.

Get it balanced Typically, a diagnosis of menopause is given only after twelve months have passed since your final period. Synthetic or bio-identical hormone replacement are commonly prescribed. B vitamins, fish oil, primrose oil, and flaxseed oil are natural treatments that may ease symptoms. Adopting brain-healthy habits becomes more important than ever to preserve cognitive function and keep your body looking young. Exercise, good sleep, great nutrition, and meditation can help.

HORMONE REPLACEMENT THERAPY

There is a huge controversy surrounding hormone replacement therapy (HRT). In 2002, the World Health Initiative Study found that the hormone replacement medication Prempro increased the risk for breast cancer, heart disease, stroke, and blood clots. The fallout was immediate and widespread, with millions of women tossing their HRT medications in the trash.

The problem with this study is that it looked at only one medication, Prempro, which is a combination of synthetic estrogen (made from horse urine), a little estrone, and a synthetic progesterone called progestin. These hormones are not the same as those produced in the human body. In addition, the estrogen in this synthetic drug was more potent than the estrogen your body produces naturally.

Today, we have come full circle on the question of HRT and there is a trend toward treating women with hormones that are identical to those produced in the body. These medications, called bio-identical hormones, can be helpful in boosting your vitality as well as protecting cognitive function. They also protect you from serious diseases, including cardiovascular disease, stroke, and Alzheimer's disease. Studies show that women who have complete hysterectomies, including taking their ovaries, without hormone replacement have double the risk for Alzheimer's disease. This confirms that these hormones are critical for brain health. In a new study from UCLA, researchers used brain scans to study the health of a group of women's brains on and off hormone replacement. Over two years, the women who did not take hormone replacement showed decreased activity in an area of the brain called the posterior cingulate gyrus, one of the first areas that die in Alzheimer's disease. The women who were taking HRT showed no reduction in this area of the brain.

Research on pain has found that women going through menopause who don't take HRT may struggle more with pain. I have noticed this in my own practice. I treat many postmenopausal women who complain of pain, whether it is chronic backaches, neck problems, or even conditions like fibromyalgia. If you are considering HRT, remember that it is highly individualized and that one treatment does not work for everyone. Just as your brain is completely unique, so are your hormones.

BALANCE LEPTIN AND GHRELIN TO CONTROL YOUR APPETITE AND LOSE WEIGHT

These two hormones may hold the key to your weight loss. Regulated by sleep, leptin and ghrelin work together to control feelings of hunger and satiety. Ghrelin levels rise to signal the brain that you are hungry, then leptin levels increase to tell your brain when you are full. Adequate sleep keeps these two hormones nicely balanced. But when you don't get enough sleep, they get out of whack and increase your appetite and your cravings for carbohydrates, cookies, and candy. See Chapter 10, "The Sleep Solution," for the latest research on how these two hormones affect your weight.

Low leptin Without enough leptin, you never feel like you've gotten enough to eat. Overweight people have high levels of leptin because their brain becomes resistant to it. The less fat on your body, the better.

High ghrelin Studies show that high levels of this hormone trick your body into thinking you are hungry and make you want to dive into the doughnuts and candy bowl as opposed to the fruit

ACTION STEP
One of the best ways to balance leptin and ghrelin is to get at least seven hours of sleep each night.

bowl. With chronically high levels of ghrelin, there's a strong possibility you are going to gain weight.

Common symptoms of low leptin and high ghrelin Overweight, obesity, overeating, and cravings for simple carbohydrates.

Get it balanced At present the treatment to balance these hormones is mostly behavioral. Get good sleep, eat small meals throughout the day so that you are not hungry and maintain a healthy blood sugar, decrease stress eating, and reduce your stress. Since leptin and ghrelin are regulated during sleep, supplements that promote sleep—such as L-tryptophan, 5-HTP, valerian, kava kava, magnesium, and melatonin—may help balance your levels.

BALANCE INSULIN TO BATTLE OBESITY AND IMPROVE HEALTH

Insulin is produced by the pancreas, primarily in response to a rise in blood sugar. One of insulin's primary functions is as a storage hormone. Its function is to take nutrients from the bloodstream and store them in the body's cells. Insulin increases the uptake of glucose into the liver and muscles for storage, as glycogen, and it also helps store excess glucose in fat cells. Since insulin is a storage hormone rather than a mobilizing hormone, it also stops the body from mobilizing and utilizing fat as a fuel source. Too much insulin stops fat burning. Eating too many simple carbohydrates, like candy, cake, or white bread, causes your blood sugar to spike, which triggers intense insulin production to remove the glucose from your bloodstream. Once insulin has removed the glucose from your blood, your blood sugar drops, causing cravings for even more sugar. It is a vicious cycle that can lead to obesity, insulin resistance, and eventually type 2 diabetes.

Insulin imbalances When this hormone is out of balance, it can lead to weight gain, delayed healing, Alzheimer's disease, strokes, heart disease, and many other problems.

Common signs of insulin imbalances Obesity, abdominal fat, diabetes, high blood pressure, and metabolic syndrome (abdominal fat, high cholesterol, and high blood pressure).

Get it balanced The most common blood test for glucose looks at the way your body is metabolizing glucose on that particular day. A better test checks your Hg A1C levels, which show how you are metabolizing glucose over a two- to three-month period. Losing weight, exercising, and taking certain medications such as insulin or glucophage can help balance your blood sugar levels. Alpha-lipoic acid, cinnamon, and ginseng have been found to help balance blood sugar. Reducing your intake of sugary sweets and simple carbohydrates can help keep insulin levels in balance.

BALANCE YOUR GROWTH HORMONES TO SLOW THE AGING PROCESS

The pea-sized pituitary gland, located at the base of the brain, produces human growth hormone. As its name implies, growth hormone fuels growth throughout childhood and into adulthood. It also helps bodily tissues and organs repair themselves for optimal function. As we enter middle age, however, the pituitary gland slows production of growth hormone, also known as IGF-1 (insulinlike growth factor-1). The reduction in growth hormone impairs the body's ability to repair itself, thus triggering cell death and aging.

A breakthrough study published in a 1990 issue of the *New England Journal of Medicine* sparked interest in growth hormone as a potential antiaging therapy. In the study, twelve men over the age of sixty were followed for a six-month period. During that time, one group received growth hormone therapy while the other group did not. The men receiving growth hormone experienced a 14.4 percent decrease in body fat and an 8.8 percent increase in lean body mass. This landmark—albeit small—study prompted a wealth of new research aiming to determine to what extent low levels of growth hormone promote the aging process and whether raising levels of growth hormone could put the brakes on aging.

Low levels of growth hormone Dr. Eric Braverman, a clinical assistant professor of integrative medicine at Weill Cornell Medical College, conducted a comprehensive review of the medical literature about growth hormone. His findings show that low levels of IGF-1 may result in the following:

- Delayed cognitive processing speed (the equivalent of ten to twenty years of aging), which leads to declines in memory, IQ, and attention span as well as mood problems, such as anxiety and depression

- Decreased blood flow to the brain
- Obesity
- Decreased muscle mass and bone density
- Cardiovascular disease, high blood pressure, and diabetes

According to Dr. Braverman's review, increasing levels of IGF-1 can help reverse these problems. Growth hormone has also been found to protect against some forms of cancer and beta amyloid, an abnormal protein found in the brain that is considered to be one of the major hallmarks of Alzheimer's disease.

> **ACTION STEP**
>
> If you are obese or have age-related problems, try lifestyle and diet changes first, then consider having your IGF-1 levels checked.

Common signs and symptoms of underactive growth hormone

Osteoporosis, muscle deterioration, memory problems, obesity, anxiety, depression, cardiovascular disease, high blood pressure, and diabetes are all potential signs of low levels of IGF-1.

Get it balanced A blood test is typically used to evaluate growth hormone levels. Growth hormone replacement is achieved with injections that can cost thousands of dollars, which makes it prohibitive for many people. The practice is considered very controversial, and some concern has been raised about a possible link between growth hormone replacement and cancer. However, based on Dr. Braverman's review, there have been no studies that have shown that growth hormone therapy increases the risk of cancer.

Take note that growth hormone injections aren't the only way to increase the amount of growth hormone in the body. Natural ways to stimulate the production of growth

> **ACTION STEP**
>
> Online at www.amenclinics.com/cybcyb, you will find a series of questionnaires for both men and women, developed by my friend and colleague Angie Meeker, doctor of pharmacy. The questionnaires will give you a sense of your own potential hormone issues. Of course, you should discuss the results of the questionnaires with your own health-care professional.

hormone include getting adequate sleep, doing intense physical activity, and eating protein at every meal, while reducing the consumption of sugar and high-glycemic carbohydrates.

The Hormone Solution

Hormone Robbers	Hormone Balancers
Low thyroid	Thyroid replacement, supplements such as iodine and selenium
Adrenal fatigue	Adequate sleep (at least seven hours), eliminated caffeine and alcohol, B vitamins, 5-HTP, phosphatidylserine, DHEA or 7-keto-DHEA
Low testosterone	Testosterone replacement, DHEA
High testosterone in women (PCOS)	Glucophage or other medications
Low estradiol	Estrogen replacement, fish oil, primrose oil, flaxseed oil
Low progesterone	Progesterone replacement
PMS	5-HTP, medications to boost serotonin, exercise, enriched nutrition, meditation, adequate sleep
Perimenopause	Hormone replacement, B vitamins, fish oil, primrose oil, flaxseed oil, exercise, meditation, enriched nutrition, adequate sleep
Menopause	Hormone replacement, B vitamins, fish oil, primrose oil, flaxseed oil, exercise, meditation, enriched nutrition, adequate sleep
Low leptin/high ghrelin	Adequate sleep, frequent small meals, 5-HTP, L-tryptophan, valerian, kava kava, melatonin
Insulin imbalances	Losing weight, exercise, alpha-lipoic acid, cinnamon, ginseng, reduced intake of simple carbs, medication

8

THE HEART SOLUTION

Use Your Brain to Strengthen
and Soothe Your Heart

Whatever is good for your heart is good for your brain,
and whatever is good for your brain is good for your heart.

Three times in my life I have had crushing chest pain, the kind of chest pain that felt like an NFL lineman was sitting on my rib cage. The first time, I was twenty-six years old and in medical school in Oklahoma. My grandfather had his second heart attack at the age of seventy-five. He was a warmhearted, kind, happy man who loved to do things for others. He had many, many friends and he had been a candy maker who owned his own shop on Wilshire Boulevard in Los Angeles for many years. The candy, and the inflammation caused by excessive sugar, likely contributed to his heart disease. I was named after him and he was my best friend growing up.

After his heart attack, Grandpa became very depressed for the first time in his life. Those who loved him were very surprised by the change. He had trouble sleeping at night, cried easily, and lost a lot of weight. The antidepressants then, in 1980, were not much help to him, and he died within a short time. At his funeral I had crushing chest pain. His loss was overwhelming and I truly sobbed for the first time in my life. What I found out later, to my sad dismay, was that people who suffer a depressive episode after a heart attack are three times more likely to die in the next two and a half years than those who do not have depression. If only I knew, I would have pushed for them to treat his depression more aggressively. As I was writing this book, my first grandchild, Elias, was born. The day of his birth I had constant thoughts of my grandfather and how important he was in my life, which, I am sure, will help drive me to be a good grandpa too, but without all the candy.

The second time I had chest pain was at age forty-five at three o'clock in the morning. I woke up holding my chest, panicked, and couldn't breathe. Before bed that night, I was reading Dean Ornish's book *Love and Survival*. In it, he wrote about a study where researchers asked ten thousand men one question, "Does your wife show you her love?" The men who answered no had significantly more illnesses and, in fact, died early. At the time, I had been in a twenty-year marriage that was filled with stress and chronic unhappiness. I had to answer the question as a definite no. The chest pain was a reflection of my unconscious mind telling me that the lack of love was killing me.

The third time I had chest pain, at age fifty-one, was during another period of grief when I had lost a very close friend. When I could no longer talk to my friend, my heart ached. I couldn't sleep, my mind raced, and the crushing pain in my chest returned. I also remember that when my other grandfather died, my father's mother used to hold her chest and cry with pain and sorrow. Grief is manifested physically, often through chest pain. After my own experiences, I researched the physical effects of grief.

Scientific studies report that grief triggers a storm of hormonal activity. Stress chemicals, such as adrenaline and cortisol, are pumped into the bloodstream. They cause the heart to beat irregularly, causing the feeling of fluttering in your chest, and they cause spasms of the blood vessels that supply the heart, also causing pain. If the heart is already compromised by atherosclerosis (fortunately for me, mine was not), it can set the stage for a heart attack by constricting blood vessels, rupturing atherosclerotic plaques, and forming blood clots or triggering dangerous abnormal heart rhythms.

In my last experience, I felt so terrible that I decided to do a SPECT scan on myself during grief. I had already done ten other scans over the years, so I had a pretty good idea of my own brain pattern. In this study, I found that my emotional brain was significantly overactive, especially in the anterior cingulate gyrus—as I was stuck on thoughts of missing my friend—and my insular cortex, an area of the brain that often sends stress signals to other parts of the body, especially the heart. I needed to calm my brain in order to soothe my heart. The brain's stress is clearly played out in every organ of the body, but most especially in the heart. Your heart and brain are completely intertwined with each other.

The brain-heart connection is beautifully and consistently displayed throughout our language.

"My heart is broken."

"You make my heart beat fast."

"I miss you with all my heart."

"He's a heartthrob."

"She's a heartbreaker."

"She ripped out my heart."

"I am so nervous that my heart is beating out of my chest."

"He's got a lot of heart."

"I don't get heart attacks, I give them."

This chapter will look at the brain-heart connection and how you can optimize it to enhance your overall heart health. Boosting brain health improves heart health. Improving heart health also enhances your brain. Let's start by examining two of the body's brain-heart systems: the autonomic nervous system and heart rate variability. Then we will look at a number of brain-heart connection robbers and boosters.

AUTONOMIC NERVOUS SYSTEM

The nerves that link the brain and the heart are part of the autonomic nervous system (ANS), which also connects the brain to other organs, such as the stomach, intestines, kidneys, and skin. Unless trained, this system functions in an involuntary, or reflexive, manner. It usually directs the activities of the body that do not require conscious control. Think of the ANS as allowing things to happen automatically or unconsciously. For example, it functions without your direction for digestion when you eat a spinach, blueberry, and walnut salad—without your having to say, "Okay, stomach and intestines, start working to get the nutrition from this brain-healthy food." And when you are at a scary movie, you don't need to tell your heart to beat faster with excitement; it just does as a result of the ANS.

The ANS is made up of two divisions—sympathetic and parasympathetic—that modulate your body's responses. These two divisions could be thought of as opposing forces. The sympathetic division signals your heart to increase its firing rate and increase the strength of muscle-cell contraction; and the parasympathetic division sends signals to slow down your heart rate and relax. The sympathetic fibers are activated in times of stress, or emergency "fight-or-flight" situations. The parasympathetic fibers slow the heart rate and allow us to "rest" and "digest."

Excessive sympathetic stimulation can cause significant heart and blood vessel problems, including angina or heart pain, high blood pressure, heart arrhythmias, and even heart attacks. Through training we can learn to calm an excessively overactive sympathetic nervous system and improve our heart health.

When I was an intern at the Walter Reed Army Medical Center, I spent a month on the cardiac intensive care unit. One night when I was on call, I was caring for an army chaplain who had a severe heart arrhythmia. We were having trouble getting his heart rhythm under control, and he was unable to sleep. The chaplain had been feeling a fair amount of anxiety because his heart problem was causing him to be medically discharged from the army. As was my habit for sleeping problems, I asked my patient if I could hypnotize him to see if it would help him sleep. With his permission, one of the nurses who wanted to watch sat in with us. He readily went into a hypnotic trance and we noticed a considerable calming of his anxiety. As I went on, the nurse touched my arm and with an astonished look in her eyes motioned for me to look at the heart rate monitor. His heart rhythm had normalized. He then fell into a peaceful sleep. My nurse friend caused quite a stir on the unit by telling everyone what had happened.

The next morning on rounds our attending, a friendly but skeptical cardiologist by the name of Bill Oetgen, asked me what happened. He was intrigued and we studied the chaplain's heart both in and out of a hypnotic trance. His heart rhythm was definitely healthier under hypnosis. We presented the case at the hospital grand rounds and published the case in the *Journal of Clinical Hypnosis*.

Balancing the sympathetic and parasympathetic tone to the heart can be healing. In a 2008 report published in the *Cleveland Clinic Medical Journal*, one hundred people who had coronary bypass surgery were studied. Fifty were put under hypnosis right after the surgery, while fifty were treated as usual without hypnosis. In the hypnosis group, there were significantly fewer complications, including heart arrhythmias, than in the control group. Hypnosis is one form of training that has a positive impact on heart health, likely through balancing the ANS. Meditation, deep relaxation therapies, guided imagery, and biofeedback are other tools for helping.

ACTION STEP

Try hypnosis, meditation, deep relaxation therapies, guided imagery, and biofeedback to improve heart health by calming the ANS.

HEART RATE VARIABILITY

Heart rate variability (HRV) is another important phenomenon to understand in optimizing the brain-heart connection. HRV is the beat-to-beat variation in heart rhythm. Most people think that a healthy heart rhythm is perfectly regular. Not so. Normally, under healthy conditions, our heart rhythm is not even; it bounces around a bit. High HRV has been associated with heart health, while low HRV has been associated with illness.

HRV issues are most obvious when mothers deliver babies. Obstetricians typically monitor the baby's HRV before delivery with scalp monitors. In a healthy baby, the heart rate varies significantly. If the baby's heart rate becomes too steady, the baby is considered to be in trouble. Lower HRV is a sign of distress. The same thing is true after we are born. Low HRV is a sign of stress and trouble for both our hearts and our brains. HRV has been found to predict survival after heart attack. Over a half dozen well-designed studies have shown that reduced HRV predicts sudden death in patients who have had a heart attack. Reduced HRV appears to be a marker of fatal heart arrhythmias. Several studies also suggest that lower HRV may predict risk of death even among individuals free of heart disease.

Several studies have suggested a link between negative emotions (such as anxiety and hostility) and reduced HRV. One research group reported an association between anxiety and reduced HRV in 581 men, while another group observed lower HRV in individuals who were "highly anxious." At least three well-designed studies have shown a relationship between high levels of anxiety and heart disease.

One critical piece of HRV is forgiveness. By holding on to hurts and anger, you lower your HRV and increase your own chances for heart problems. Learn-

ACTION STEP

Hostility, anger, depression, loneliness, frustration, sleep deprivation, obesity, diabetes, air pollution, and chronic stress all decrease HRV. Positive emotion, gratitude, appreciation, forgiveness, holding your puppy, listening to soothing music, smelling lavender, losing weight, exercising, and eating more fruits and vegetables have scientific evidence showing they increase HRV and overall health. Your brain's decisions can improve your heart!

ing to let go and forgive those who have hurt you is one way to allow your heart's rhythm room to expand.

My best friend as a youngster grew up in a war zone. Will's mother could never let go of hurts, while his father had the temper from hell, especially when he drank. The constant screaming and chaos had a profoundly negative effect on everyone in the family. Will frequently suffered from panic attacks and headaches, and missed many days at school. Will hated his father for the bruises he put on his mother, and he was horrified whenever the police showed up at his door. For decades, Will's own intimate relationships suffered, as he had trouble trusting anyone.

Then, years later, Will's dad had open-heart surgery. After the surgery, his dad became psychotic and saw little green men talking to him. I was called to help. As part of my evaluation, I scanned Will's dad. His scan showed a large defect in the area of his left temporal lobe, a finding often consistent with violence. When I asked his father if he had ever had a brain injury, he said, "By God, Danny, I did. When I was twenty years old, I was driving an old milk truck. It was missing its driver's-side rearview mirror, so I had to put my head out of the window to look behind me and one day when I was doing that my head hit a wooden pole and knocked me unconscious. After the injury I had more problems with my memory and my temper."

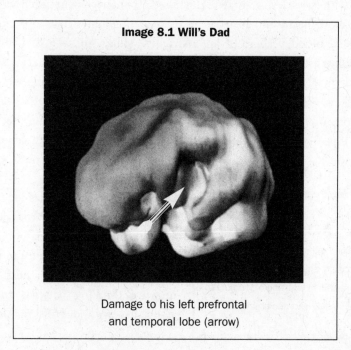

Image 8.1 Will's Dad

Damage to his left prefrontal
and temporal lobe (arrow)

Seeing the scans and hearing about the brain injury caused Will and everyone in the family to look at their dad in a different light. With treatment, Will's father did much better. For years, it was easy to say that Will's dad was a bad person, but when you look at his behavior through the lens of brain imaging, a new world of understanding, help, and forgiveness opens up. Will's heart and life also opened up after he could forgive his father, rather than rigidly holding on to the idea of how much he hated him.

BRAIN–HEART CONNECTION ROBBERS

Decreased blood flow I often say that whatever is good for your heart is good for your brain, and whatever is bad for your heart is bad for your brain. Blood flow is critical to both organs and critical to your survival. Anything that decreases blood flow to your heart, brain, or body decreases healthy function. Smoking, excessive caffeine, excessive stress, certain medications or abuse drugs, and a lack of exercise all have the potential to damage brain-heart health.

Excessive stress Constant exposure to stress hormones kills cells in the brain's memory centers and also decreases HRV and heart health. Research has found that higher self-ratings of anxiety and stress within a week were associated with lower levels of HRV. Having stress-management practices is critical to both brain and heart health. Stress hormones may also constrict narrowed blood vessels. In an instructive study from Duke University, researchers asked fifty-eight men and women with coronary artery disease to wear portable monitors for two days. They were asked to write in their diaries what they were doing and feeling. Tension, frustration, and other negative emotions often led to heart monitor recordings that pointed to decreased blood flow in the arteries to the heart. This decreased blood flow can cause a heart attack.

ACTION STEP

Eliminating bad brain habits, exercising, and taking fish oil can be very helpful in boosting blood flow to the heart and brain.

Depression Many studies report that depression increases the risk of heart attacks and sudden death. Getting depression treated promptly and effectively is critical to heart health. The negative thinking patterns that are associated with depression also decrease HRV.

Grief As discussed earlier, grief can send stress signals to the heart, causing vasospasm and abnormal heart rhythms. Finding effective ways to deal with grief may save your life. In one study, Dr. Ivan Mendoza of Caracas, Venezuela, found that when he reviewed 102 cases of sudden death in people ages thirty-seven to seventy-nine, thirteen of the deaths occurred on the anniversary of a parent's death. Ten of the sudden deaths occurred in men, who typically internalize their feelings, and four of the thirteen died at the same age their parent did. Learning to deal with grief through talking, crying, processing your feelings, and correcting bad thinking habits can save your life.

Anxiety disorders Panic attacks, phobias, fears, obsessions, and compulsions all increase stress on your heart and increase the chances for heart problems. Mitral valve prolapse, a condition where the mitral valve in the heart works inefficiently, has long been known to be associated with anxiety.

Untreated ADD Being late all the time, not completing tasks, always putting things off until the last minute; being distracted, inattentive, and disorganized; having relationship problems; seeking conflict; and having school, work, or relationship problems are all symptoms commonly associated with ADD. Always living on the edge or being upset with someone puts a strain on your brain and your heart. A Mayo Clinic study found that people who have ADD use nonpsychiatric medical services three times more than the general population.

Constant excitement In a world where we are literally thrilling ourselves to death by overdoing video games, scary movies, texting, e-mail, and computer time, we are decreasing the health of our brain and heart. The body needs time for rest and reflection. It is okay to tone down all of the high-stimulus activities.

Relationship problems Trouble with the important people in your life predisposes people to depression, anxiety, and heart problems. There is solid scientific research that working on your relationships can help heal depression and soothe your heart. Or, in my own case—as I discussed in the introduction to this chapter—after my first wife and I had seen eight therapists, the

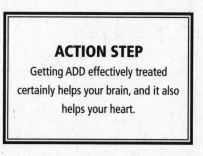

ACTION STEP

Getting ADD effectively treated certainly helps your brain, and it also helps your heart.

chest pain was telling me it was time to move on. My heart has been much healthier with the right partner.

Dementia Heart disease in its many forms, such as hypertension, heart attacks, and heart arrhythmias, all increase the risk of Alzheimer's disease and other forms of dementia. Taking care of your heart is also a very positive step toward taking care of your brain.

Inflammation Chronic inflammation from any cause constricts blood flow to the heart and to the brain. Many scientists now think it is one of the major causes of both cardiovascular disease and Alzheimer's disease. Homocysteine and C-reactive protein tests are laboratory measures of inflammation. Taking steps to decrease inflammation, such as eating right and taking fish oil, are critical to the health of every system in your body.

Blood sugar abnormalities Diabetes and blood sugar abnormalities are deadly because they eventually cause your small blood vessels to become brittle and break, causing strokes, dementia, and heart attacks. Making sure you exercise and have a brain-body–healthy diet is critical to the brain-heart connection.

Doctors have known for decades that too much carbohydrate-laden foods like white bread and cornflakes can be detrimental to heart health. In an important new study, researchers showed how these high-carbohydrate foods increase the risk for heart problems. Dr. Michael Shechter of Tel Aviv University and colleagues visualized exactly what happens inside the body when the wrong foods for a healthy heart are eaten. He found that foods with a high glycemic index distended brachial arteries for several hours. Elasticity of arteries anywhere in the body can be a measure of heart health. But when aggravated over time, a sudden expansion of the artery wall can cause a number of negative health effects, including reduced elasticity, which can cause heart disease or sudden death. Hold the ice cream and Frosted Flakes.

Dr. Shechter says, "Doctors know that high-glycemic foods rapidly increase blood sugar. Those who binge on

---

ACTION STEP

To prevent rapid increases in blood sugar levels, stick to foods like oatmeal, fruits and vegetables, legumes, and nuts, which have a low-glycemic index and are also great for your brain.

these foods have a greater chance of sudden death from heart attack. Our research connects the dots, showing the link between diet and what's happening in real time in the arteries."

Obesity As we saw in Chapter 3, "The Weight Solution," excess fat is associated with inflammation, more stored toxins in the body, hypertension, and dementia. HRV has also been found to be low in obese individuals. Paying attention to decreasing the fat on your body will help your brain and your heart.

Excessive alcohol In small to moderate amounts, alcohol is reported to be good for your heart and, some studies even suggest for your brain. HRV is improved with small amounts of wine, but not beer or hard liquor. The problem, of course, is not with a little bit of alcohol, it is with a lot. Daily drinking is associated with a smaller brain, which means poorer decision making, stress, and heartache. In a fascinating study from the Harvard School of Public Health on the preventable causes of death, alcohol use caused 90,000 deaths a year from road traffic and other injuries, violence, chronic liver disease, cancers, alcohol-use disorders, stroke, arrhythmias, and hypertensive disease. On the other hand, alcohol was reported to have averted 26,000 deaths due to its positive effect on heart health. On balance, it seems that less alcohol is better.

Unbalanced hormones Low testosterone levels in men and low estrogen levels in women have been associated with lowered HRV and heart disease. See Chapter 7, "The Hormone Solution," to make sure your hormones are properly balanced.

BRAIN-HEART CONNECTION BOOSTERS

Love and positive emotion It is well established that chronic anger and negative emotion can have a damaging effect on your brain and your heart, while positive emotion can improve HRV and overall brain and heart health. Focus on what you love about your life and those around you, and your heart will be healthier and happier. I have seen many patients throughout the years who have told me that they are pessimists so they will never be disappointed. My response after understanding the brain-heart connection is that they may never be disappointed but they are also likely to die earlier.

Laughter Laughter is another form of positive emotion that can influence your brain, heart, and blood-vessel function. In a unique study, researchers from the University of Maryland found that while watching funny movies, such as *There's Something About Mary,* nineteen out of twenty people had increased blood flow to the heart. Conversely, watching stressful movies, such as the opening scene from *Saving Private Ryan,* decreased blood flow in fourteen out of twenty people. Specifically, blood flow decreased by about 35 percent after experiencing stress, while blood flow increased by 22 percent after laughing, which is equivalent to what happens after a fifteen- to thirty-minute workout.

The ability of blood vessels to expand is known as vasodilation and is a sign of heart health. Decreased blood flow limits the body's ability to react to physical or emotional stress and results in an increased risk of heart attacks and strokes. Past studies have found that stress hormones like adrenalin and cortisol, which are released when a person is stressed, may harm the body by suppressing the immune system and constricting blood vessels. On the other hand, laughing causes the body to release chemicals called endorphins, which may counteract the effects of stress hormones and cause blood vessels to dilate. In a similar manner, laughing may also boost the immune system and reduce inflammation, which is thought to increase the risk of various health problems.

Meditation and yoga Our heart beats faster when we inhale and slower when we exhale. Most meditation and yoga techniques have us exhale slowly, which can slow our heart rate and calm our entire body. This is a wonderful technique to calm anxiety and increase HRV. Meditation on a regular basis helps to increase both brain and heart health. Meditation and yoga both have strong scientific evidence that they can help decrease blood pressure.

One of my patients from our retired NFL player study told me that he was worried about his memory, which was leading to significant anxiety. He was currently a professional speaker and had experienced several moments where his mind would go blank while he was speaking. He noticed that the feeling of anxiety was escalating. I told him that before his talks, he should take ten deep breaths, focusing on exhaling each breath very slowly. And, when his

> ### ACTION STEP
> Getting control of your breathing is often the first step to getting control of your heart and mind.

mind went blank during a talk, to just take a moment and exhale slowly. Anxiety causes your heart to race and your mind to go blank. He told me later that this simple technique was very helpful to him.

Hand warming A fascinating biofeedback technique that increases HRV and deepens relaxation is learning how to warm your hands with your brain. By directing attention to your hands with warm mental images, such as putting your hands in front of a warm fire, holding a cup of hot green tea, holding your partner's warm skin, or sitting in a hot tub, many people can actually increase the temperature in their hands and induce a generalized relaxed brain and body state.

Whenever we are stressed, our hands get cold because blood is shunted away from our hands and feet to the large muscles of our shoulders and hips, so we can fight or run. Learning to warm your hands counteracts the stress response and increases parasympathetic tone and relaxation. There are a number of studies that report lowered blood pressure with hand warming. In one study from Korea, hand warming was used to treat patients with hypertension. A significant decline of the systolic blood pressure by 20.6 mmHg and of the diastolic blood pressure by 14.4 mmHg was observed in the treatment group.

Hypnosis As I wrote earlier in this chapter, hypnosis can be a very powerful tool to enhance heart health and deep brain relaxation, especially in our fast-paced society. When I was a student of hypnosis at the University of California, Irvine, School of Medicine, under the direction of Donald Shafer, M.D., I saw videos of hypnotic masters changing their own blood-flow patterns. One video featured an East Indian physician in a hypnotic trance who put a needle through a vein in her hand and then withdrew it. The vein was bleeding from both sides. Then, under her control, she made the bleeding stop on one side, then made it bleed again, then made the other side stop and bleed again, then made both sides stop. It was an amazing display of brain-body control. This gave me the idea of hypnotic trances, relaxation, and blood-vessel control. As an intern, whenever I had a difficult time drawing blood from a patient, I would put them in a light trance, which made it easier for both of us.

Ability to regulate emotion Having control over your thoughts and feelings is a key skill in enhancing mood and emotion. A study from Brazil also reports that this skill is essential in regulating HRV and heart health. When you allow your thoughts to run wild in your brain, you may set off a panic attack, with your heart racing, chest pain, and blood pressure spiking. Learning how to manage them using the techniques outlined in Chapter 13, "The ANT Solution," will help your brain and heart.

Exercise Physical activity has a positive effect on blood flow to the brain and helps to strengthen the heart. See Chapter 5, "The Exercise Solution," for more information.

Fish oil Taking fish oil has been found to be good for your heart and your brain. A number of studies report that taking fish oil and boosting omega-3 fatty acids helps to raise HRV, which we have seen is good for both brain and heart health. There is also strong scientific evidence that omega-3 fatty acids may reduce high cholesterol and triglycerides in the blood, decrease the risk of sudden cardiac death, and decrease blood pressure.

Proper hormone levels Balanced hormones are essential for both brain and heart health.

WARM HANDS EQUAL A WARM HEART

Take a moment to feel your hands. Feel the energy and temperature in your hands. As I mentioned earlier, there is a simple biofeedback technique that involves hand warming. When you intentionally learn how to warm your hands with your brain, by directing your thoughts to warming images, such as putting your hands in front of a fire . . . your body goes into a relaxed state.

There is scientific evidence that using this technique can help you lower your blood pressure and decreases anxiety. There is also new evidence that when your partner holds something warm, such as your warm hand, he or she trusts you more and feels closer to you and more giving. Cold hands have the opposite effect.

Lawrence Williams, Ph.D., assistant professor at the University of Colorado at Boulder, and John A. Bargh, Ph.D., professor of psychology at Yale University, conducted two studies on undergraduate students to assess how hand temperature affects emotions. They found that holding warm things may actually make people view others more favorably and may also make people more generous.

The first study included forty-one college students with an average age of

18.5. A tester met each participant in the lobby of the building where the tests were being conducted. In the elevator on the way up, the tester casually asked the participant to hold his cup of coffee while he recorded some information on his clipboard. The participant did not know the coffee was part of the experiment. Half the participants were asked to hold a cup of warm coffee and half were asked to hold a cup of iced coffee.

Once in the testing room, participants were given a packet of information on an unknown person described with words like *intelligent, skillful, industrious, practical,* and *cautious.* Participants were then asked to evaluate the person's personality using a questionnaire. Participants who had held the warm coffee were much more likely to score the pretend person as warmer than those who had held the iced coffee.

"When we ask whether someone is a warm person or cold person, they both have a temperature of 98.6," Bargh, coauthor of the paper, said. "These terms implicitly tap into the primitive experience of what it means to be warm and cold."

In the second experiment, fifty-three participants were asked to hold either a hot or a cold therapeutic pad. Participants thought their role was to evaluate the product. After the "test," they were offered a reward for themselves or a treat for a friend. The people who had held the warm pad were more likely to choose the reward for the friend.

"It appears that the effect of physical temperature is not just on how we see others, it affects our own behavior as well," Bargh says. "Physical warmth can make us see others as warmer people, but also cause us to be warmer—more generous and trusting—as well. At a board meeting, for instance, being willing to reach out and touch another human being, to share their hand, those experiences do matter although we may not always be aware of them."

These studies are so interesting because we know that when our hands are cold we are more likely to be anxious and fearful, traits that decrease intimacy and closeness to others.

Here's a simple exercise to bring heartfelt closeness in your intimate relationships. When holding your partner's hand, imagine warm, loving energy going from your hand to hers. With each exhale, send warm and intentional thoughts of love and gratitude. Do this for just a few minutes a day and soon you will begin to notice a positive difference in your relationship. I have seen in our imaging studies that the act of focusing loving, grateful energy can be very powerful.

The brain-heart solution lies in understanding that taking care of your brain is helping to love your heart, and caring for your heart is absolutely essential in caring for your brain.

The Heart Solution

Heart Robbers	Heart Boosters
Hostility, anger	Positive emotion, love, gratitude, appreciation
Grief	Ability to regulate mood and emotion
Relationship problems, loneliness	Connection
Frustration	Forgiveness
Chronic stress, need for excitement	Meditation/yoga
Depression	Hand warming
Anxiety	Hypnosis
ADD	Holding a puppy
Sleep deprivation	Healthy sleep
Obesity	Losing weight
Diabetes/blood sugar spikes	Soothing music
Air pollution	Smelling lavender
Decreased blood flow from any cause	Exercise
Poor diet	Eating more fruits and vegetables
Dementia	Fish oil
Inflammation	Laughter
Excessive alcohol	Limited alcohol
Unbalanced hormone levels	Balanced hormone levels

9

THE FOCUS AND ENERGY SOLUTION

Boost Your Energy to Stay on Track Toward Your Goals

And what is a man without energy? Nothing—nothing at all.

—MARK TWAIN

Dwayne, forty-five, one of my close friends, came to the clinic for a scan. His energy had been waning, and his mind felt older than he liked. He had trouble concentrating, was starting to mix up names, was more forgetful, and was struggling with mental fatigue throughout the day, especially midafternoon and evening. He was working two jobs, one of which was being a psychotherapist in the evening. His wife was becoming very frustrated with him, as he had no time or emotion to give her. When we performed a brain SPECT scan on Dwayne, it showed overall decreased activity in his brain.

Dwayne had a slew of bad brain habits. He rarely got more than five hours of sleep, drank eight to ten cups of coffee a day, did not exercise, and mostly had a fast-food diet on the run. Dwayne had sent me plenty of patients for scans, so when he saw his own brain, he knew something had to change. "But I can't stop the caffeine," he said. "I will not be able to work at night. I will be a mess."

"That is only your distorted thought as a justification of the caffeine," I said. Because of our relationship and the fact that Dwayne was a psychotherapist who understood my work, I could be candid with him. "You do not want to go through the pain of withdrawal, so you rationalize that it is easier to continue to poison yourself. Not that smart."

"No, seriously, I will fall apart without the caffeine," he replied.

"Is that true?" I asked. "Can you absolutely know that it is true?" I was

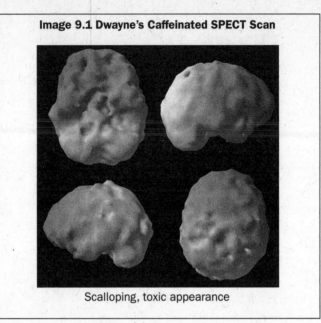

Image 9.1 Dwayne's Caffeinated SPECT Scan

Scalloping, toxic appearance

borrowing a phrase from the work of my friend Byron Katie, who wrote *Loving What Is*, a book that teaches people to question their own thoughts.

Dwayne thought for several moments, then said, "I guess I really don't know, but something has got to change."

Dwayne realized that his thoughts were only setting him up to fail, and he agreed to cut back on his caffeine use, get better sleep, and get on a brain-healthy diet. A month later, I got an excited call from Dwayne. He told me he had completely cut out the caffeine and that he was sleeping and eating better. "I feel ten years younger," he said. "You were right, thank you." I love Dwayne's story, because it highlights how the little lies that we tell ourselves are ruining the health of our brains and our bodies. You can have better energy and focus by paying attention to the health of your brain.

Another friend, Ted, called me late at night complaining of feeling sad, overwhelmed, unfocused, and tired. This was very unusual for Ted, whom I had known for fifteen years. He had just had a physical, and the doctor found nothing to explain why he felt so bad. I asked him if his doctor ordered a testosterone level. He said no. I told him to have his doctor order a total and free testosterone level. Both results came back very low. Testosterone replacement caused a marked positive change in my friend's health and overall energy level. As you saw in Chapter 7, "The Hormone Solution," when testosterone

Image 9.2 Ted's Low-Testosterone SPECT Scan

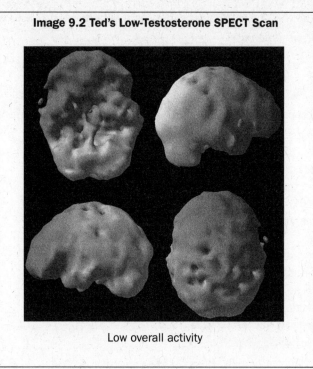

Low overall activity

levels are low, both men and women are more prone to low energy, poor concentration, depression, low libido, and memory problems.

Your energy and focus are dependent on the health of your brain. In order to stay on track toward your goals and to have the best body possible, it is critical to optimize your brain so that you can be focused and energetic. Our "bad brain habits" on a daily basis are hurting our ability to concentrate and to feel the energy we need to achieve our goals for a better body. We need energy to get our butts out of bed and off the couch in order to be physically active. We need energy to help us deal with daily stress. We need energy to cook nutritious meals rather than opting for fast food because we're too tired to cook. We need laser-sharp focus to plan what we are going to do once we arrive at the gym. We need focus to help us grocery shop and plan what we are going to make for breakfast, lunch, and dinner. The goal is to wake up every day with the focus to know what you need to do to get the body you want and the energy to do it.

In this chapter, we will look at the focus and energy solution to help you live a healthier, more vibrant life. We will look at the "focus and energy robbers" and the "focus and energy boosters," plus develop a focus and energy solution all of us can use.

FOCUS AND ENERGY ROBBERS

Focus and energy robbers fall into a number of different categories, including these:

Inherited brain disorders
Infectious causes
Hormonal issues
Low or erratic blood sugar states from any cause
Anemia
Brain trauma
Environmental toxins
Medications
Chronic stress
Untreated past emotional trauma
Bad brain habits

Let's look at some of these in greater detail.

Inherited brain disorders These include illnesses, such as attention deficit disorder (ADD), some forms of depression, anxiety disorders, and obsessive-compulsive disorder. These disorders tend to run in families. Of course, there are many environmental factors that can make these problems better or worse, but there is a definite inherited vulnerability to them.

ADD is the classic focus and energy problem. The energy issue can be too much, such as hyperactivity or restlessness, or too little, which is often associated with a subtype of ADD called inattentive ADD. Both types almost always start in childhood, but the inattentive type, which is more common in girls, is often missed because the students are not disruptive like their hyperactive brethren, often appear spacey, and may have low energy. In addition, symptoms common to both types of ADD include distractibility,

> ### ACTION STEP
> To ease ADD symptoms, try exercise, an elimination diet, and supplementation with fish oil, zinc, acetyl-l-carnitine, and SAMe.

disorganization, trouble being on time, poor handwriting, and being too sensitive to touch, smells, and light.

Dietary interventions may be helpful for ADD. As noted earlier, a study from Holland reported that children who were put on an elimination diet and ate only lean protein, fruits, vegetables, rice, and pear juice had the same positive response rate they had when given Ritalin, a common medication for ADD. Exercise has also been found to be helpful. Certain supplements such as fish oil, zinc, acetyl-l-carnitine, B_6, and magnesium have also been found to be helpful for some people with ADD (see Appendix C, "The Supplement Solution," for more information), while others do better with medications, such as Ritalin, Adderall, or Provigil.

Our brain imaging work has taught us that illnesses such as ADD, anxiety, and depression are not single or simple disorders, and all of them have multiple types. Knowing which type you have is essential to getting the right help. You can see my books *Healing ADD* and *Healing Anxiety and Depression* for more detailed information.

Julie, fifty-four, came to see me for low energy and problems with focus. She was also disorganized, easily distracted, often late or in a hurry, and frequently in conflict with her husband. Her general lab work, including her hormone levels, was normal, plus she had had the primary problems since grade school. Her teachers always told her parents that if only she tried harder, she would do better. I have noticed on brain SPECT scans that the harder people with ADD try, the worse their brains look. Typically, we do two brain SPECT scans on our patients, one at rest and one when they are doing a concentration task. At rest, the ADD person's brain often looks fine, but when they try to concentrate, there is often decreased activity, especially in the front part of the brain in the PFC, which is often responsible for sustained attention. We published a recent study that reported this drop-off of activity helps to predict a positive response to stimulant medication over 80 percent of the time.

Julie's scan showed decreased PFC activity with concentration compared to rest, which meant the harder she tried, the worse it got for her. On treatment, which included fish oil, a healthy diet, exercise, acetyl-l-carnitine, and SAMe, she did much better, especially in the areas of her energy and focus.

Untreated depression and anxiety disorders are also commonly associated with low energy and trouble focusing. A persistent sad mood, in combination with sleep problems, appetite issues (either too much or too little), and persistent negative thoughts, including feelings of hopelessness, helplessness, or worthlessness, tension, fear, and dread, are common symptoms of anxiety and

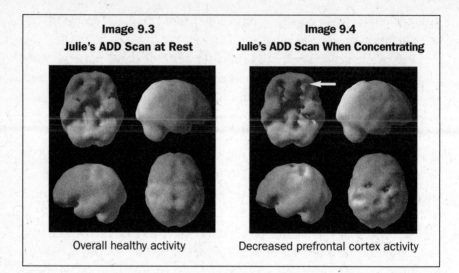

Image 9.3	Image 9.4
Julie's ADD Scan at Rest	Julie's ADD Scan When Concentrating
Overall healthy activity	Decreased prefrontal cortex activity

depression and need to be explored. Untreated depression actually doubles people's risk for Alzheimer's disease. Chapter 15, "The Brain Health Solution," explores this issue in more depth.

Infectious causes Infections, such as chronic fatigue syndrome or Lyme disease, rob people of their energy and focus. When I first started in private practice, chronic fatigue syndrome (CFS) was often thought of as a "crock" illness. There is not a single reliable test to diagnose CFS, so many physicians thought these patients were "psychiatric" and sent them to me. I hated when that happened. It seemed that whenever a doctor did not know what to do for a patient, he or she would label the mysterious illness as "psychosomatic" and send the patient to a psychiatrist or psychologist. When I scanned my first group of ten or so CFS patients, I was horrified at the level of damage I saw on the scans.

Joan was referred to me by her family physician, who thought her "fatigue and trouble focusing" was all in her mind. The limited tests her doctor did came back normal. Joan's brain SPECT scan showed severe overall decreased activity (Image 9.5).

This level of damage is not caused by negative thinking or past emotional trauma (although neither of those things helps a brain). Likely, there are many causes of CFS, which need to be worked up by a competent professional. But if you feel terrible and someone says it is all in your head, they may be right. It may be an illness or an infection that affects your brain, which was the case with Joan. In recent years, we have also seen that the brain is often, although

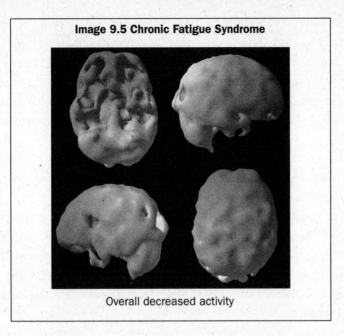

Image 9.5 Chronic Fatigue Syndrome

Overall decreased activity

not always, affected by Lyme disease. Other infections, such as meningitis or HIV, can also seriously negatively impact the brain.

Hormonal issues As you can see from Ted's story, low hormone levels can seriously affect energy levels, focus, and brain function. Some of the worst scans I have seen have been low-thyroid scans. There is a group of scientific studies showing severe low activity with hypothyroidism. Low estrogen levels have been associated with decreased brain activity, as well, especially in the area of the brain that makes people more vulnerable to Alzheimer's disease. Chapter 7, "The Hormone Solution," discusses hormones in detail.

Low or erratic blood sugar states from any cause Things like hypoglycemia, poor diet, or diabetes may have a significant negative effect on energy and focus. This is one reason I tell my employees not to have candy out on their desks for others to grab when they walk by. These people are looking for love in the wrong place. Most people know that when you eat a sugar load, you may have a blood sugar spike and then a blood sugar lull. A

ACTION STEP
Eat small meals that include at least some protein throughout the day to avoid blood sugar spikes and crashes.

recent television piece on the Obama administration showed that many of his staffers had M&Ms on their desks. I was horrified that the White House would not have better eating guidelines for their staff. Don't you want the country's business performed by people who can focus and have great energy? I applaud the Obamas for planting a vegetable garden, but the president's smoking and the plentiful candy are not great brain-healthy examples.

Anemia Anything that lowers your red blood cell count, such as anemia, causes you to feel tired and unfocused. Excessive alcohol use causes red blood cells to become enlarged and inefficient. Hold the alcohol.

I once had a close friend who complained of feeling scattered, tired, and depressed. Her scan looked like she was an alcoholic or a drug addict, but I had known her for many years and knew that this was not the case. In working up medical causes of fatigue, we discovered she had pernicious anemia from a vitamin B_{12} deficiency (Image 9.6). After treatment, her brain looked much, much better and she felt like her old energetic and focused self.

Brain trauma Physical injuries, strokes, lack of oxygen, or other trauma can cause serious brain damage and affect energy and focus.

My sister Mary is a very successful insurance agent and has been a mem-

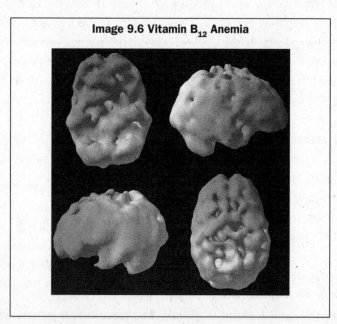

Image 9.6 Vitamin B$_{12}$ Anemia

ber of the high-producing insurance agent organization Million Dollar Roundtable for the past twenty-eight years. In 1994, she lost her husband, Oscar, to stomach cancer, which was very stressful for Mary and her four children. Now as a single mother, Mary was chronically stressed. Fifteen months later, she was in a car accident. After-

> **ACTION STEP**
>
> If you experience any form of brain trauma, it is critical that you adopt a brain-healthy program to enhance brain function.

ward, she noticed problems with her focus, follow-through, energy, drive, and motivation. Her scan showed damage to the left side of her brain. The death of Oscar and the accident had drained all of her brain reserve.

Getting on a brain-healthy program, including supplements—such as fish oil, acetyl-l-carnitine, and ginkgo biloba to enhance overall brain function—and intense exercise along with cognitive retraining made a huge difference for her. Both of her follow-up scans have shown significant improvement.

Environmental toxins Toxins, such as mold exposure, can cause trouble. In 1998, a colleague of mine named Carolyn moved into a home that had been flooded at one time. Very soon after she and her family moved in, they started experiencing health issues. For example, Carolyn suffered from numerous bouts of bronchitis, and she kept getting skin rashes. Over the next couple of years, her symptoms worsened. Carolyn, who had worked as a therapist for years, found that she could no longer focus on what her patients were saying and couldn't think clearly enough to offer them appropriate treatment plans. She often felt anxious and sometimes couldn't tell right from left, which made it very difficult for her to drive.

Her youngest son was in high school at the time, and he kept telling her that he couldn't focus or concentrate well enough to study at home. So he would head over to a friend's house, where he had no problem hitting the books. At home, he had no energy to get going in the morning, and he started racking up tardies at school. Whenever he spent the night at a friend's house, though, he felt energetic, popped up out of bed with no problem, and easily made it to school on time.

> **ACTION STEP**
>
> If your home has ever been flooded or had water damage, check for mold.

By 2001, Carolyn knew there was something very wrong, but she didn't know what. One day, she saw a feature about toxic mold on TV and suspected that this might be the problem. She set up an appointment with a doctor to get tested for allergies to mold, and she hired a mold inspector to check the house. The tests came back positive—mold was the culprit. She and her family moved out of the house that year and never went back. Her children have recovered well for the most part, but Carolyn still hasn't returned to work and lives with residual sensitivities. She says she has good days when her brain functions well and bad days when she has trouble focusing and thinking.

Medications Many medications, including chemotherapy, beta-blockers, antianxiety pills, antidepressants, and painkillers, can sap energy or make it more difficult to focus. Most cancer treatments, such as chemotherapy and radiation therapy, not only kill cancer cells but also kill normal cells. After someone goes through chemotherapy, radiation, or both, their brain scans often show a toxic appearance, meaning their brains have been affected as well. Many post-chemotherapy or -radiation patients complain of low energy, poor concentration, memory problems, and a general lowering of cognitive ability. Understanding this and caring for these brains is absolutely essential to having the best brain and body possible. Many cancer chemotherapy medications go straight to the brain, and they target not only dividing cancer cells but also any normal brain cells that are dividing. While the problem area is targeted and destroyed, there are always "innocent bystanders" caught in the crossfire.

Angelo came to the Amen Clinics for a repeat scan after he was aggressively treated for leukemia. We had seen him five years earlier for problems in his marriage. This time he complained of memory problems, trouble concentrating, and low energy. His SPECT scan showed significant toxicity and lower overall activity not seen on his prior scan. On our brain recovery program, he felt much better and his energy and ability to focus improved.

Chronic stress As you saw with the example of my sister Mary, chronic stress can lead to focus and energy problems.

Untreated past emotional trauma Any trauma from the past that still haunts you is yet another energy and focus robber and is important to get treated.

Bad brain habits Too much caffeine, alcohol, or sugar; drug use; lack of exercise; poor sleep; poor diet; and negative thinking patterns make concentration and focus much worse. Drinking large amounts of alcohol—four or more glasses of wine or the equivalent in hard liquor on a daily basis—raises the risk of dementia. New research shows that even moderate amounts of alcohol have

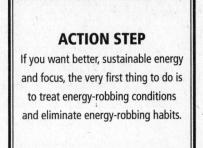

ACTION STEP

If you want better, sustainable energy and focus, the very first thing to do is to treat energy-robbing conditions and eliminate energy-robbing habits.

negative effects on the brain. One study found that people who drink three times a week have smaller brains than do nondrinkers.

New research using brain scans confirms that marijuana use harms the brain. In a study appearing in the *Journal of Psychiatric Research,* researchers showed that heavy marijuana use among young adults and adolescents may affect normal brain development, interrupting an important process called myelinization. With myelinization, brain cells are coated with a protective sheath that increases the brain's processing speeds. The process, which isn't completed until about age twenty-five, starts at the back of the brain and works forward, making the PFC the last area to gain the protective covering. This explains why the subjects in this study showed abnormalities in their PFC and temporal lobes, the areas of the brain involved with decision making, attention, executive functioning, memory, and language. With a brain that hasn't developed properly, it is harder to stay focused and make the best decisions for your health.

FOCUS AND ENERGY BOOSTERS

My mother is known as the Energizer Bunny. At age seventy-eight, she can outgolf, outshop, outcook, and outentertain people half her age. She can go from morning to late at night with a great attitude and a big heart. She has seven children, twenty-one grandchildren, and eight great-grandchildren. She is someone I can call at the last minute and tell I want to bring five people over for dinner, and she will then tell me what to pick up at the store. She has amazing energy, a great attitude, and is always ready to play and have fun. Her lifestyle boosts her energy. She exercises regularly by playing golf, doesn't drink coffee or smoke, rarely drinks alcohol, and eats healthfully.

ACTION STEP

Here is a typical lab panel I order for my patients who struggle with issues of energy and focus to rule out medical causes that may be contributing to the problem. It is a good idea to discuss this panel with your health-care provider.

- Complete blood count—to rule out anemia, inefficient red blood cells, or too little or too many white blood cells
- Fasting chemistry metabolic panel—to check the health of the kidneys, liver, and blood glucose levels
- B_{12}—deficiency is a common cause of anemia and lethargy
- Folate—an essential brain nutrient
- 25-hydroxy vitamin D—low levels are commonly seen with depression, memory problems, and immune system problems
- C-reactive protein—a measure of inflammation
- Homocysteine—a measure of inflammation
- Lipid panel
- Fasting insulin
- Hemoglobin A1C to check risk for diabetes
- Two-hour postmeal glucose—for those suspected of low blood sugar or hypoglycemia
- Thyroid panel with TSH, free T3, free T4, thyroid antibodies gland, and thyroid antibodies hormone
- DHEA-S
- Free and total serum testosterone for men and women
- Estradiol and progesterone for women over forty-five years of age
- Food-allergy testing
- Fatty acid profile to check levels of omega-3 fatty acids

The first step to getting the energy and focus you need is to eliminate and treat the focus and energy robbers described above. At the same time, develop and maintain a brain-healthy lifestyle described in this book, make sure to get adequate sleep, eat a brain-healthy diet to maintain a level blood sugar throughout the day, exercise four or five times a week, use a stress-reduction program (because anxiety and stress rob us of energy and concentration), and test and optimize your hormone levels.

Even though it sounds odd, meditation in particular is one of the best energy boosters. Researchers from our laboratory and others around the

world have demonstrated that meditation enhances activity in the brain's
PFC, even to the point of boosting the
number of brain cells. The better your
PFC functions, the more focused and
energetic you feel. Spend ten minutes
every day meditating to boost your
energy. See Chapter 11 for simple meditation techniques.

> **ACTION STEP**
>
> If you want better energy, meditate.
> Just a few minutes a day will
> improve your energy.

Certain foods are energy boosters, especially those that are low in calories
and high in fiber (from fruits, vegetables, beans, and whole grains) and protein. Since I was young, my mother was a follower of the innovative physician Dr. Henry Bieler, who emphasized diet and lifestyle for disease
prevention. In 1965, he wrote *Food Is Your Best Medicine*, where he discussed
the pH balance in the body, with an alkaline pH being positive for the body
and an acidic pH being harmful. If the body is too acidic, it withdraws alkaline minerals, such as calcium and magnesium, from bones and soft tissues to
maintain balance. An acidic body is a breeding ground for disease and results
from consuming too much sugar, caffeine, alcohol, and red meat. From a psychiatric standpoint this makes sense, as anything that lowers magnesium can
make people feel anxious, agitated, uptight, and stressed. Dr. Bieler's Broth
was a staple for my family. It consists of squash, string beans, celery, parsley,
fresh herbs, and water.

Green tea is another potential energy booster. It has about half the caffeine as coffee, plus theanine, which helps people feel focused. There is scientific evidence that green tea helps keep weight off, boosts exercise ability, helps
muscles recover faster from workouts, and improves attention span.

In addition, there are a group of supplements with good scientific evidence of their helping boost mood, concentration, and energy. Stay away from
caffeinated energy drinks, as they boost the stress hormone cortisol and can
make you fat. Caffeine supplements are also associated with addiction, tolerance (where you need to take more and more to get the same result), and
withdrawal. Green tea, in moderation, is okay because the theanine content
helps to balance the effects of the caffeine.

My favorite supplements to boost focus and energy are B_3 (niacin),
B_6 (pyridoxine), green tea leaf extract, rhodiola, ginseng, ashwagandha,
L-tyrosine, DL-phenylalanine, ginkgo biloba, SAMe, and small amounts
of caffeine. See Appendix C, "The Supplement Solution," for more information.

The Focus and Energy Solution

Energy Robbers	Energy Boosters
Any brain problems	Overall brain-healthy program
Brain trauma	Focus on brain protection
Poor sleep	Adequate sleep (at least seven hours)
Low blood sugar	Frequent small meals with at least some protein to maintain healthy blood sugar
Poor diet	Brain-healthy diet
Alcohol/drug abuse	Freedom from alcohol or drugs
Depression	Treatment for depression
Anxiety	Meditation for relaxation and to boost the PFC
Chronic stress	Stress-reduction plan
Lack of exercise	Exercise
Hormone problems (i.e., thyroid, testosterone, estrogen, cortisol)	Optimized hormone levels
Medical problems, such as B_{12} deficiency	Treatment of any underlying medical problems
Medications such as Xanax or OxyContin	Fish oil to decrease inflammation and enhance blood flow
Diabetes	Diet and exercise
Environmental toxins	Great ventilation and elimination of any toxins
Any systemic inflammation	Anti-inflammation program, including fish oil, healthy diet, and folic acid, and for some, low-dose ibuprofen or baby aspirin
Chemotherapy	Supplements, such as vitamins B_3 and B_6, L-tyrosine, DL-phenylalanine, green tea leaf extract with L-theanine, Panax ginseng, rhodiola, ashwagandha, SAMe, and a small amount of caffeine
Excessive caffeine	When you want a caffeine boost, get it from tea, which has been shown to help keep off weight, boost exercise ability, ease muscle recovery from workouts, and improve attention span and relaxation

PART FOUR

CHANGE YOUR BRAIN, INCREASE LOVE AND VITALITY

10

THE SLEEP SOLUTION

Rest Your Brain for a Slimmer
Shape and Smoother Skin

Sleep plays a major role in preparing the body and
brain for an alert, productive, psychologically
and physiologically healthy tomorrow.

—James Maas, Ph.D., *Power Sleep*

You know how bad you look and feel after a night of poor sleep. You feel like your head is glued to the pillow, and you can barely muster the energy to get out of bed. You shuffle to the bathroom, turn on the light, and come face-to-face with puffy bags and dark circles under your eyes. You head outside for your usual thirty-minute jog but stop after ten minutes because you feel whipped. Then you head to work, where you snap at your coworkers and customers because you are in a foul mood. It isn't a pretty picture, is it?

Good sleep is essential for optimal brain and body health. It is involved in rejuvenating all the cells in your body, gives brain cells a chance to repair themselves, and activates neuronal connections that might otherwise deteriorate due to inactivity. It is also necessary if you want to have glowing skin, high energy, a sunny mood, excellent health, and stable weight. Unfortunately, as many as seventy million Americans have trouble sleeping. If you are one of them, your brain and body could be in trouble.

ARE YOU GETTING ENOUGH SLEEP?

Many Americans aren't getting the sleep they need. According to the 2009 Sleep in America Poll, Americans are averaging only six hours and forty minutes of sleep on workdays and school nights. People tend to squeeze in an extra twenty-seven minutes of sleep on weekends. Even more disturbing, the percentage of people getting less than six hours of sleep has risen from 12 percent in 1998 to 20 percent in 2009, while the percentage of Americans getting a good eight hours a night has decreased from 35 percent in 1998 to 28 percent in 2009. The numbers reveal that getting a good night's sleep is becoming little more than an elusive dream for many Americans. Chronic sleep problems affect millions of us. Temporary sleep issues are even more common and will affect almost every one of us at some point in our lifetime.

AVERAGE SLEEP REQUIREMENTS BY AGE

Age Range	Number of Hours of Sleep
1–3 years old	12–14 hours
3–5 years old	11–13 hours
5–12 years old	10–11 hours
13–19 years old	9 hours
Adults	7–8 hours
Seniors	7–8 hours

Sources: National Sleep Foundation, National Institute of Neurological Disorders and Stroke

Think about your own sleep habits. When was the last time you drifted off to sleep easily, slept soundly all night long, and woke up feeling refreshed and alert? When was the last time you hopped out of bed in the morning raring to go? When was the last time you sat down to watch a movie and didn't nod off? If you aren't getting adequate sleep, your brain and body are at risk.

Sleep troubles come in many varieties. Do you have trouble falling asleep? Do you go to sleep easily but wake up repeatedly throughout the night? Do you find it hard to drag yourself out of bed in the morning? Do you or your significant other snore? All of these problems can lead to decreased brain function and a second-rate body. Getting less than six hours of sleep a night has been associated with lower overall brain activity, which can affect your weight, your skin, your mood, your health, and your athletic performance.

ACTION STEP

Stop trying to convince yourself that you need only five hours of sleep each night. Be aware of the basic sleep requirements for your age group.

WHY LOSING SLEEP CAN MAKE YOU FAT

You probably thought that your cravings for candy and cookies were just a sign of mental weakness and a lack of willpower on your part. You may be wrong. An expanding body of evidence has shown that sleep deprivation is associated with weight gain and obesity. Here's what researchers from around the nation have discovered about sleep and your weight.

According to a study from the University of Chicago, people who are sleep deprived eat more simple carbohydrates than people who get adequate sleep. The researchers studied twelve healthy men in their twenties and found that when the men slept only four hours a night, they were more likely to choose candy, cookies, and cake over fruit, vegetables, or dairy products.

For this study, which appeared in the *Annals of Internal Medicine*, researchers also looked at two hormones—leptin and ghrelin—that are regulated by sleep and involved in appetite. As discussed earlier, leptin and ghrelin work together to control feelings of hunger and satiety. Ghrelin levels rise to signal the brain that you are hungry, then leptin levels increase to tell your brain when you are full. The researchers measured the levels of leptin and ghrelin before the study, after two nights of only four hours of sleep, and after two nights of ten hours of sleep. After four hours of sleep, the ratio of ghrelin jumped 71 percent, compared to a night when the men slept for the longer period of time. This made the men feel hungrier and drove them to consume more simple carbohydrates. As explained in an earlier chapter, eating simple carbs sends blood sugar levels skyrocketing then plummeting, which saps energy and leaves you feeling fatigued.

In a study published in the *American Journal of Clinical Nutrition*, researchers had people sleep for five and a half hours for two weeks and then eight and a half hours for another two weeks at random. Then they measured how many snacks the subjects munched during their stays in the sleep laboratory. When the people slept only five and a half hours, they consumed an average of 221 more calories in high-carbohydrate snacks than when they got eight and a half hours of sleep.

This pattern occurs in the real world, too, not just in researchers' sleep labs. According to the 2009 Sleep in America Poll, people who are having trouble sleeping are almost twice as likely to chow down on sugary foods and simple carbs, such as potato chips, to help them make it through the day. They are also more inclined to skip breakfast or other meals, which puts your blood sugar levels on a roller-coaster ride that's bad for brain function and often leads to poor nutrition choices later in the day.

Sleeping less makes you eat more sugary junk foods rather than fruits, vegetables, and whole grains. It also makes you eat more calories overall, which increases your risk of gaining weight and becoming obese. A study from researchers at Case Western University tracked the sleeping habits and weight fluctuations of 68,183 women for sixteen years. The women were divided into three categories—those who slept seven hours a night, those who logged six hours of sleep, and those who got five hours or less of sleep. *They found that the women who slept five hours or less gained the most weight over time and were the most likely to become obese.* The women who slept only six hours a night were more likely to pack on extra weight than the women who got seven hours of shut-eye.

Dozens of other studies point to a connection between a lack of sleep and weight gain or obesity. For example, researchers at the University of Warwick, England, reviewed data from more than 28,000 children and more than 15,000 adults and found that sleep deprivation almost doubles the risk of obesity for adults and children. Another study conducted by researchers at Stanford University found that people who sleep less have higher body mass index (BMI) levels.

The Stanford University study also found lower leptin levels and higher ghrelin levels in people who sleep less. The researchers examined a thousand people, measuring their sleep habits, their sleep on the night before the exam, and their leptin and ghrelin levels. They found that people who consistently slept five hours or less per night had on average 14.9 percent more ghrelin (which stimulates appetite) and 15.5 percent lower leptin (which tells your brain you are full) than people who slept eight hours a night. These studies show that when you don't get enough sleep, you feel hungrier and don't feel full regardless of how much you eat, so you eat more, which makes you fat!

So, if dodging sleep can make you fat, can getting adequate sleep help you lose weight? Editors at *Glamour* magazine decided to put this notion to the test with an unscientific—yet fascinating—study. They enlisted seven female readers and gave them one simple task: sleep at least seven and a half hours each night for ten weeks. In addition, they were instructed not to make any significant changes in their diets or exercise routines

---

ACTION STEP

If you are trying to drop excess weight, spend more time in bed.

during the ten weeks. The results were amazing. All seven women lost weight, with the weight loss ranging from six pounds to an astonishing fifteen pounds.

GET MORE SLEEP FOR SKIN THAT GLOWS

We often talk about getting our "beauty sleep," and we couldn't be more accurate with that description. Getting adequate sleep actually does far more for your skin than a medicine cabinet filled with wrinkle creams, moisturizers, acne treatments, and antiaging serums. With the right amount of sleep, your skin will look younger, smoother, and more refreshed. When you try to get by on little sleep, you set yourself up for premature aging of the skin, dark circles under the eyes, even acne. Here's how sleep can benefit your skin.

Rejuvenate the skin. Cell regeneration is a process during which old, dead skin cells are replaced with fresh new cells. This process goes on at all times within the body, but it happens more quickly at night so you generate more new skin cells while you sleep than at any other time. As we get older, cell replacement slows down, which makes sleep even more crucial if you want to delay the thin, saggy skin that comes with age.

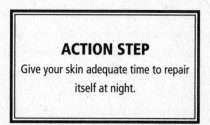

ACTION STEP

Give your skin adequate time to repair itself at night.

Reverse skin damage. On a daily basis, your skin is faced with elements, including the sun's harmful UV rays, secondhand smoke, and other environmental pollutants, which cause premature aging and damage. While you sleep, your skin repairs itself from this daily damage.

Prevent acne. As we sleep, the brain regulates the body's hormones, including androgens, which stimulate the production of sebum, or oil, in glands located in the skin. When hormones are balanced, sebum production is regulated to help keep skin looking clear and smooth. Hormonal imbalances can cause too much sebum production, which can lead to acne.

LOSE SLEEP AND YOU LOSE FOCUS AND WILLPOWER

People who get less than seven hours of sleep a night have lower activity in the prefrontal cortex and temporal lobes, which are involved in memory

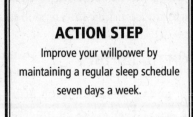

ACTION STEP

Improve your willpower by maintaining a regular sleep schedule seven days a week.

and learning. This limits the ability to pay attention, learn, solve problems, and remember important information. These are all vital skills you need if you want to tackle a new dance routine, learn a new sport, learn to cook brain-healthy recipes, or remember to take your medications. Considering this, it is no surprise that sleep-deprived individuals struggle to maintain a healthy body.

HIT THE SACK FOR PEAK ATHLETIC PERFORMANCE

It should come as no surprise that lack of sleep hinders athletic performance. Anyone who has ever exercised or played sports while sleep deprived knows that it is tough to be at your best on the court, on the field, or in the gym.

Research shows us that sleep deprivation impairs motor function, which makes you less coordinated and more likely to strike out at bat or shank your drive on the golf course. Reaction times are slowed, so you don't get to the ball fast enough. The reduced cognitive functioning associated with lack of sleep means that you may not make the best on-court decisions or may not remember the new steps you learned the week before in your ballroom dancing class. Plus, you tend to feel tired faster because sleep deprivation negatively affects glucose metabolism.

On the other hand, getting a good night's sleep can give your game a boost. That's according to researchers at Stanford University who looked at the relationship between sleep habits and athletic performance in six male Stanford basketball players. The researchers measured the subjects' sprint times as well as free-throw and three-point shooting percentages. For the first two weeks, the college players maintained their regular sleep habits; for the second two weeks, they were told to get as much extra sleep as possible. After the extended sleep period, the athletes were faster and more accurate shooters. The average

ACTION STEP

To help you fall asleep faster, avoid exercising or playing sports close to bedtime.

sprint time decreased by one second, free-throw shooting improved by about 10 percent, and three-point shooting increased by more than 10 percent. The extra sleep offered another performance bonus: The test athletes reported having more energy.

A follow-up study involving students on Stanford's men's and women's swim teams showed similar improvements. They swam faster, reacted quicker off the blocks, improved turn time, and increased kick strokes after a two-week period of extended sleep.

Sleep may offer other benefits to athletes at every level—from the NBA's MVP to the weekend golfer to the company softball player. Research from Harvard Medical School suggests that after initial training—whether it is learning how to execute your NBA team's offensive plays, how to hit a chip shot, or how to swing a bat—the brain continues to learn while you sleep. This indicates that sleeping can make you a better athlete.

LACK OF SLEEP WORSENS YOUR MOOD

In a 2007 survey from the Better Sleep Council, 44 percent of workers admitted that when they are sleep deprived, they are more likely to be in an unpleasant or unfriendly mood. In general, people who are tired due to lack of sleep tend to feel irritable and don't have the energy to do much of anything. Curling up on the couch to watch TV or thumbing through a magazine might be all the energy you can muster after a sleepless night. Studies

> ### ACTION STEP
> Make sleep a priority in your life rather than an afterthought.

show that decreased motivation due to poor sleep makes you more likely to skip family events, work functions, and other recreational activities. Social connections help keep the brain young, so missing out on get-togethers and events due to fatigue can dampen your mood and prematurely age your brain. This can be especially troublesome for seniors because a lack of social connections and bonding can speed up the brain's aging process.

Plus, when you are sleep deprived, you are less inclined to exercise or get intimate with your significant other, which deprives your brain and body of feel-good chemicals that boost your mood. If you want to improve your mood, improve your sleeping habits.

SLEEP DEPRIVATION IS HAZARDOUS TO YOUR HEALTH

Skimping on sleep can affect your health in more ways than you might imagine. It can even stunt growth in young people. Growth hormones produced in the brain are typically generated as we sleep. If youngsters don't get enough sleep, they may not produce enough of the hormones to fuel growth. Chronic sleep loss is also associated with a number of poor lifestyle choices as well as brain-related conditions and disorders that put your physical and mental health at risk.

Bad lifestyle habits When you don't get enough sleep, you are inclined to gulp more caffeine, smoke more, exercise less, and drink more alcohol. Studies show that sleep-deprived adolescents are also more likely to drink alcohol, smoke marijuana, and use other drugs than those who get enough sleep.

Type 2 diabetes Sleep deprivation can put you at risk for this serious condition. In a sleep study with healthy volunteers, those who got only 5.5 hours of bedtime experienced insulin resistance and impaired glucose tolerance—two precursors of diabetes—after just two weeks.

Depression Sleep deprivation has been linked to mood problems and depression in a number of scientific studies. One study published in the journal *Sleep* found that sleep problems are an early sign of depression and that treatment of sleep issues may protect individuals from developing the disorder. Similarly, researchers at the University of Rome who studied children between the ages of seven and eleven suffering from depression found that 82 percent of them reported having problems sleeping. Another study shows that insomnia in adolescents is a significant risk factor for depression later in life. Among the elderly, sleep deprivation may prolong bouts of depression.

Anxiety Research indicates that chronic sleep problems make you more vulnerable to the development of anxiety disorders.

ADD Sleep disturbances are very common in children and adults with ADD. Many have a harder time falling asleep, spend less time in the restorative rapid eye movement (REM) stage of sleep, and sleep fewer hours overall than people who don't have the disorder. Restless nights tend to worsen ADD symptoms.

Alzheimer's disease Research has found that people with sleep apnea may be more likely to develop Alzheimer's disease and that sleep apnea may worsen cognitive impairment in people with dementia. Treating sleep apnea has been shown to improve cognitive function in people with this disease.

> **ACTION STEP**
> Get treated for sleep apnea immediately.

Parkinson's disease People who thrash around while sleeping—a condition called REM sleep behavior disorder—may face a higher risk of developing Parkinson's disease, according to a study in the journal *Neurology*.

Stroke Sleep apnea significantly increases the risk of stroke.

Psychosis People can become psychotic from lack of sleep. I noticed this when I was chief of Community Mental Health at Fort Irwin in the Mojave Desert. Fort Irwin houses the National Training Center that teaches desert warfare to soldiers. The troops used to spend days at a time in war games without much sleep. As a result, after being awake for three days in a row, a number of soldiers began to hear voices and become paranoid.

Some time ago, my uncle started having problems with his memory—he couldn't remember where he parked the car and was forgetting people's names. The whole family was really concerned, so he went to the doctor and came back with a diagnosis of Alzheimer's disease. He was devastated. His brain SPECT scan showed severe decreased activity in the back half of his brain, a finding consistent with severe memory problems, but also consistent with what we have seen with severe sleep apnea. On testing, he was diagnosed with severe sleep apnea. Treatment helped his cognitive abilities improve significantly. This story shows how critical it is to get treated for sleep problems. But most people suffering from lack of sleep neglect to seek help. They don't view it as a medical problem and choose to simply live with it. That could be a life-threatening mistake.

DANGEROUS CONSEQUENCES OF SLEEP DEPRIVATION

Sleep deprivation slows reaction times, clouds judgment, affects vision, impairs information processing, and increases aggressive behavior. All of this

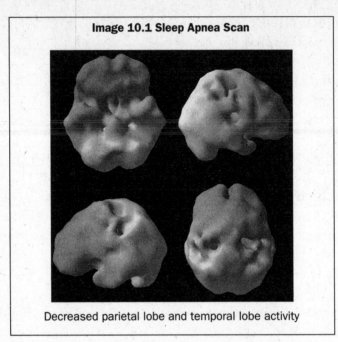

Image 10.1 Sleep Apnea Scan

Decreased parietal lobe and temporal lobe activity

adds up to danger on America's highways. According to the National Highway Traffic Safety Administration (NHTSA), drowsiness and fatigue cause more than 100,000 traffic accidents each year, causing 40,000 injuries and 1,550 deaths. The National Sleep Foundation estimates the numbers are much higher: 71,000 injuries and more than 5,500 deaths a year. One reason why the NHTSA's statistics may be low is that fatigue is often underreported as a contributing factor to a crash. In more than half of the reported fatigue-related crashes, young drivers are at the wheel.

Every day, millions of people hit the road while feeling drowsy. More than half of the respondents in the 2009 Sleep in America Poll reported having driven while drowsy in the past year, and 28 percent admitted to nodding off or falling asleep behind the wheel. Night-shift workers, people with untreated sleep apnea, and young people—particularly men—between the ages of sixteen and twenty-nine are especially likely to drive while feeling sleepy. Fatigue has also played a role in many airplane, train, and boating crashes, some of them deadly.

WHAT CAUSES SLEEP DEPRIVATION?

In our hectic, 24-7 society, I could just as easily ask "What doesn't cause sleep deprivation?" There are a seemingly endless number of reasons why millions of us are missing out on a good night's sleep. Here is a list of just a few of the many things that may cause sleep troubles.

- Medications: many medications, including asthma medications, antihistamines, cough medicines, and anticonvulsants, disturb sleep.
- Caffeine: too much caffeine from coffee, tea, chocolate, or some herbal preparations—especially when consumed later in the day or at night—can disrupt sleep.
- Alcohol, nicotine, and marijuana: although these compounds initially induce sleepiness for some people, they have the reverse effect as they wear off, which is why you may wake up several hours after you go to sleep.
- Restless legs syndrome: A nighttime jerking or pedaling motion of the legs that drives a person's bed partner crazy (as well as the person who has it).
- Women's issues: pregnancy, PMS, menopause, and perimenopause cause fluctuations in hormone levels that can disrupt the sleep cycle.
- Thyroid conditions
- Congestive heart failure
- Chronic pain conditions
- Untreated or undertreated psychiatric conditions such as obsessive-compulsive disorder, depression, or anxiety
- Alzheimer's disease: dementia patients "sundown" or rev up at night and wander.
- Chronic gastrointestinal problems, such as reflux
- Men's issues: benign prostatic hypertrophy causes many trips to the bathroom at night, which interrupts slumber.
- Snoring: snoring can wake you or your sleepmate, or everyone in the house if it is really loud.
- Sleep apnea: with this condition, you stop breathing for short periods of time throughout the night, which robs you of restful sleep and leaves you feeling sluggish, inattentive, and forgetful throughout the day.
- Shift work: nurses, firefighters, security personnel, customer

> **ACTION STEP**
> Take stock of the things in your life that might be causing you to toss and turn at night.

service representatives, truck drivers, airline pilots, and many others toil by night and sleep by day. Or, at least, they try to sleep. Shift workers are especially vulnerable to irregular sleep patterns, which leads to excessive sleepiness, reduced productivity, irritability, and mood problems.

- Stressful events: the death of a loved one, divorce, a major deadline at work, or an upcoming test can cause temporary sleep loss.
- Jet lag: international travel across time zones wreaks havoc with sleep cycles.

WHO'S AT RISK FOR POOR SLEEP?

Nobody is immune to sleep problems—they can affect anyone at any time of life. A study presented at the American Psychiatric Association's annual meeting in 2007 analyzed the sleep habits of more than 79,000 adults and revealed that about one-third of moms aren't getting adequate sleep. As a child psychiatrist, I work with a lot of troubled kids, and I notice that their moms are usually drained and exhausted. They work so hard to help their children succeed that they tend to neglect their own needs. I think moms need to do a better job of taking care of themselves, and that starts with getting a good night's sleep.

Dads have their own problems getting enough shut-eye. According to the same study mentioned earlier, about 27 percent of married dads and more than 30 percent of unmarried dads reported getting insufficient sleep.

Sleep deprivation is rampant among teens. Researchers have found that when kids hit their teen years, their sleep cycles change, making them more inclined to go to sleep later and wake up later. That makes it especially tough for teens to be up and alert for those early 7 a.m. start times at some schools. A study from 1997 found that when a high school switched from a 7:15 a.m. start time to an 8:40 a.m. start time, students reported getting more sleep and feeling less tired during the day. They also got higher grades and were less likely to have feelings of depression. A 2009 study found that later school start times increased the number of hours teens slept during the week and decreased the number of car accidents involving teen drivers in the area by 16.5 percent.

College students are also plagued by sleep troubles. According to a study published in the *Journal of American College Health*, 33 percent of college students reported taking longer than thirty minutes to fall asleep, and 43 percent woke up more than once a night. Since college students usually have more control over their schedules, encourage them to schedule more afternoon classes rather than early-morning classes.

Sleep disturbances are also common on the other end of the age spectrum. The notion that older people don't need as much sleep is a common misconception. Studies show that seniors need the same seven to eight hours a night as other adults. As part of the normal aging process, however, Grandma and Grandpa are likely to experience more unsettled sleep. As you get older, sleep patterns tend to change, and you typically find it harder to fall asleep and stay asleep. This can speed up the brain's aging process at a time when you really want to hang on to every brain cell you have.

TIPS TO HELP YOU GO TO SLEEP AND STAY ASLEEP

Here are twelve ways to make it easier to drift off to dreamland and get a good night's sleep. Remember that we are all unique individuals, and what works for one person may not work for another. Keep trying new techniques until you find something that works.

1. Maintain a regular sleep schedule—going to bed at the same time each night and waking up at the same time each day, including on weekends. Get up at the same time each day regardless of sleep duration the previous night.
2. Create a soothing nighttime routine that encourages sleep. A warm bath, meditation, or massage can help you relax.
3. Some people like to read themselves to sleep. If you are reading, make sure it isn't an action-packed thriller or a horror story—they aren't likely to help you drift off to sleep.
4. Don't take naps! This is one of the biggest mistakes you can make if you have insomnia. Taking naps when you feel sleepy during the day compounds the nighttime sleep cycle disruption.
5. Sound therapy can induce a very peaceful mood and lull you to sleep. Consider soothing nature sounds, soft music, wind chimes, or even a fan.
6. Drink a mixture of warm milk, a teaspoon of vanilla (the real stuff, not imitation), and a few drops of stevia. This increases serotonin in your brain and helps you sleep.
7. Take computers, video games, and cell phones out of the bedroom

and turn them off an hour or two before bedtime to allow time to "unwind."

8. Don't eat for at least two to three hours before going to bed.

9. Regular exercise is very beneficial for falling asleep and staying asleep, but don't do it within four hours of the time you hit the sack. Vigorous exercise late in the evening may energize you and keep you awake.

10. Don't drink any caffeinated beverages in the late afternoon or evening. Also avoid chocolate, nicotine, and alcohol—especially at night. Although alcohol can initially make you feel sleepy, it interrupts sleep.

11. If you wake up in the middle of the night, refrain from looking at the clock. Checking the time can make you feel anxious, which aggravates the problem.

12. Use the bed and bedroom only for sleep or sexual activity. Sexual activity releases many natural hormones, releases muscle tension, and boosts a sense of well-being. Adults with healthy sex lives tend to sleep better. When you are unable to fall asleep or return to sleep easily, get up and go to another room.

NATURAL TREATMENTS TO HELP YOU SLEEP BETTER

Because of our sleep problems, doctors are prescribing sleep medications that can affect your moods and memory at alarming rates. These medications are also increasingly prescribed for children of all ages. A study that appeared in a 2007 issue of *Sleep* showed that 81 percent of children who saw a medical professional for sleep-related problems were given a prescription. In my practice, my primary course of action isn't doling out a prescription. I first encourage my patients to eliminate anything that might interfere with sleep, such as caffeine, alcohol, or reading Stephen King before bedtime. I also try natural supplements and treatments. Here are some of the natural remedies I recommend.

> **ACTION STEP**
>
> Before you reach for the sleeping pills, try hypnosis. It has been proven to work and has no side effects.

ACTION STEP

If you have trouble sleeping, keep a sleep journal and track what time you go to sleep, how long it takes to fall asleep, how often you wake up, what time you get up in the morning, how you feel upon waking, how much energy you have throughout the day, and any daytime naps. Make a copy of the following sleep journal entry and fill it in daily.

MY SLEEP JOURNAL

Day/Date _____

(Answer the following questions in the morning.)
Last night, my bedtime ritual included: _____
(List things like a warm bath, meditation, reading, etc.)
Last night I went to bed at: _____ pm/am
Last night I fell asleep in: _____ minutes
Last night, I woke up: _____ times
During those times, I was awake for: _____ minutes
Last night, I got out of bed: _____ times
Things that disturbed my sleep: _____
(List any physical, mental, emotional, or environmental factors that affected your sleep.)
I slept for a total of: _____ minutes
I got out of bed this morning at: _____ am/pm
Upon waking, I felt: __refreshed __groggy __exhausted

(Answer the following questions at night.)
During the day, I fell asleep or napped: _____ times
During my naps, I slept for: _____ minutes
During the day, I felt: __refreshed __groggy __exhausted
My caffeine consumption: _____ amount _____ time of day
Medications or sleep aids I took: _____

Hypnosis

As a medical student, I saw someone get hypnotized, and I found the process so fascinating that I took a whole month's training on it. As an intern at Walter Reed Army Medical Center, a military hospital with 1,200 beds, I worked with many patients who were having trouble sleeping and wanted sleeping pills. It is easy to understand how people might have a tough time getting a decent night's sleep in such a huge, noisy hospital. On the nights I was on call, I would ask the patients if I could try hypnotizing them rather than give a sleeping pill. Almost everybody said yes, and it worked. I prescribed considerably fewer sleeping pills than my colleagues.

Hypnosis is a very powerful technique. I worked with one veteran who was a World War II hero. He had helped smuggle Jewish people out of Germany to safety. In his later years, he developed Parkinson's disease and found it difficult to sleep at night. The night I was on call he wanted a sleeping pill. I asked him if I could try to hypnotize him instead. He agreed and when I put him in a trance, his tremor stopped. Parkinsonian tremors usually stop when a person falls asleep, but his tremor stopped before he actually went to sleep.

When I told my attending neurologist, Bahman Jabbari, about it the next morning he rolled his eyes and looked at me as if I were the dumbest person on the planet. Later, I repeated the exercise in front of him and it worked. He was so amazed that we filmed our patient going into a hypnotic trance and coauthored a paper on it. That became one of my first professional papers.

Hypnosis can even help people with post-traumatic stress disorder (PTSD) get better sleep. People with PTSD often have trouble sleeping. In a study from Israel, one group of fifteen patients was given a daily prescription sleeping pill while the second group of seventeen patients underwent hypnotherapy twice a week. After two weeks, the hypnosis group showed improvement in sleep quality. The improvements were still evident a full month later, too, showing that hypnosis has lasting benefits.

At one point during my internship, I was having trouble sleeping myself. Many of my patients were dealing with very serious medical conditions and some even died. Coping with that level of responsibility was hard for me. I care very deeply about what happens to my patients, and it was making me anxious and keeping me up at night. That's when I started doing self-hypnosis to help me sleep. I figured if it works for my patients, it should work for me too. With time, I became so proficient at it that I could put myself to sleep in under one minute. To help others, I created a hypnosis CD specifically for sleep disorders that can be ordered through the Amen Clinics website (www.amenclinics.com).

Bright Light Therapy

Bright light therapy is a technique that promotes better sleep in people who suffer from seasonal affective disorder (SAD), more commonly known as winter blues. We see many people with this condition in our clinic in Tacoma, Washington. It is also very common in Alaska and Canada, where some regions get only a few hours of daily sunlight during the winter, and the lack of light can cause sleep disturbances. Bright light therapy, in which a person sits in front of a strong light that has the same wavelengths as the sun for thirty minutes, can reset sleep patterns. In my experience, I have found that bright light therapy works best in the morning.

Natural Supplements for More Restful Sleep

When sleep deprivation isn't relieved by other methods, I prescribe natural supplements, such as L-tryptophan, 5-HTP, valerian, kava kava, magnesium, and melatonin. Some of these natural interventions may also be helpful during periods of temporary insomnia due to stress, jet lag, trying to sleep in a new environment, or doing shift work. See Appendix C, "The Supplement Solution," for more information.

The Sleep Solution

Sleep Robbers	Sleep Enhancers
Any brain problems	Brain health
Brain trauma	Focus on brain protection
Low blood sugar	Frequent small meals with at least some protein to maintain healthy blood sugar
Caffeine	No caffeine
Poor diet	Enriched diet
Alcohol, drug abuse	Freedom from alcohol and drugs
ADD	Effective treatment for ADD
Some forms of depression	Journaling when sad or anxious, treatment
Anxiety	Meditation or self-hypnosis for relaxation
Negative thinking	Killing the ANTs (automatic negative thoughts)
Alzheimer's disease	Sleep aids, especially melatonin
Sleep apnea	Treatment for sleep apnea
Hormonal fluctuations	Balanced hormones
Thyroid conditions	Treatment for thyroid conditions
Chronic pain	Exercise
Chronic stress	Stress-reduction plan
Too much TV, video games, computers	Technology turned off a few hours before bedtime
	Soothing sounds
	Bright light therapy
	Supplements such as melatonin, L-tryptophan, 5-HTP, valerian, kava kava, and magnesium

11

THE STRESS SOLUTION

Relax Your Brain to Reduce Your
Wrinkles and Improve
Your Immune System

Stress is nothing more than a socially acceptable form of mental illness.
—Richard Carlson, Ph.D.

Maria was in her forties when she came to our offices for help. She was unhappy because her belly had gotten fat, and she had been struggling for years to lose the weight. She was also under constant stress. Her mother had suffered a stroke several years earlier, and Maria had taken on the role of caretaker. On top of that, her son had started acting out. Maria was spending so much time caring for the others in her family that she had been neglecting her own health and well-being for too long. I told her something that I tell many of my patients, "You need to put on your own oxygen mask first before you help others." What I mean by this is you need to look out for yourself first so you can be healthy enough take care of the people you love. Thanks to some stress-management techniques and a renewed focus on her own needs, Maria lost the abdominal fat and fared much better in taking care of her mother and son.

Stress is a normal part of everyday life. Bad traffic, a big deadline at work, a fight with your spouse—there are hundreds of things that can make us feel stressed out. When the event passes, so does the stress, and we can breathe a big sigh of relief. With chronic stress, however, there is no relief. Stemming from family discord, financial hardships, health issues, work conflicts, or school trouble, chronic stress can be unrelenting. And it affects far too many of us. In a recent poll by the American Psychological Association, a whopping

80 percent of Americans said the weakened economy is causing them significant stress. That spells trouble for your brain and body.

THE BRAIN–BODY RESPONSE

Don't get me wrong. A little stress can be a good thing. When stress hits, the brain tells your body to start pumping out adrenaline (epinephrine) and cortisol, two hormones released by the adrenal glands (located above the kidneys). Within seconds, your heart starts to pound faster, your breathing quickens, your blood courses faster through your veins, and your mind feels like it is on heightened alert. You are ready for anything—running away from a would-be mugger, giving a speech in front of a roomful of peers, or taking an exam.

These stress hormones are the primary chemicals of the fight-or-flight response and are especially useful when you face an immediate threat, such as a rattlesnake in your front yard (which happened to me once). What's amazing is that the human brain is so advanced that merely imagining a stressful event will cause the body to react to the perceived threat as if it were actually happening. You can literally scare your body into a stress response. The brain is a very powerful organ.

Brief surges of stress hormones are normal and beneficial. They motivate you to do a good job at work, study before a test, or pay your bills on time. The problem with stress in our modern world is not these short bursts of adrenaline and cortisol. The problem is that for many of us, the stress reactions never stop—traffic, bills, work, school, family conflict, not enough sleep, health issues, and jam-packed schedules keep us in a constant state of stress. Take note that it isn't just the bad stuff in life that makes us stressed. Even happy events, such as having a baby or getting a promotion, can be major stressors. Take a look at the following lists of just some of the many events and situations that can cause stress.

Negative Events That Cause Stress

- Death of a loved one
- Getting laid off
- Getting divorced
- Unwanted pregnancy
- Miscarriage
- Financial problems

- Being involved in a lawsuit
- Having health problems
- Having a sick relative
- Caring for an ailing family member
- Having a mental disorder or living with someone who has one
- Problems at work
- Problems at school

Positive Events That Cause Stress

- Getting married
- Having a baby
- Starting a new job
- Getting a promotion
- Moving to a new home
- Transferring to a new school
- Going to college
- Having a bestselling book

HOW CHRONIC STRESS HARMS THE BRAIN

Chronic stress constricts blood flow to the brain, which lowers overall brain function and prematurely ages your brain. A series of studies published in the journal *Psychoneuroendocrinology* looked at long-term exposure to stress hormones, especially cortisol, and its effect on brain function in people of varying age groups. The research showed that older adults with continuously high levels of cortisol performed worse on memory tests than older adults with moderate to low cortisol levels. The older adults with high cortisol levels also had a 14 percent smaller hippocampus, the area of the temporal lobes involved with memory. The hippocampus is part of the stress response system and is responsible for sending out signals to halt the production of cortisol once a threat has vanished. But when the number of brain cells in the hippocampus is depleted, it no longer sends out this signal, which results in the release of even greater amounts of cortisol.

Researchers found that short, temporary spikes in cortisol had a negative—although temporary—effect on young adults' thinking and memory skills. In young children and teenagers, the research showed that kids with lower socioeconomic status had higher average stress hormone levels than the other children. As a group, these studies reveal that chronic stress impairs the brain function of people of all ages.

Excessive amounts of cortisol affect other areas of the brain, too. Canadian researchers used functional brain imaging studies to show that exposure to stress hormones is associated with decreased activity not only in the hippocampus, but also in the amygdala, part of the emotional brain and the prefrontal cortex. As a result, chronic stress has negative consequences for both cognitive function and emotional balance.

It gets even worse. An ongoing overload of cortisol reduces brain reserve, which makes you more vulnerable to the many physical effects of stress. When stress hurts your brain, it can also ravage your body.

HOW CHRONIC STRESS MAKES YOU LOOK OLDER

If you have crow's-feet, wrinkles, sagging jowls, or thinning skin, don't blame it on your parents. New research shows that environmental factors—including chronic stresss—rather than genetics, may be at fault. In a fascinating study involving identical twins, environmental factors were found to make people look older than they really are. For the study, which was published on the *Plastic and Reconstructive Surgery* journal's website, a panel of plastic surgeons examined digital photos of 186 pairs of identical twins who had attended the Twins Festival in Twinsburg, Ohio, in 2006 and 2007. The physicians attempted to determine the age of each individual based on their facial features. What they found is that individuals who had experienced stressful events tended to look older than their siblings who had led more stress-free lives. For example, twins who were divorced looked almost two years older than their siblings who were married, single, or even widowed. One of the study's authors cited the presence of stress as one of the common denominators in the twins who looked older.

ACTION STEP

Before you spend hundreds of dollars on wrinkle removers, consider that your skin problems may be due to stress as opposed to the natural aging process.

Other scientific evidence shows that chronic stress can mimic the effects of aging to make you look and feel like you've aged beyond your years. According to a 2009 study of 647 women, the physical effects of chronic stress were found to be similar to the effects of smoking, being obese, or being ten years older than their actual age. The study looked at the association between perceived stress levels and the length of telomeres, the protective caps located on the ends of chromosomes. The longer the caps are, the more protection they provide. The shorter they are, the less protection provided.

Telomeres naturally shorten over time as we age, eventually becoming so short that they trigger cell death. In this study, the women with higher levels of perceived stress had shorter telomeres than women with low-level stress, indicating premature aging.

You can see the effects of stress-induced aging by simply looking in the mirror. With natural aging, your skin begins to lose collagen and elastin, two proteins that provide support and elasticity for a more youthful appearance. Stress causes collagen and elastin to break down prematurely, which leads to sagging skin and wrinkles. Unfortunately, wrinkles aren't the only skin problem that comes with unrelenting stress. Since chronic stress toys with your hormones, it can also lead to acne breakouts regardless of your age.

HOW CHRONIC STRESS MAKES YOU SICK

Your body responds to the way you think, feel, and act. Because of this brain-body connection, whenever you feel stressed, your body tries to tell you when something isn't right. For example, high blood pressure or a stomach ulcer might develop after a particularly stressful event, such as the death of a loved one. Chronic stress weakens your body's immune system, making you more likely to get colds, flu bugs, and other infections during emotionally difficult times. It has also been implicated in heart disease, hypertension, and even cancer. In fact, too much stress can actually kill you.

In a 2004 issue of *Psychological Bulletin*, a team of psychologists published findings from a thorough review of nearly three hundred scientific studies linking chronic stress and the immune system. According to their analysis, the studies, which dated from 1960 to 2001 and involved 18,941 test subjects, show incontrovertible evidence that stress causes changes in the immune system. What they found is that short-term stress temporarily boosts immunity, but chronic stress weakens the immune system, making people more vulnerable to common ailments and serious diseases. In particular, the elderly and people who are already suffering from an illness are more susceptible to changes in the immune system due to chronic stress.

A recent study in the *Journal of Immunotoxicology* reported that it isn't just the stress you are feeling today that harms your ability to fight off disease. It indicates that exposure to chronic stress early in life makes you even more vulnerable to a depressed immune system throughout your lifetime.

Also, when you are feeling stressed, you may not take care of your health as well as you should. You may not feel like exercising, eating nutritious foods, or taking medicine that your doctor prescribes. Abuse of alcohol, tobacco, or other drugs may also be a sign of chronic stress. These behaviors stand in the way of your goal to get a body you love.

HOW STRESS STRETCHES YOUR MIDSECTION

Your boss is handing out pink slips. You just had a fight with your teenage daughter. You are late for an appointment. How do you react? You may try to calm your nerves with chocolate, ice cream, French fries, or potato chips (or all of the above). And there's a scientific reason why. Stress and the stress hormone cortisol are linked to increases in appetite and cravings for carbs and sweet stuff that can make you fat.

Two studies that appeared in *Physiology & Behavior* investigated the effect of stress on the foods people choose to eat and the amount of food they consume. The results were just what you might expect. The first experiment found that stress causes people to turn away from healthy low-fat foods, such as grapes, in favor of high-fat fare like M&Ms. In the second experiment, researchers looked at changes in food consumption among men and women. They found that people on a diet—especially women—were the most likely to eat more when they were stressed out.

Animal studies show us that chronic stress is a recipe for dangerous weight gain. One study out of Georgia State University showed that when hamsters faced repeated stress over a thirty-three-day period, they overate, gained weight, and in particular, gained a significant amount of abdominal fat, also known as visceral fat. This type of fat, which gives people an apple shape rather than a pear shape, is the worst kind of fat because it surrounds vital organs and is associated with a number of serious diseases, such as cardiovascular disease and diabetes.

Another study, conducted by researchers at Georgetown University Medical Center, found that chronic

> **ACTION STEP**
>
> If you are having trouble losing weight, consider stress as a factor. In addition to eating a nutritious diet and exercising, learn some stress-management skills.

stress combined with a high-fat, high-sugar diet leads to abdominal obesity in mice due to a neurotransmitter called neuropeptide Y (NPY). The brain releases NPY directly into the fatty tissue in the abdomen. The researchers exposed the mice to cold water or aggression to create a stressful environment. The chronic stress stimulated the release of NPY in the abdominal fat and increased its growth by 50 percent in just two weeks. After three months, an expanding belly wasn't the only physical change the mice experienced. They also displayed symptoms typically associated with metabolic syndrome, including high blood pressure, inflammation, high cholesterol, glucose intolerance, and more. What this study shows us is that chronic stress packs on even more abdominal fat than you might experience from a high-fat, high-sugar diet alone—and it does it faster.

Adolescents and teens are also vulnerable to weight gain from stress. A study in the *Journal of Adolescent Health* that looked at data from 1,011 adolescents and their mothers found that the more stressors in their lives, the more likely they were to have weight troubles.

Living with stress on a daily basis makes you more likely to have issues with your weight for a number of other reasons. For example, chronic stress usually goes hand-in-hand with a lack of sleep, something that pumps up cortisol production and throws your appetite-control hormones out of balance. This leads to overeating, cravings for sugary treats, and a greater tendency to store fat. The fact that chronic stress can make you feel tired and achy means you are less inclined to exercise, which can make the numbers on the scale start to rise. Stressful situations also make many of us reach for comfort foods as a way to soothe our emotions. All of these things make it harder to beat the battle of the bulge.

IS STRESS MAKING YOU INFERTILE?

As mentioned, I have been interested in medical hypnosis since medical school. When I was a psychiatric intern, I hypnotized many of my patients and staff who requested help. My favorite story from that year was when I helped a nurse get pregnant. As my reputation for using medical hypnosis grew, a very pretty nurse came to me and asked if I could help her get pregnant. That was an interesting request, I thought to myself. She told me that she and her husband had been trying to get pregnant for four years, and it wasn't happening. Every time they had sex, she would start to cry and get really upset at the thought of not being pregnant. She figured that her stress was interfering with conception.

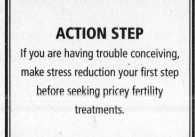

ACTION STEP

If you are having trouble conceiving, make stress reduction your first step before seeking pricey fertility treatments.

I explained to her that her fallopian tubes (the tubes between her ovaries and uterus) were wrapped in smooth muscle and that stress hormones were probably clamping shut the tubes, making it much harder for her to get pregnant. I put her in a hypnotic trance with deep relaxation suggestions focused on her lower abdomen and also made a hypnosis tape for her to listen to after she made love with her husband. Three months later she was pregnant.

It was such a joyful experience to see that healing the brain-body connection could be so helpful to this couple. The one mistake I made was telling my wife that I helped a really pretty nurse at work get pregnant. Just kidding.

It is clear that too much stress affects the way your body functions, including its ability to reproduce. Scientific evidence shows that chronic stress causes hormonal changes that disrupt reproductive function.

The same way that stress prematurely ages your body and skin, it also speeds up the aging process of your reproductive system. For women, it is harder to conceive as age advances, whether the aging is natural or stress induced. Women aren't the only ones who suffer from infertility due to stress. Researchers in India have found that emotional stress damages sperm cells. In addition to causing problems for natural conception, elevated stress levels also impact the success of fertility treatments, such as in vitro fertilization (IVF).

A 2005 study published in *Human Reproduction* investigated the effects of stressful life events on IVF treatment. The researchers asked 809 women to complete a questionnaire about stressful and negative life events during the twelve months prior to undergoing fertility treatment. Women who became pregnant following treatment reported fewer stressful events than women who didn't conceive. The researchers concluded that stress may reduce the chances of a successful outcome following IVF treatment.

There's a commentary I love in the same journal from a psychologist on the faculty at UNED University in Madrid, Spain. He is convinced that stress is to blame for many cases of infertility and suggests that stress reduction should be the first course of treatment for infertility rather than expensive and invasive treatments, such as IVF. It makes sense to me—stress reduction poses no side effects and doesn't involve any of the ethical or religious quandaries that come with some fertility treatments.

HOW STRESS PLAYS TRICKS WITH YOUR MENTAL HEALTH

Chronic stress drains your emotional well-being and is associated with anxiety, depression, and Alzheimer's disease, all of which can affect your body. Stress activates the limbic system of the brain, which is your emotional center. If you experience some form of emotional trauma—say, you are involved in a car accident or you are raped—your emotional system becomes very active, which can make you more upset and depressed. After experiencing a trauma, some people develop post-traumatic stress disorder (PTSD), which means the stress never goes away.

On July 16, 2003, thirty-three-year-old Steven was working in a bike shop in Santa Monica, California. The bicycle repair mechanic decided to visit the local farmers' market for lunch. As Steven arrived at the market, eighty-seven-year-old George Russell Weller lost control of his 1992 Buick LeSabre and plowed through the open-air market. Hearing the screams and commotion, Steven looked up and saw Weller's car heading straight for him. Steven thought he was going to be hit, but at the last moment, he managed to jump out of the way of the oncoming car.

Steven was one of the lucky ones that day—ten people were killed, and more than fifty were injured. A former Gulf War veteran, he used the medical skills he had learned in the military to help save the wounded around him. In spite of his efforts, one woman died in his arms. Traumatized, Steven headed back to work. For months after the horrific accident, he couldn't sleep and he couldn't stop shaking.

To help Steven, we used a treatment technique called eye movement desensitization and reprocessing (EMDR). This technique involves patients bringing up emotionally troubling memories while their eyes follow a trained therapist's hands moving horizontally back and forth. Following a specific protocol, the clinician helps the patient minimize negative thoughts and reactions about the traumatic event. After just one treatment, Steven started showing improvement, and after only eight hours of treatment, his shaking subsided and he felt significantly better.

The concept of EMDR sounds simple, but it is not a do-it-yourself therapy. It is important that EMDR be performed by a trained therapist. You can contact the EMDR International Association at www.emdria.org for more information and a list of certified EMDR therapists.

A 2008 study from the Rand Corporation reported that one in five soldiers returning from Iraq and Afghanistan have symptoms of post-traumatic stress disorder or major depression. As more of our soldiers begin returning from Iraq, we can expect many of them to suffer with this chronic stress disorder.

Common Signs and Symptoms of Stress

- Frequent headaches or migraines
- Gritting or grinding teeth
- Stuttering or stammering
- Tremors or trembling lips or hands
- Neck ache, back pain, or muscle spasms
- Light-headedness, faintness, dizziness
- Hearing ringing, buzzing, or popping sounds
- Frequent blushing or sweating
- Cold or sweaty hands or feet
- Dry mouth or problems swallowing
- Frequent colds, infections, or herpes sores
- Rashes, itching, hives, goose bumps
- Unexplained or frequent allergy attacks
- Heartburn
- Stomach pain or nausea
- Constipation or diarrhea
- Difficulty breathing or sighing
- Sudden panic attacks
- Chest pain or heart palpitations
- Frequent urination
- Poor sexual desire or performance
- Excessive anxiety, worry, guilt, or nervousness
- Increased anger, frustration, or hostility
- Depression, frequent or wild mood swings
- Increased or decreased appetite
- Insomnia, nightmares, or disturbing dreams
- Difficulty concentrating, racing thoughts
- Trouble learning new information
- Forgetfulness, disorganization, or confusion
- Difficulty in making decisions
- Feeling overwhelmed
- Frequent crying spells or suicidal thoughts
- Feelings of loneliness and worthlessness
- Little interest in appearance or punctuality
- Nervous habits, fidgeting, or feet tapping
- Increased irritability or edginess
- Overreaction to petty annoyances
- Increased number of minor accidents
- Obsessive or compulsive behavior
- Reduced work efficiency or productivity
- Lies or excuses to cover up poor work
- Rapid or mumbled speech
- Excessive defensiveness or suspiciousness
- Problems in communication or sharing
- Social withdrawal or isolation
- Constant fatigue or weakness
- Frequent use of over-the-counter drugs
- Weight gain or loss without diet
- Increased smoking
- Increased alcohol or drug use
- Excessive gambling or impulse buying

Source: The American Institute of Stress

WHO'S VULNERABLE TO STRESS?

Unfortunately, everyone is vulnerable to the effects of chronic stress. It can attack you at any stage of your life. When chronic stress hits you or someone in your circle, everybody suffers. You've heard of the trickle-down economic theory; there's also a trickle-down stress theory. When the boss is stressed out, everybody at work is stressed out. When your spouse is stressed out, everybody in the family is stressed out.

It happened in my own family when I was growing up. My father owned a chain of grocery stores with a colleague. When I was fourteen years old, he decided to sell the stores to a much larger grocery group, Arden-Mayfair. Going to work for someone else was a big mistake for my dad. He is a very independent person. He hated it and was under a lot of stress. He was miserable and not a lot of fun to be around. Stress often runs downhill.

CALMING THE STRESS IN YOUR LIFE
SO YOU CAN HAVE A BETTER BODY

In my practice, I deal with so many patients who suffer severe stress. Most of the time, it is because no one has ever taught them stress-management skills. When I show them that there are better ways to deal with stress, they do a much better job at it. Here are sixteen different ways to help you calm stress so you can have better skin, better immunity, and a trimmer figure. Pick four or five ways that you like the best.

1. Meditate or pray on a regular basis. Decades of research have shown that meditation and prayer calm stress and enhance brain function. At the Amen Clinics, we performed a SPECT study on a Kundalini Yoga form of meditation called Kirtan Kriya in which we scanned eleven people on one day when they didn't meditate and then the next day during a meditation session. For the meditation, the participants recited the following simple sounds known as the five primal sounds: "sa," "ta," "na," "ma," with "aa," the end of each sound, considered to be the fifth sound. The meditation involved touching the thumb of each hand to the index finger while chanting "sa," the middle finger while chanting "ta," the ring finger while chanting "na," and the pinkie finger while chanting "ma." The sounds and fingering were repeated for two minutes out loud, two minutes whispering, four minutes silently, two minutes whispering, and two minutes out loud.

Figure 11.1

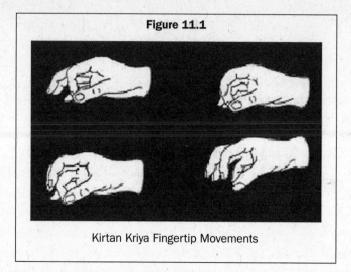

Kirtan Kriya Fingertip Movements

The brain imaging scans taken after the meditation showed marked decreases in activity in the left parietal lobes, which showed a decreasing awareness of time and space. They also showed significant increases in activity in the prefrontal cortex, which showed that meditation helped to tune people in, not out. We also observed increased activity in the right temporal lobe, an area that has been associated with spirituality.

My friend Andy Newberg at the University of Pennsylvania also used brain SPECT imaging to study the neurobiology of meditation, in part because it is a spiritual state easily duplicated in the laboratory. They scanned nine Buddhist monks before and during prolonged meditation. The scan revealed distinctive changes in brain activity as the mind went into a meditative state. Specifically, activity decreased in the parts of the brain involved in generating a sense of three-dimensional orientation in space. Losing one's sense of physical place could account for the spiritual feeling of transcendence, being beyond space and time. They also found increased activity in the prefrontal cortex, associated with attention span and thoughtfulness. Meditation seemed to tune people in, not out. Another functional brain imaging study of transcendental meditation (TM) showed calming in the anterior cingulate and basal ganglia, diminishing anxiety and worries and fostering relaxation.

The benefits of meditation go far beyond stress relief. Studies have shown that it also improves attention and planning, reduces depression and anxiety, decreases sleepiness, and protects the brain from cognitive decline associated with normal aging. In a study from researchers at UCLA, the hippocampus and frontal cortex were found to be significantly larger in people who meditate regularly. Meditation has also been found to aid in weight loss, reduce muscle tension, and tighten the skin.

Many people think it takes years of practice to learn how to meditate. It doesn't. A fascinating Chinese study from my friend neuroscientist Dr. Yiyuan Tang showed that people who received just twenty minutes of daily meditation training for five days showed a significant decrease in stress-related cortisol. You don't need to devote big chunks of time to the practice of meditation, either. In my clinical practice, I often recommend meditation as an integral part of a treatment plan. Many of my patients have reported back that they feel calmer and less stressed after just a few minutes of daily meditation.

If the whole concept of meditation seems a little too New Age for you, take note that you can do it just about anywhere anytime. You don't have to sit cross-legged on the floor or burn incense or any of those things you might associate with meditation. If you are at work, you can simply close the door to your office, sit in your chair, close your eyes, and relax for a few moments. At home, you can sit on the edge of your bed after you wake up and spend a couple of minutes calming your mind. Try the following Relaxation Response for a simple introduction to meditation.

The Relaxation Response

One of the simplest ways to meditate and reduce stress is a technique called the Relaxation Response, developed by Herbert Benson, M.D., at Harvard Medical School. I encourage you to set aside ten to twenty minutes today to try it. The following is the technique outlined in Dr. Benson's book *The Relaxation Response*.

Directions

Sit quietly in a comfortable position.

Close your eyes.

Deeply relax all your muscles, beginning at your feet and progressing up to your face. Keep them relaxed.

Breathe through your nose. Become aware of your breathing. As you breathe out, say the word "one" (or some other relaxing word you choose) silently to yourself. For example, breathe in . . . out, "one," in . . . out, "one," etc.

Continue for ten to twenty minutes. You may open your eyes to check the time, but do not use an alarm. When you finish, sit quietly for several minutes, at first with your eyes closed and later with your eyes opened. Do not stand up for a few minutes.

Do not worry about whether you are successful in achieving a deep level of relaxation. Maintain a passive attitude and permit relaxation to occur at its own pace. When distracting thoughts occur, try to ignore them by not dwelling upon them and return to repeating "one." With practice, the response should come with little effort. Practice the technique once or twice daily, but not within two hours after any meal, since the digestive processes seem to interfere with the elicitation of the Relaxation Response.

Prayer, too, offers many of the same health and stress-relief benefits as meditation. Physicians Larry Dossey (*Healing Words*), Dale Matthews (*The Faith Factor*), and others have written books outlining the scientific evidence of the medical benefits of prayer and other meditative states. Some of these benefits include reduced feelings of stress, lower cholesterol levels, improved sleep, reduced anxiety and depression, fewer headaches, more relaxed muscles, and longer life spans. People who pray or read the Bible every day are 40 percent less likely to suffer from hypertension than others.

A 1998 Duke University study of 577 men and women hospitalized for physical illness showed that the more patients used positive spiritual coping strategies (seeking spiritual support from friends and religious leaders, having faith in God, praying), the lower the level of their depressive symptoms and the higher their quality of life. A 1996 survey of 269 family physicians found that 99 percent believed prayer, meditation, or other spiritual and religious practice can be helpful in medical treatment; more than half said they currently incorporate relaxation or meditation techniques into treatment of patients.

2. Take a yoga class. Yoga is an ancient and venerated form of stress relief. Many yoga classes promote mental calmness, self-awareness, and a focus on being in the present moment—all of which bring about a sense of relaxation and well-being. Yoga has solid scientific evidence that it can be helpful for reducing high blood pressure, altitude sickness, anxiety, arthritis, asthma, carpal tunnel syndrome, depression, epilepsy, heart disease, lung diseases, substance abuse, and boosting your quality of life. Yoga has become so popular that you can find classes geared to all ages and all ability levels.

3. Learn to delegate. People often have jam-packed schedules that leave little or no breathing room. Trying to race from one activity to the next while meeting work, school, and family obligations can become overwhelming. In our modern society, it seems like being busy is a sort of badge of honor. Ask anyone what they have planned for the day, and it is likely they'll respond by telling you how incredibly busy they are. "I'm finishing a project for work, hosting a dinner party, making the kids' costumes for the school play, volunteering at church, and going to my book group." Phew! It can make you stressed out just thinking about all that.

News flash! You don't have to accept every invitation, take on every project, or volunteer for every activity that comes your way. Two of the greatest life skills you can learn are the art of delegation and the ability to say no. Too often, just to please others, we agree to do things without first asking ourselves if the request fits into our own lives. Many people say yes without first processing the request through their prefrontal cortex. When someone asks you to do something, a good first response would be "Let me think about it." Then you can take the time to process the request to see if it fits with your schedule, desires, and goals. When you have too much on your plate, delegate.

4. Practice gratitude. If you want your brain to work better, be grateful for the good things in your life. Psychologist Noelle Nelson and I did a study on gratitude and appreciation. She was working on a book called *The Power of Appreciation* and had her brain scanned twice. The first time she was scanned after thirty minutes of meditating on all the things she was thankful for in her life. After the "appreciation meditation," her brain looked very healthy.

Then she was scanned several days later after focusing on the major fears in her life. One of her fears was about what would happen if her dog got sick and she couldn't work. She had a string of frightening thoughts: "If my dog got sick, I couldn't go to work because I would have to stay home to care for him. . . . If I didn't go to work, however, I would lose my job. . . . If I lost my job, I wouldn't have enough money to take my dog to the vet and he would likely die. . . . If the dog died, I would be so depressed I still wouldn't be able to go back to work. . . . Then I would lose my home, and be homeless."

I scanned her brain after she mulled on these thoughts. Her frightened brain looked very different from her healthy gratitude brain and showed seriously decreased activity in two parts of her brain. Her cerebellum had completely shut down. The cerebellum, also called the little brain, is involved in physical coordination, such as walking or playing sports. New research also suggests that the cerebellum is involved in processing speed, like clock speed on a computer and thought coordination or how quickly we can integrate new information. When the cerebellum is low in activity, people tend to be clumsier and less likely to think their ways out of problems. They think and process information more slowly and get confused more easily.

The other area of her brain that was affected was the temporal lobes, especially the one on the left. The temporal lobes are involved with mood, memory, and temper control. Problems in this part of the brain are associated with some forms of depression, but also dark thoughts, violence, and memory problems. In Noelle's scans, when she practiced gratitude, her temporal lobes looked healthy. When she frightened herself with negative thinking, her temporal lobes became much less active. Negative thought patterns change the brain in a negative way. Practicing gratitude literally helps you have a brain to be grateful for.

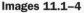

Images 11.1–4

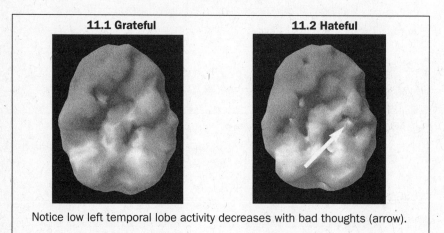

Notice low left temporal lobe activity decreases with bad thoughts (arrow).

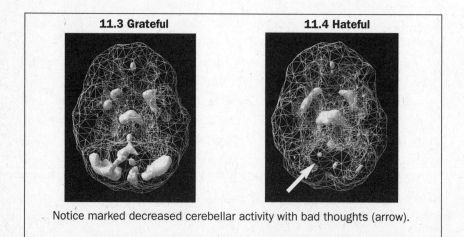

Notice marked decreased cerebellar activity with bad thoughts (arrow).

Focusing on the good things in your life can make you happier regardless of your circumstances, according to decades of research from Dr. Martin Seligman, the renowned director of the University of Pennsylvania Positive Psychology Center. Seligman promotes the fascinating concept of positive psychology, which is based on the theory that happiness isn't the result of good genes, rather that it can be cultivated. In his book *Authentic Happiness,* he writes that showing gratitude on a daily basis is one of the keys to increasing your sense of joy, happiness, and life satisfaction.

Here is a quick gratitude exercise you can try. Write down five things you are grateful for every day. Use the form provided, make copies of it, or just use a notepad to write down the things you are grateful for. The act of writing helps to solidify them in your brain. In my experience, when depressed patients did this exercise every day, they actually needed less antidepressant medication. Other researchers have also found that people who express gratitude on a regular basis are healthier, more optimistic, make more progress toward their goals, have a greater sense of well-being, and are more helpful to others. Doctors who regularly practice gratitude are actually better at making the correct diagnoses on their patients.

Five Things I'm Grateful for Today

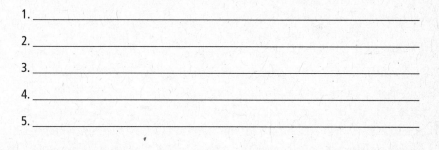

1. _____

2. _____

3. _____

4. _____

5. _____

5. Get enough sleep. Getting adequate sleep enhances your ability to fight stress. Read Chapter 10 to review the many ways sleep helps the brain.

6. Get moving. Physical activity is a big stress reliever. Read Chapter 5 to learn more about why exercise is the single most important thing you can do for your brain.

7. Learn to warm your hands using only your mind. See Chapter 8, "The Heart Solution," for more details.

8. Practice diaphragmatic breathing. The simple act of breathing delivers oxygen to your lungs, where blood picks it up and takes it to every cell in your body. Breathing also eliminates waste products, such as carbon dioxide, from the body. When there's too much carbon dioxide in your system, it can cause stressful feelings of disorientation and panic. Brain cells are particularly sensitive to oxygen, as they start to die within four minutes when they are deprived of oxygen. Even the slightest changes in oxygen content can alter the way you feel.

Diaphragmatic breathing, in which you direct and control your breathing, has several immediate benefits. It calms the basal ganglia, the area of the brain that controls anxiety, helps your brain run more efficiently, relaxes your muscles, warms your hands, and regulates your heartbeat.

Here's how you do it. As you inhale, let your belly expand. This pulls the lungs downward, which increases the amount of air (and oxygen) available to your lungs, body, and brain. When you exhale, pull in your belly to push the air out of your lungs. This allows you to expel more air, which in turn encourages you to inhale more deeply. Keep breathing in this fashion, and stressful feelings may diminish.

Diaphragmatic Breathing Exercise

Try this simple three-step exercise to make sure you are breathing deeply enough.

Lie on your back and place a small book on your belly.

When you inhale, make the book go up.

When you exhale, make the book go down.

Here's another breathing tip that can soothe stress. Whenever you feel stressed out, take a deep breath, hold it for four to five seconds, then slowly blow it out (take about six to eight seconds to exhale completely). Take another deep breath (as deep as you can), hold it for four to five seconds, and blow it out slowly again. Do this about ten times and odds are that you will start to feel very relaxed.

9. Listen to soothing music. Music has healing powers that can bring peace to a stressful mind. Of course, it depends on the type of music you listen to. Listening to music that has a calming effect, such as classical music or ambient sounds, has been shown to reduce stress and calm anxiety. Other types of music may be stress-inducing and destructive. I believe it is no coincidence that the majority of teens who end up being sent to residential treatment facilities or group homes listen to more heavy-metal music than other teens. Music that is filled with lyrics of hate and despair may encourage those same mind states in developing teens. What your children listen to can hurt them or help them. Teach them to love classical music when they are young.

ACTION STEP

I use music in my own life to help calm stress. Here's a list of some of my favorite recordings that I personally find healing. You may want to try listening to them too.

- Don Campbell, *Mozart as Healer: Classial Healing for the New Millennium, Essence: The Ambient Music of Don Campbell,* and *Healing Powers of Tone and Chant*
- Compiled by Joan Z. Borysenko and Don Campbell, *Inner Peace for Busy People: Music to Relax and Renew*
- Michael Hoppé, *Solace*
- David Lanz, *Beloved*
- Dean Evenson, *Arctic Refuge: Gathering of Tribes* (with various artists), *Ascension to Tibet, Healing Dreams* (with Scott Huckabay), *Healing Sanctuary, Music for the Healing Arts, Native Healing, Peace Through Music* (with various artists)

---

10. Surround yourself with the sweet smell of lavender. Your deep limbic system is the part of your brain that directly processes your sense of smell. It is also the emotional center of your brain, which means that smells can have a big impact on your mood. The scent of lavender has been used since ancient times for its calming, stress-relieving properties. This popular aroma has been the subject of countless research studies, which show that it reduces cortisol levels and promotes relaxation and stress reduction.

One remarkable study that appeared in the journal *Early Human Development* examined two groups of mothers giving their babies a bath. The first group used lavender bath oil; the second didn't. The first group of moms appeared more relaxed, smiled more, and touched their babies more often during the bath than the second group of moms. Their babies cried less and spent more time in deep sleep following the bath. The first group of moms and their infants also had significantly lower cortisol levels than the second group, which didn't use lavender bath oil.

You can find this natural stress reliever in the form of oils, candles, sprays, lotions, sachets, and potpourri. Many other scents, such as geranium, rose, cardamom, sandalwood, and chamomile, are considered to have a calming effect that reduces stress.

11. Rehearse or practice situations that cause stress. Nobody is completely immune to stress. Everybody gets stressed out about something from time to time. For many people, things like speaking in public, going on a job interview, or going to an event where you don't know anybody can make your palms sweat and your heart race. In these cases, you can benefit from a little practice. The more you do something, the less stress inducing it becomes.

12. Live in the present. The notion of living in the present is a simple concept, but it is one of the hardest to implement. Many of us dwell on the past, holding grudges about things that happened years or even decades ago, stewing over a fight with a colleague, or feeling bad about things that happened to us in high school. You could be lying on a warm, sunny beach while on vacation, but inside your head, you are fuming about a comment your significant other made the week before. Equally common are those of us who fret about the future, worrying about bad things that *might* happen. In Eckhart Tolle's extraordinary book *The Power of Now,* he encourages readers to shed the pains of the past, stop fearing the future, and live in the present moment. He believes that the present is all we really have, that we can't change the past, and that it is what we're doing right now that shapes our future.

13. Practice self-hypnosis. Like meditation and prayer, self-hypnosis is a powerful tool to balance brain function and decrease stress. When I'm feeling overly stressed, I use the same self-hypnosis exercise I wrote about in Chap-

---

ACTION STEP

In principle, I agree that it is a good idea to live in the present. Worrying about the past and fretting about the future only add to your stress. However, through SPECT imaging, I have found that when people think about happy memories from the past, it enhances brain function. Instead of erasing your past completely, make sure the version of it that runs through your head has a positive spin.

ter 10, "The Sleep Solution." However, instead of drifting off to sleep at the end of it, I stay in my "special place" for about ten or fifteen minutes, then come back to full consciousness. It usually makes me feel very refreshed and relaxed. This is one of my favorite stress busters.

14. Avoid substances that harm your brain. Consuming caffeine, eating sugary snacks, drinking alcohol, and smoking are some of the most common—and unfortunately, some of the worst—ways to deal with stress. Duke University researcher James Lane, Ph.D., has been studying the effects of caffeine on stress for more than a decade. According to his findings, caffeine disrupts a natural process that keeps stress under control. When ingested, caffeine prevents the release of adenosine, a chemical that regulates bodily functions. Normally, when we get stressed, adenosine levels rise to reduce the body's response to stress.

With caffeine, however, adenosine is suppressed so your body's response to the stress is heightened. Lane's body of research shows that consuming caffeine increases stress hormone levels when people are faced with stressful events or tasks. Basically, this means that drinking a large caffe latte before a test or a big meeting will only amplify any feelings of stress you might have experienced normally.

People often reach for a glass of wine or alcohol to calm the effects of stress. Research, however, shows that in many people, drinking actually induces stress and elevates stress hormone levels. Alcohol also lowers overall blood flow and activity in the brain, which diminishes your ability to cope with stress.

The same goes for smoking. When smokers get stressed, they tend to light up in search of relief. But inside the body, it is another story. Nicotine causes your blood pressure to rise and your heart rate to increase, which are signs of increased stress. And like alcohol, smoking causes blood vessels to constrict, which reduces the amount of oxygen going to the brain and subsequently lowers brain function.

Numerous studies have shown that when unrelenting stress hits, it causes many of us to look for solace in a big bowl of Ben & Jerry's Chunky Monkey, a fistful of M&Ms, or a bag of Oreo cookies. Unfortunately, high-fat foods can also trigger stressful reactions. Researchers at the University of

> **ACTION STEP**
>
> When you feel stressed, skip the alcohol, cigarettes, and candy. They lower brain function and ultimately increase stress.

Calgary examined stress reactions in two groups of students. The first group ate a high-fat breakfast while the second group noshed on a low-fat meal. Two hours later, the test subjects went through a series of stressful tasks. In each of the tasks, the group that gorged on the high-fat meal showed higher stress reactions than the second group.

15. Laugh more. There is a growing body of scientific literature suggesting that laughter counteracts stress and is good for the immune system. It is no joke! One study of cancer patients found that laughter reduced stress and improved cell activity associated with increased resistance to the disease.

According to the University of California, Irvine's Professor Lee Berk, "If we took what we know about the medical benefits of laughter and bottled it up, it would require FDA approval." Laughter lowers the flow of dangerous stress hormones that suppress the immune system, raise blood pressure, and increase the number of platelets, which cause clots and potentially fatal coronary artery blockages. Laughter also eases digestion and soothes stomachaches, a common symptom of chronic stress. Plus, a good rollicking guffaw increases the release of endorphins, which makes you feel better and more relaxed. Laughter truly may be the best medicine when it comes to stress relief.

The average child laughs hundreds of times a day. The average adult laughs only a dozen times a day. Inject more humor into your everyday life. Watch comedies (this could be a helpful form of TV), go to comedy clubs, go to humorous children's plays, read joke books (my favorite is *The Far Side* by Gary Larson, which is pretty sick, but I am a psychiatrist after all), and swap jokes with your friends and coworkers.

I can't stress enough (pun intended) how important it is to learn to laugh at yourself too. When you drop the milk jug and it goes splashing across the kitchen floor, when you call a business associate by the wrong name, or when you stumble over your words while teaching a class, be the first to chuckle at yourself. When you stop taking yourself so seriously, your stress levels will subside.

16. Seek help for chronic stress. If you are chronically stressed, it may be a good idea to see a psychotherapist to talk about your problems and learn better stress-management skills. Many people have a negative attitude about seeing a psychotherapist, but I think of them as life consultants. When a great business has troubles, it is likely to deal with the problems head-on and find the best consultants to help. We should behave the same way in our personal lives. In dealing with stress, I often refer people to biofeedback therapists, hypnotherapists, and people who do a form of psychotherapy called eye movement desensitization and reprocessing, or EMDR, which helps them deal with anxiety, past traumas, and performance enhancement.

SUPPLEMENTS THAT CALM STRESS

Some supplements may be helpful in soothing stress, including B vitamins, L-theanine, GABA, St. John's wort, 5-HTP, magnesium, and valerian. Take these under the supervision of your health-care professional. Just because something is natural does not mean it is completely innocuous. See Appendix C, "The Supplement Solution," for more information. You can also get more detailed information online at www.amenclinics.com/cybcyb.

The Stress Solution

Stress Inducers	Stress Relievers
Any brain problems	Brain-healthy lifestyle
Poor sleep	Adequate sleep, at least seven hours
Alcohol/drug abuse	Freedom from alcohol or drugs
Caffeine	Limited caffeine
Depression	Treatment for depression
Anxiety	Meditation for relaxation
Lack of exercise	Physical activity, including yoga
Smoking	Quitting smoking
	Diaphragmatic breathing
	Soothing music
	Calming scents like lavender
	Self-hypnosis
	Laughter
	Stress-reduction plan
	B vitamins, L-theanine, GABA, St. John's wort, 5-HTP, magnesium, and valerian

12

THE MEMORY SOLUTION

REMEMBER WHAT YOU NEED

TO DO EVERY DAY

One need not be a chamber to be haunted,
One need not be a house;
The brain has corridors surpassing
Material place.
—EMILY DICKINSON, "GHOSTS"

John was sixty-five years old and had type 2 diabetes. The directions from his doctor were clear: Exercise, eat a healthy diet, and take your medicine. But he kept forgetting. He would regularly go out for doughnuts and coffee laden with cream and sugar. And he often forgot to take his medicine unless his wife handed it to him. Frustrated, his wife would chastise him, and he would promise to do better. The diabetes was stealing healthy blood flow to his brain, especially to his prefrontal cortex (impulse control and short-term memory) and the inside of his temporal lobes (where information gets into long-term memory). Even though John knew what to do, he often forgot and reverted back to his habitual behavior. And it cost him dearly. Over time, he lost his eyesight and had both legs amputated. His skin looked much older than he was, and he was significantly overweight.

A healthy body requires a good memory. You need to remember what to do every day to keep yourself healthy and NOT forget. This is different from willpower, where urges and cravings overtake your prefrontal cortex. Memory is being able to hold a plan in your mind so that you can consistently pursue your goals and make them happen. Memory requires focus to get the information into your brain and then, once inside, the information needs to get into the brain's long-term storage bins. Some people have a deterioration of memory as they age; some never had a very good memory. Either way, you can improve your memory if you improve the overall health of your brain and your body.

Considering Alzheimer's disease is expected to triple in the next twenty-five years, it is critical for all of us to think about and optimize our memory centers. I have seen this disorder ravage families, making everyone feel stressed and look older than they are. In this chapter, I will help you understand the different types of memory, specific memory problems, what to do about them, and how to boost your overall memory.

TYPES OF MEMORY

Memory is a recording of one's experiences stored in the brain—be it an interesting conversation, a piece of information, a "memorable scene," or a notable event. There are three types of memories differentiated by the time lapse between the experience and the recall of that experience. Each type of memory activates different brain areas when one attempts to recall it.

Working memory resides in the frontal lobe and lasts less than a minute. This form of memory is commonly referred to as one's attention span and lasts up to one minute before being erased. Trying to memorize a dance step someone just showed you is an example of working memory.

Short-term memory resides on the inside of the temporal lobes in an area called the hippocampus and lasts a few minutes to a few weeks before being erased. When you try to recall the dance step you learned in last week's dance class, these brain areas are activated. Not all of your moment-to-moment experiences activate short-term memory. Only those experiences that are novel, interesting, or that you intended to remember will sufficiently stimulate nerve cells in this area of the brain to record them.

Long-term memory can last a lifetime. Scientists are not yet certain which brain areas are directly involved in long-term memory, but likely they are scattered across many areas of the brain. When you try to recall the name of your first dance teacher when you were a child, you are accessing your long-term memory.

MEMORY BOOT CAMP

In order to have the best memory possible, you need to keep your brain and body healthy, work your memory on a regular basis, and treat any memory problems early.

Exciting research suggests that new learning and doing the same old thing in a different way can help your brain stay healthy and young. Boring is not only, well, boring, it is also potentially harmful to the long-term well-being of your brain. In several new scientific studies, people who do not engage in regular learning activities throughout their lives have a higher incidence of Alzheimer's disease.

The brain is like a muscle. The more you use it, the more you can continue to use it. New learning makes new connections in the brain, making you sharper and more efficient. No learning actually causes the brain to disconnect itself. Unlike a muscle, however, the brain gets easily bored and requires new and different challenges to stay healthy. Once the brain really learns something, such as how to navigate the streets of your hometown, it uses less and less energy to accomplish the task. To keep active, the brain needs a constant stream of new challenges. New adventures, new sites, and new skills encourage brain health. Here are three fantastic ways to keep your brain young.

1. Foreign immersion Going on a cooking vacation to Italy, unless you have done it several times before, is a perfect way to keep your brain young. Travel to new lands, especially ones filled with fascinating history and sites, keeps the brain learning and working at optimal efficiency. In addition, going to different cultures often involves a new language, which really pushes the linguistic and memory centers of the brain. If you also add another skill, such as cooking—as long as you do not drink too much wine—there is an even greater benefit. Likewise, consider traveling to a new city nearby, watching a foreign film, going to an international restaurant, or listening to new music; these also expose the brain to new experiences. Learning enhances cells in the hippocampus, a part of the emotional and memory center of the brain.

2. New paths A simpler, cheaper exercise closer to home is to start taking new and different ways to and from work each day. Going the same old way each time puts the brain on automatic pilot, which does nothing positive for it. Look for ways to vary your commute or drive. For example, from time to time, take some side streets rather than the highway to see other neighborhoods. New navigation routes enhance the brain's parietal lobes, which are involved in direction sense. Driving the scenic route home may help to decrease your stress level, which will have a global positive effect on the brain.

3. Move it Exploring new exercises is perhaps one of the most powerful ways to keep the brain young. One of my favorite exercises for the brain is dancing.

Exercise by itself boosts blood flow to the brain and helps keep it young. When you add in a coordination exercise to music, such as learning a new dance step, it boosts the cerebellum and temporal lobes, which are two of the major processing and learning centers in the brain. It gives the brain an extra boost. But go light on the wine spritzers—drinking ruins the positive effect.

DON'T IGNORE MEMORY PROBLEMS

Memory problems are typically considered an issue for the elderly. In my experience as both a child and adult psychiatrist, however, I have seen memory problems across the life span. They commonly appear in children with learning disorders, in teens and adults who smoke marijuana, in adults with depression and substance-abuse problems, and in the cognitive decline that occurs with aging and many forms of dementia. In assessing memory problems, it is important to consider

- Medical causes, such as low thyroid or B_{12} deficiencies
- Medications that interfere with memory, such as antianxiety medicines like Xanax or painkillers like OxyContin
- Brain illnesses, such as depression or ADD
- Early stages of Alzheimer's disease
- Excessive stress—stress hormones have been found to kill cells in the hippocampus
- Lack of sleep or sleep apnea
- Postanesthesia—some people react negatively to general anesthesia and complain of subsequent memory problems
- Environmental toxins, such as finishing furniture or painting your car in a closed garage
- Drug and alcohol abuse

UNDERSTANDING AND TREATING MEMORY LOSS

The predominant cause of memory loss is a family of diseases called Alzheimer's disease and related disorders (ADRD), which includes but is not limited to Alzheimer's disease, vascular dementia, Parkinson's disease, and frontal lobe dementia. In addition to ADRD, many other conditions cause memory loss. For simplicity, the following tables list the major causes of memory loss, the appropriate treatment, and the possible results of treatment.

TABLE 12.1 ALZHEIMER'S DISEASE AND RELATED DISORDERS		
Disease	**Treatment**	**Result of Treatment**
Alzheimer's disease, thought to be caused by beta-amyloid plaque formation and excessive tau proteins in brain cells, as well as inflammation	Medications or supplements to boost the neurotransmitter acetylcholine, to boost blood flow to the brain, or to modulate the neurotransmitter glutamate. Exercise and mental exercise can also help.	Stabilization and sometimes improvement
Frontal lobe dementia, thought to be caused by excessive tau proteins	No established treatment	Usually not helpful
Parkinson's disease (PD), thought to be caused by cell death in the areas of the brain that produce the neurotransmitter dopamine	Medications or supplements to enhance the neurotransmitter dopamine in the brain. Certain brain surgeries have been found to help the tremor associated with PD.	Stabilization and often improvement
Vascular disease caused by either small or large strokes or some form of insufficient blood flow to the brain	Treat illnesses and risk factors, such as diabetes, hypertension, and heart disease.	Stabilization and often improvement

TABLE 12.2 OTHER CAUSES OF MEMORY LOSS AND DEMENTIA		
Disease	**Treatment**	**Result of Treatment**
ADD	Exercise, higher-protein, lower-carbohydrate diet, and stimulant supplements or medications	Improvement
Alcohol dependence	Alcohol cessation	Improvement if caught early enough
Anxiety	Hypnosis, biofeedback, relaxation therapies such as meditation, correcting negative thought patterns, and antianxiety supplements or medications	Improvement
Brain infections	Intravenous antibiotics	Improvement if caught early enough
Cancer	Diagnose and treat	Frequent improvement
Cancer chemotherapy	Cognitive rehabilitation, hyperbaric oxygen treatment, supplements and medication	Frequent improvement

Disease	Treatment	Result of Treatment
Depression	Correcting negative thought patterns, exercise, fish oil, and antianxiety supplements or medications	Improvement if caught early enough
Diabetes	Diet, exercise, supplements, and medications	Improvement if caught early enough
Drug abuse	Drug cessation	Improvement if caught early enough
Fatigue	Diagnose cause and treat	Frequent improvement
Head injury	Cognitive rehabilitation, hyperbaric oxygen treatment, supplements, and medication	Frequent improvement
Hydrocephalus	Shunt	Frequent improvement
Medications	Adjust medication	Improvement if caught early enough
Metabolic problems	Diagnose etiology and treat	Improvement if caught early enough
Thyroid disease	Thyroid hormone	Improvement if caught early enough
Vitamin B_{12} deficiency	Vitamin B_{12} replacement	Improvement if caught early enough
Vitamin D deficiency	Vitamin D replacement	Improvement if caught early enough

MEDICAL TESTS TO CONSIDER
FOR EVALUATING MEMORY PROBLEMS

When a person is suffering from memory problems, the following tests may be useful in evaluating the problem:

- Urinalysis
- Liver function tests
- Homocysteine level
- 25-hydroxy vitamin D level
- Thyroid function tests
- HIV
- Apolipoprotein E genotype
- For males, a testosterone level
- If sleep problems are present, a sleep study to rule out sleep apnea
- Complete blood count
- Folic acid test
- Vitamin B_{12} level
- Blood glucose level
- Syphilis screening
- Erythrocyte sedimentation
- Fasting lipid panel
- For females after menopause, an estradiol level
- Brain SPECT imaging

After looking at 55,000 brain scans, there is no doubt in my mind that the lights in the attic dim with age unless we actively work to keep the brain healthy. In looking at our database of scans spanning the life span from three to a hundred years old, it is clear that the normal brain has fewer and fewer resources with age. There is less blood flow that brings oxygen and glucose to nourish neurons and that takes away waste products, and there are fewer antioxidants for protection against free-radical formation and lower hormone levels to keep it young. This is the fate of the typical brain. However, your brain does not have to succumb to age at the same rate as others'. There are simple things you can do today to prevent disease and keep your brain healthy for as long as possible.

In order to stay healthy, the brain and body has to repair itself on a constant basis. It is not like a car that you can take into a garage when it needs a tune-up or when it has to have a part replaced. Your brain and body have mechanisms to repair damage as a result of the normal wear and tear of life. The hardware of the brain—neurons, dendrites, axons, synapses, and others—must be cared for. The brain has to maintain its 100 billion neurons to consistently function well. If the number of neurons in any cortical circuit decreases by more than a third—as is the case in Alzheimer's disease—the circuit can no longer compensate for the loss, and symptoms appear.

Diseases of aging in the brain typically cause the following problems:

- Reduce the number of brain cells, such as in Alzheimer's disease.
- Reduce the number of connections between cells, which happens when there is depression or a lack of mental or physical exercise.
- Impair the generation of electrical activity, which can happen if one consumes three or more alcoholic drinks at a time.
- Disrupt cell machinery to produce energy, which happens in Parkinson's disease, diabetes, or chemotherapy and radiation therapy for cancer.
- Damage axons to slow the speed of signals in the brain, such as in hypertension, heart disease, strokes, and head trauma.

KNOW AND REDUCE YOUR RISK FOR THE
DISEASES OF BRAIN AGING

The following list contains the risk factors for diseases of brain aging. The numbers in parentheses indicate how significant the risk factor is. For example, 2.0

means there is twice the risk of having a problem; 4.0 means the risk is quadrupled. Check the ones that apply to you.

1. _____ (3.5) one family member with Alzheimer's disease or other cause of dementia
2. _____ (7.5) more than one family member with Alzheimer's disease or other dementia
3. _____ (2.0) a single head injury with loss of consciousness for more than a few minutes
4. _____ (2.0) several head injuries without loss of consciousness
5. _____ (4.4) alcohol dependence or drug dependence in past or present
6. _____ (2.0) major depression diagnosed by a physician in past or present
7. _____ (10) stroke
8. _____ (2.5) heart (coronary artery) disease or heart attack (myocardial infarction or MI)
9. _____ (2.1) high cholesterol (hyperlipidemia)
10. _____ (2.3) high blood pressure (hypertension)
11. _____ (3.4) diabetes
12. _____ (3.0) history of cancer or cancer treatment
13. _____ (1.5) seizures in past or present
14. _____ (2.0) limited exercise (less than twice a week or less than thirty minutes per session)
15. _____ (2.0) less than a high school education
16. _____ (2.0) jobs that do not require periodically learning new information
17. _____ (2.3) smoking cigarettes for ten years or longer
18. _____ (2.5) have one apolipoprotein E4 gene (if known)
19. _____ (5.0) have two apolipoprotein E4 genes (if known)
20. _____ (38) over eighty-five years old
    _____ **Total Score** (Add up the scores in parentheses for all items checked.)

Interpretation:

If the score is 0, 1, or 2, then you have low risk factors for developing the brain diseases of aging.

If the score is 3, 4, 5, or 6, then you have a moderate risk for developing the diseases of aging and prevention should be taken seriously.

If the score is greater than 6, then prevention strategies should be part of your everyday life.

GENETIC RISK FACTORS

A family history that includes memory problems is a cause for concern and preventive action. This is especially true for people who have a first-degree relative (mother, father, brother, or sister) with Alzheimer's disease, stroke, or Parkinson's disease. Several genes are associated with Alzheimer's disease and other causes of memory problems, especially the E4 version of the apolipoprotein E (apoE) gene on chromosome 19. Everyone has two apoE genes, and if one of them—or worse, two of them—is apoE4, that person's chances of getting memory problems is quite high. Of course, apoE genes alone are not dangerous; we need them to function, but the E4 type increases our risk for age-related problems. There are three versions of the apoE gene: E2, E3, and E4, and it is the last one that is the culprit. As with all genes, we inherit one copy from each parent, and any one person could have the following combination:

E2/E2, E2/E3, E2/E4
E3/E3, E3/E4 or
E/4, E/4.

If a person has two E4 genes, it means he received one from each parent. For about 15 percent of the general population, at least one of their two apoE genes is the E4 gene. People who have no apoE4 gene at all have only a 5 to 10 percent chance of developing Alzheimer's disease after age sixty-five, whereas people with one apoE4 gene have about a 25 percent chance. Given the increase in risk of problems with this gene, it would be wise to know your apoE genotype.

ALCOHOL AND DRUG ABUSE

Alcohol is a double-edged sword. It can increase the risk for stroke, heart disease, and possibly Alzheimer's disease. Five percent of all strokes in the United

States are alcohol related. Four or more drinks a day increase risks for stroke and heart disease, while one drink every few days actually reduces these risks (presumably by increasing HDL cholesterol, which clears other types of cholesterol that cause hardening of the arteries).

Clearly, drug abuse damages the brain. There are more than a hundred brain imaging studies that demonstrate that drug abuse—including cocaine, methamphetamines, marijuana, heroin, and other opiates—diminishes brain function and damages neurons. One of the first things I learned from doing brain imaging on a wide variety of psychiatric patients was that drug abuse damages the function seen on SPECT scans. I have made several posters on the effects of drugs on brain function that hang in more than fifty thousand schools, prisons, and drug-abuse treatment centers nationwide. Recently, it was found that cocaine inhibits a part of cells involved in energy production, a finding that has also been linked to Parkinson's disease.

Reducing the risk of aging from alcohol and drug abuse is simple—stop using the things that harm brain function. If drinking is a problem, I recommend stopping altogether and seeking treatment if needed. If it is not a problem, limit it to no more than one to two normal-size drinks a week.

CANCER AND CANCER TREATMENT

In addition to cancers that invade the brain and can cause dementia, some *treatments* for cancer get into the brain and can also cause dementia. However, there are few studies on this issue. One of the studies done examined the effect of chemotherapy in a hundred women with breast cancer. Dr. F. S. van Dam of the Netherlands Cancer Institute found that women who received chemotherapy plus tamoxifen were four to eight times more likely to develop cognitive impairment than early-stage breast cancer women who had not received chemotherapy. A 1995 review of children who are long-term survivors of cancer, particularly brain cancer and leukemia, showed that the two most common long-term effects of radiation therapy and chemotherapy are cognitive and hormonal impairment. Surprisingly, they found that the cognitive impairment is progressive and not static. Anything you do to decrease the risk of cancer, such as exercising, eating more fruits and vegetables, decreasing stress and stopping smoking, will also help your brain stay healthy.

CARDIOVASCULAR DISEASE

All forms of cardiovascular disease increase brain aging. The heart and blood-vessel system delivers blood and nutrients to the brain. Whatever is good for the heart is good for the brain. Whatever is bad for the heart and blood-vessel system is bad for the brain. Forms of cardiovascular disease include atherosclerosis, coronary artery disease, congestive heart disease, heart rhythm problems, high cholesterol, and hypertension.

The most effective way to prevent cardiovascular problems is to prevent the diseases that produce them. Exercise and diet are important factors that you have some control over. You can also investigate your family history. If it includes heart disease, stroke, diabetes, or high cholesterol, then you should consult your physician and ask her to screen for these conditions at the appropriate age of risk for the condition or, in general, after the age of forty. An annual screening after the age of fifty is extremely wise. Regular cardiovascular exercise for thirty minutes or more goes a long way to improving lipid metabolism to reduce lipid deposits in blood vessel walls. The main focus of your diet should be to not overdo it on saturated fats that are high in the bad cholesterols and that contribute to the fatty deposits in the blood vessels that cause atherosclerosis. Foods high in saturated fats include butter, cheese, cookies, doughnuts, pastries, ice cream, fatty meat, etc.

CEREBRAL VASCULAR DISEASE
(BRAIN BLOOD VESSEL DISEASE)

The risk of developing serious brain problems in a person who has a stroke is six to ten times greater than that in the general population. Even a stroke smaller than a pencil-head eraser increases the risk for dementia four- to twelve-fold.

A stroke is a single, damaging attack, but the risk factors that lead to a stroke, such as high blood pressure, smoking, heart disease, and diabetes, develop over a long time. You can reduce your stroke risk by taking the following simple steps:

- Keep blood pressure under control. Check your blood pressure often, and if it is high, follow your doctor's advice on how to lower it. Treating high blood pressure reduces the risk for both stroke and heart disease.

- Stop smoking. Cigarette smoking is linked to increased risk for stroke and heart disease. The risk of stroke for people who have quit smoking for two to five years is lower than that for people who still smoke.
- Exercise regularly. Exercise makes the heart stronger and improves circulation. It also helps control weight. Being overweight increases the chance of high blood pressure, atherosclerosis, heart disease, and adult-onset (type 2) diabetes. Physical activities like walking, bicycling, swimming, and tennis lower the risk of both stroke and heart disease. Talk with your doctor before starting a vigorous exercise program. See Chapter 5, "The Exercise Solution."
- Eat a healthy, balanced diet and control diabetes. If untreated, diabetes can damage the blood vessels throughout the body and lead to atherosclerosis. See Chapter 4, "The Nutrition Solution."

The warning signs for stroke include sudden numbness or weakness in the face, arm, or leg, especially on one side of the body; sudden confusion, trouble speaking, or understanding; sudden trouble seeing in one or both eyes; sudden trouble walking, dizziness, loss of balance, or coordination; sudden severe headache with no known cause. If you suspect that either you or someone you know is having a stroke, call 911 immediately even if the symptoms seem to have gone away. Sometimes the warning signs last for only a few minutes and then they disappear, but that does not mean the problem is resolved. You could have had a transient stroke, called a transient ischemic attack (TIA), and although it doesn't last long, it is a symptom of a greater medical problem. Don't ignore a TIA—see your doctor right away.

DEPRESSION

Depression has been associated with increased risk for dementia. A prior history of medically treated depression can be associated with a threefold increase in this risk. In an impressive study, Drs. Yaffe and Blackwell from the University of California, San Francisco, studied the association between depression and cognitive decline. As part of an ongoing prospective study, they evaluated 5,781 elderly women. They studied them at baseline and four years later, using tests of depression, memory, and concentration. At baseline, 211 (3.6 percent) of the women had six or more depressive symptoms. Only 16 (7.6 percent) of these women were receiving treatment, which meant 92.4 percent of depressed women in the study were not being treated. Increasing symptoms of depression was associated with worse performance at baseline and follow-up on all tests. Women with three to five symptoms of depression were at 1.6 greater odds for cognitive deterioration, while women with six or more symptoms of depression were at 2.3 greater odds for problems, more than double the risk. They concluded that depression in older women is associated with both poor cognitive function and subsequent cognitive decline.

It is critical to note that most psychiatric diseases in general are, in effect, brain diseases. Schizophrenia, for example, has been shown to affect the frontal and temporal lobes, and depression has shown decreased activity in the frontal lobes. These illnesses are also exacerbated by chronic stress; increased stress hormones have been shown to kill cells in the hippocampus.

Early treatment is essential to stave off the ravages of psychiatric illnesses. Our work with SPECT teaches us that with appropriate treatment, the brain becomes more balanced and works in a much more efficient way. Treatment can involve medication, psychotherapy, supplements, or a combination of all three. Medication and supplements work by altering certain neurotransmitters in the brain—for example, antidepressants that enhance serotonin, norepinephrine, or dopamine. Psychotherapy has also been shown recently to affect neurotransmitter systems and enhance activity seen on SPECT scans.

DIABETES

Diabetes damages almost every organ, including the brain, by making blood vessels hard and brittle. This increases the likelihood of stroke, heart disease, and hypertension, all of which increase aging problems for the brain. In diabetes there is a failure to keep blood sugar (glucose) at appropriate levels, which impairs memory and other cognitive functions. Sometimes, the treatment of diabetes lowers blood glucose too much (hypoglycemia), which can also impair memory and other cognitive functions.

People with a family history of diabetes should have an Hg A1C and fasting blood glucose test once a year after the age of forty. Also, if symptoms of increased urination, increased thirst, or increased appetite develop, then fasting blood glucose should be checked for diabetes. One of the most effective preventions against diabetes is exercise, which improves insulin's ability to regulate blood glucose. Although there are many reasons why daily exercise is better than exercise only every three days, the available data suggest that exercising at least every three days helps protect against diabetes and a number of other illnesses. Diets high in refined sugars increase the risk of diabetes.

LACK OF EDUCATION

A number of studies that attempted to identify risk factors for dementia have noted an inverse relationship between education and dementia—the more education, the less dementia. This is a controversial risk factor because educational background and achievement can introduce a number of other factors that generally affect health and opportunity. Despite the controversy, there is significant evidence to support the idea that education (and increased mental activity) produces a functional reserve in the brain, which can provide protection against developing dementia. The philosophy of use it or lose it is very much at play in the brain. The more it is challenged and stimulated (without overdoing it, which leads to the harmful effects of stress), the more ability it will have during aging.

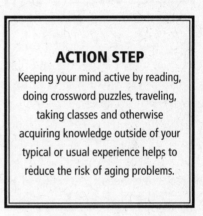

ACTION STEP

Keeping your mind active by reading, doing crossword puzzles, traveling, taking classes and otherwise acquiring knowledge outside of your typical or usual experience helps to reduce the risk of aging problems.

No one that I am aware of has studied whether or not learning disabilities and other conditions, such as ADD, which often leads to school failure, are associated with dementia. My strong suspicion is that there is a connection. Any condition that negatively impacts brain function can put the brain at risk for other problems later on. I believe we should aggressively treat children and teens with school problems so that they will stay in school and, hopefully, grow to love learning and be the lifelong learners they need to be in order to help protect their brains.

HIGH HOMOCYSTEINE LEVELS

Homocysteine is an amino acid regulated by folic acid in red blood cells. If elevated, homocysteine increases risks for coronary artery disease, stroke, and dementia. The risk is largely eliminated for homocysteine levels of 10 or below. High homocysteine levels in the blood increase LDL cholesterol, which narrows the coronary blood vessels. A study of persons who required opening up of

---

ACTION STEP

If your homocysteine levels are high, consider taking a supplement with B_6, B_{12}, and folic acid.

---

their coronary arteries by a procedure called coronary angioplasty showed that homocysteine levels higher than 11 could be treated with folic acid (1 mg), vitamin B_{12} (400 mg), and vitamin B_6 (10 mg) to reduce the levels to about 7. This homocysteine reduction helped prevent renarrowing of the coronary arteries after the angioplasty surgery and halved the chance that these blood vessels would close up again and require another angioplasty surgery. High homocysteine levels can also make blood clot more easily than it should, increasing the risk of blood-vessel blockages and stroke or heart attack.

Homocysteine is normally changed into other amino acids for use by the body. If your homocysteine level is too high, you may not have enough B vitamins to help this process. Most people with a high homocysteine level don't get enough folate (also called folic acid), vitamin B_6 (pyridoxine), or vitamin B_{12} in their diets. Replacing these vitamins helps return homocysteine levels to normal. Other possible causes of a high homocysteine level include low levels of thyroid hormone, kidney disease, psoriasis, some medicines, or inherited deficiencies in the enzymes used to process homocysteine in the body.

HORMONES

Estrogen Deficiency Induced by Menopause

Six of ten studies showed that women who took estrogen had a lower risk for Alzheimer's disease (AD). The best of these studies was the Baltimore Longitudinal Study of Aging, where 472 women who were going through menopause or had completed it were followed for up to sixteen years. Women who never used estrogen during the study were twice as likely to develop dementia.

This study and others showing beneficial effects of estrogen have been contradicted by reports from the Women's Health Initiative, discussed in Chapter 7, which found that women who used Premarin (an estrogen made from horse ovaries) were twice as likely to develop AD as non-estrogen users. However, the Women's Health Initiative study did not examine the risk of AD using forms of estrogen made by the human ovary, such as estradiol. Evidence suggesting that these more natural forms of estrogen for women may still reduce AD risk and provide other benefits comes from the largest study ever done on the severest form of estrogen deficiency—hysterectomy with removal of the ovaries. This study of 100,000 women who participated in the 1986 National Mortality Followback Survey found that women with a hysterectomy were twice as likely to develop dementia. What one can conclude from this complex maze of seemingly contradictory research findings is that women should avoid Premarin and other forms of estrogen that are not made by the human ovary. However, severe reductions in female estrogen hormones are equally harmful and should be treated.

There is a large body of basic scientific research demonstrating sound reasons why estrogen, in the right amount, protects the brain, the blood vessels, and the bones. Human forms of estrogen, taken in the smallest amounts needed to keep blood estradiol levels from falling too low in women after menopause, are reasonably safe and have not, to date, been demonstrated by the Women's Health Initiative or any other study to be harmful. If there is a family history of dementia, then it is worth having a blood estradiol test after menopause to determine if you have estrogen deficiency. You can then evaluate with your doctor whether low-dose estradiol or other natural estrogens would be worth taking.

The situation is more complex in women with a family history of both AD and breast or uterine cancer, because some studies have found that estrogen use increases the risk of these two cancers. Whether low-dose estradiol significantly increases the risk of heart disease or stroke in women without symptoms is more controversial. The relative benefits of taking low-dose estradiol after menopause (reduced risk of AD and osteoporosis) may be greater than the relative risks (increased risk of endometrial cancer, breast cancer, and maybe stroke and heart disease), but the decision regarding treatment depends on your personal history and the risk factors for each of these diseases.

Although not all studies agree, estrogen use after menopause appears to significantly reduce AD risk. Estrogen use in estrogen-deficient women can also improve verbal fluency and possibly verbal short-term memory. Evista is a form of estrogen that is reported to be safer to take in women with increased risk of breast or uterine cancer.

TESTOSTERONE DEFICIENCY IN MALES

Testosterone levels normally start to decline after age fifty. By age eighty, testosterone levels are 20 to 50 percent of their younger adult values. Low testosterone levels may increase dementia risk. A case-control study involving 83 AD patients and 103 normal volunteers of similar age showed significantly reduced total testosterone levels in AD males. However, until a well-designed group study is done, it is not certain whether or not testosterone deficiency is a risk factor for AD.

Men who have or have had prostate cancer treatment or men fifty years and older may develop cognitive impairment due to testosterone deficiency, which can be checked by a blood test. Symptoms including difficulty with vision not due to eye problems, difficulty remembering locations or faces or other objects of interest, breast enlargement, or a change in the distribution of body hair should alert men to check for testosterone deficiency.

PARKINSON'S DISEASE

Parkinson's disease (PD) is caused by the loss of dopamine-producing cells. There is a significant connection between PD and AD. There is no known cure for PD, but with early detection there are medications that help with the symptoms. It has also been suggested that coenzyme Q10, a powerful antioxidant, along with high doses of vitamins C and E, may be helpful in delaying the need for stronger and stronger medications. Vitamin B$_6$ increases the production of dopamine and may be helpful early in the disease process. The natural hormone melatonin, which regulates sleep, has been found to reduce tremors and protect against free-radical damage on dopamine neurons. Fish oils and flaxseeds, which contain omega-3 fatty acids, have nerve-nourishing effects that can boost dopamine.

SEIZURES AND SEIZURE MEDICATION

About 125,000 Americans develop epilepsy every year. Thousands more experience isolated seizures that may or may not happen again in the future. Recurring seizures are defined as epilepsy. Treatment of epilepsy has improved dramatically in recent years. Seizures can often be controlled, and chances of long-term remission are improving all the time. However, seizures and certain antiseizure medications can have a negative effect on brain function and be associated with dementia. During seizures there is dramatic increased activity, and then in the in-between period there is significant decreased activity. Antiseizure medications work by increasing inhibition in the brain. If this is done too enthusiastically—as with the older antiseizure medications like Dilantin and phenobarbital—it can cause overall decreased activity and damage the healthy cells around the seizure-promoting ones.

Obviously, seizure disorders need to be vigorously treated. Once a person is seizure-free for two years, however, many neurologists start to taper the antiseizure medications to see how much is needed. Also, newer antiseizure medications, such as Trileptal, are less likely to cause too much overall inhibition of brain function. If you are taking antiseizure medication and notice memory problems, that is a symptom that the temporal lobes may be calmed too much. The most common cause of seizures in someone with epilepsy is not taking seizure medication as prescribed. For some people whose seizures cannot be controlled with medication, there is the option of surgery to remove the damaged tissue. Sometimes it is possible to identify a certain action or event that will always produce seizures in sensitive people. Seizure "triggers" include flickering lights, breathing very quickly and deeply, drinking an excessive amount of fluid, and even, in very rare cases, reading or listening to a certain piece of music. Sleep deprivation (like staying up all night studying) may produce seizures; so may excessive use of alcohol or withdrawal from certain drugs. Excessive sugar has also been implicated, and ketogenic diets, which eliminate sugars, have been found to be helpful.

SLEEP APNEA

Obstructive sleep apnea—a condition associated with loud snoring, stopping breathing entirely for brief periods many times during the night, and chronic tiredness—can cause cognitive impairment. In our clinic we have seen hundreds of people with sleep apnea and they uniformly have troubled brains, especially in the areas associated with memory. In one brain SPECT study of obstructive sleep apnea, researchers found significantly reduced activity in the left parietal lobe. Reduced left-parietal-lobe activity can impair comprehension, making it difficult to understand conversations or read books. Treatment of the sleep apnea with nasal continuous positive airway pressure (CPAP), a machine that pushes air at a high pressure through the nasal passageways, completely reversed the impaired brain activity in these patients. Sleep apnea should be evaluated and treated as early as possible.

SMOKING

Cigarette smoking is the number one cause of preventable deaths in the United States, accounting for nearly 500,000 deaths per year. It accounts for 12 percent of all the strokes in the United States and is therefore a major risk

ACTION STEP

Stop smoking now! To help you quit, consider hypnosis, nicotine gum or patches, and the antidepressant Wellbutrin.

factor for dementia. Smoking is also a risk for lung, stomach, and bladder cancer, as well as hypertension and heart disease. Nicotine constricts small blood vessels in all of the organs of the body, including the brain, and prematurely ages everything.

Obviously, stop smoking. I know this is often much easier said than done. Over the years, I have helped many people stop smoking and I have found that no one program works for everyone. Hypnosis is effective for some; the use of nicotine patches or gum works for others; the medication Wellbutrin (bupropion), a dopamine-enhancing antidepressant, is helpful for others; and some respond to group therapy. In my experience, it is usually a combination of treatments that is needed.

Keeping your memory healthy is critical to your efforts to get a better body and vice versa. In order to keep your memory healthy, you need to keep your body healthy as well. As you have seen, the strategies are simple—stop polluting your body, eat good food, exercise your mind and body, and treat disease early.

SUPPLEMENTS TO ENHANCE MEMORY

The rational use of supplements can also be very helpful for your memory. Ginkgo biloba, phosphatidylserine (PS), sage, vinpocetine, curcumin, and huperzine A have been shown to be helpful to enhance memory. Medications that have also been found to help memory include Namenda, Aricept, Exelon, and Reminyl. See Appendix C for more information on supplements and also visit www.amenclinics.com.

The Memory Solution

Memory Robbers	Memory Boosters
Any brain problems	Overall brain-healthy program
Brain trauma	Focus on brain protection
Poor sleep	Adequate sleep (at least seven hours)
Low blood sugar	Frequent small meals with at least some protein to maintain healthy blood sugar
Poor diet	Enriched diet
Alcohol/drug abuse	Freedom from alcohol or drugs
Depression	Treatment for depression
Anxiety	Meditation for relaxation and to boost the PFC
Lack of exercise	Exercise
Lack of mental exercise	Lifelong learning
Excessive TV or computer	Limited TV and computer
Hormone problems (i.e., thyroid, testosterone, estrogen, cortisol)	Optimized hormone levels
Medical problems, such as B_{12} deficiency	Treatment of any underlying medical problems
Medications such as Xanax or OxyContin	Fish oil to decrease inflammation and enhance blood flow
Diabetes	Diet and exercise
Alzheimer's disease	Alzheimer prevention plan described above
Stroke	Stopping smoking
Postanesthesia loss	Overall brain-healthy program
Environment toxins	Great ventilation and elimination of any toxins
Any systemic inflammation	Anti-inflammation program, including fish oil, healthy diet, folic acid, or some low-dose ibuprofen or baby aspirin
Chemotherapy	Cancer prevention diet, lots of fruit and veggies
	Supplements include ginkgo, huperzine A, PS, sage, curcumin, and vinpocetine

13

THE ANT SOLUTION

Think Your Way to Being
Thinner, Younger, and Happier

Don't believe every negative thought that goes through your brain.

"I will never lose weight."

"I can't help being fat—my whole family is fat."

"It is my wife's fault I'm fat—she always puts too much food on my plate."

"Dieting is useless—I'm just going to gain all the weight back."

"I'm a failure because I can't lose weight."

"I'm stressed out, so I have to eat."

"I have always had a sweet tooth—I will never be able to stop eating chocolate."

"It is too hard to stick to a diet."

"I have never been a good sleeper."

"I don't have to count calories, I already know it all."

"I don't need a lot of sleep—I can just drink more coffee to stay awake."

"My memory is terrible, but that is normal since I'm forty-five."

"I'm certain I will get Alzheimer's disease because my dad has it."

"There is nothing I can do to prevent wrinkles."

"Everybody over fifty has bags under their eyes."

"I don't want to go to the doctor because I know she will find something wrong."

"My kids are always getting colds, so it is normal that I get them, too."

"I just know I'm going to get cancer one day."

"I have no control over my high blood pressure—taking medication is the only option."

Do any of these thoughts sound familiar? If so, you have been lying to yourself. These kinds of thoughts are LIES, and they prevent you from getting the body and the brain you want. The good news is you don't have to believe every stupid lie that goes through your head. Even better, you can talk back to the lies. How many of you were good at talking back to your parents as teenagers? I was excellent! You need to be good at talking back to yourself.

Most of us never give thinking a second thought (pun intended). Thinking comes naturally to all of us. In all our years of education, nobody ever teaches us how to think, what to think, or what not to think. For many of us, it is a free-for-all in our minds, with random thoughts racing through without any rhyme or reason. For others of us, we get stuck on the same repetitive negative thoughts and can't get rid of them. Is this good for our brains? No! Is this good for our bodies? No! Our negative thinking has taken control of our brains, and we need to take control back. It is time for boot camp for your thinking. Improved brain function, a better figure, enhanced moods, greater immunity, and glowing skin will be your reward.

HOW THOUGHTS AFFECT YOUR BRAIN AND BODY

Did you know that your thoughts are so powerful that they cause physical reactions in your brain and body? It is true. Bad, mad, sad, hopeless, or helpless thoughts release chemicals that make you feel bad. Your hands get cold, you start to sweat more, your heart rate quickens and flattens (low heart rate variability is associated with negative thinking and heart disease . . . which isn't good for your health), you breathe faster and more shallowly, and your muscles tense up. These awful, miserable, negative thoughts make your brain and body work less efficiently. On the other hand, happy, positive, hopeful, loving thoughts release chemicals that make you feel good. Your hands feel warmer, you sweat less, your heart rate slows and becomes more variable (which is a good thing), your breathing slows and deepens, and your muscles relax. These effects take place immediately and make your brain and body function better.

How do we know the body reacts to our thoughts? Biofeedback instruments, such as those used for lie detector tests, tell us so. How do we know that the brain reacts to our thoughts? We know this thanks to brain imaging studies. Previously, I told you about a study we did comparing the effects of negative thoughts and gratitude on brain function. The results were astounding. The scans showed that gratitude and positive thinking enhanced brain function. That makes it easier for you to make the best decisions regarding your diet and overall health. Negative thinking, however, caused serious decreases

---

ACTION STEP

Your thoughts matter. If you want to feel good, think good thoughts.

---

in activity in the cerebellum and temporal lobes, especially the left temporal lobe. When activity in the cerebellum is low, it is harder for you to think and process information quickly—definitely not something you want to happen when you have to decide whether or not to accept that third glass of wine your host just offered you or if you want the supersize version of your meal that the fast-food cashier just suggested.

Decreased activity in the temporal lobes is associated with mood, memory, and temper-control problems. Feelings of depression, difficulty remembering important information, and violent acts may occur. These pose serious consequences for your body. Depression has been linked to being overweight or obese. If you don't have a good memory, you will not remember all the things you need to do to maintain good health. And violence can lead to bodily injury. Ouch!

Several other studies confirm these findings. Researchers at the National Institute of Mental Health conducted an intriguing study about the affects thoughts have on brain function. They looked at brain activity in ten healthy women under three different conditions: when they were thinking happy thoughts, neutral thoughts, and sad thoughts. During the happy thoughts, the women demonstrated a cooling of their emotional brain, and they felt better. During the sad thoughts, there was a significant increase in the emotional brain's activity, which is consistent with depression. Another neuroimaging study from Canadian researchers found that sadness and negative emotions significantly influence in a negative way brain function and brain plasticity.

MEET THE ANTS:
AUTOMATIC NEGATIVE THOUGHTS

ANTs (automatic negative thoughts) are the negative thoughts that enter your head throughout the day, make you feel bad, and prevent you from adopting healthy behaviors. They sabotage your healthy eating plans, diminish your desire to exercise, destroy your self-esteem, and make you feel rotten.

I came up with the concept of ANTs as a way to help my younger patients understand the notion of negative thoughts. One day, I came home to an ant invasion in my kitchen. There were thousands of the creepy crawlers every-where. I grabbed the bug spray and started spraying to kill them. As I was spraying them, I thought, "These ants are just like the thoughts inside my patients' brains." A few ants aren't a big deal, but when you have an infestation, it spoils your day. The ANTs in your head are just the same. A negative thought here and there isn't too troublesome, but if you have thousands of awful thoughts, it makes you feel awful.

In our high school course Making a Good Brain Great, we teach a session on ANTs. The students find it one of the most valuable parts of the class. They are fascinated to learn that they don't have to believe every thought they have, and they are shocked that nobody has ever taught them this concept before. We have heard from the students that the idea that they can put a stop to their negative thoughts is very empowering and helps them believe that they can control their thoughts rather than letting their thoughts control them.

In my practice, I have identified nine "species" of ANTs that can steal your happiness and ruin your life:

1. All or nothing
2. Always thinking
3. Focusing on the negative
4. Thinking with your feelings
5. Guilt beating
6. Labeling
7. Fortune-telling
8. Mind reading
9. Blame

Let's look at each ANT species more closely.

1. All or nothing These are the ANTs that infest your brain when you think that everything is all good or all bad. It is the same as black-or-white thinking. If you stick to your exercise plan for a month, you think you are the most dis-ciplined person on the planet. If you miss a day at the gym, you think you have no discipline and give up and go back to being a couch potato. A better approach is to acknowledge that you didn't do your daily workout and then get back on track the following day. One slipup doesn't mean you should give up entirely.

2. Always thinking This is when you think in words that overgeneralize, such as *always, never, every time,* or *everyone.* Consider some of the thoughts at the beginning of this chapter: "I will never lose weight," "I have always had a sweet tooth—I will never be able to stop eating chocolate," "My kids are always getting colds, so it is normal that I get them, too." This kind of thinking makes you feel like you are doomed to fail at eating right and staying healthy. It is as if you have no control over your actions or behaviors.

3. Focusing on the negative This ANT makes you see only the negative aspects of situations even when there are plenty of positives. "I know I lost ten pounds, but I wanted to lose fifteen, so I'm a failure" is an example of this type of thinking. Focusing on the negative makes you more inclined to give up on your efforts. Putting a positive spin on this same thought— "Wow! I lost ten pounds. I'm on my way to my goal of fifteen pounds"— encourages you to keep up the good work and makes you feel pretty good about yourself.

4. Thinking with your feelings "I feel like my skin is never going to clear up." Thoughts like this occur when you have a feeling about something, and you assume it is correct, so you never question it. Feelings can lie too. Look for evidence. In this example, schedule an appointment with a dermatologist to find out if there's anything you can do to improve your skin.

5. Guilt beating Thinking in words like "should," "must," "ought to," and "have to" are typical with this ANT, which involves using excessive guilt to control behavior. When we feel pushed to do things, our natural tendency is to push back. That doesn't mean that guilt is all bad. There are certainly things in life that we should and shouldn't do if we want to have the best body possible: "I want to eat the chips and guacamole at the party, but I should have the raw carrots instead" or "I feel like staying in bed, but I should do my workout." Don't mistake these for guilt-beating ANTs.

6. Labeling When you call yourself or someone else names or use negative terms to describe them, you have a labeling ANT in your brain. A lot of us do this on a regular basis. You may have said one of the following at some point in your life: "I'm a loser"; "I'm a failure"; or "I'm lazy." The problem with calling yourself names is that it takes away your control over your actions and behaviors. If you are a loser, a failure, or lazy, then why bother trying to change your behaviors? It is as if you have given up before you have even tried. This defeatist attitude can be ruinous for your body.

Beware of the Red Ants

These last three ANTs are the worst of the bunch. I call them the red ANTs because they can really sting.

7. Fortune-telling Predicting the worst even though you don't know what will happen is the hallmark of the fortune-telling ANT. You probably have these ANTs in your brain if you've ever said anything like "I know I'm not going to be able to stick with an exercise program"; "I'm going to cheat if I try to diet"; "I just had a biopsy. I'm sure it is cancer, and I'm going to die." The problem with fortune-telling is that your mind is so powerful it can make happen what you see. So when you are convinced that your biopsy will bring bad news, you get stressed about it, which depresses your immune system and increases your odds of getting sick. In fact, chronic stress has been implicated in a number of diseases, including cancer.

Nobody is safe from fortune-telling ANTs, not even me. Several years ago, I wrote an article for *Parade* magazine called "How to Get Out of Your Own Way." After the article was published, my office received more than ten thousand letters asking for more information about self-defeating behavior. The media got wind of the response, and I was invited to appear on CNN. It was a great opportunity for me to get the word out about the work we do here at the Amen Clinics, but I had never been on TV before, and I was nervous—*really* nervous.

I was sitting in the "green room" right before I went on and all of a sudden, I had a panic attack. I couldn't breathe, my heart was racing, and I wanted to get the heck out of there. Thankfully, I treat people with this problem. I told myself the same things I tell my patients: "If you are having a panic attack in a safe situation, don't leave, or panic will rule your life. Slow down your breathing. Write down your thoughts and what kind of ANTs they are." So I stayed put, took a deep breath, and grabbed a pen to write down my thoughts: "I'm going to forget my name"—fortune-telling. "I'm going to stutter"—fortune-telling. "Two million people are going to think I'm stupid"—fortune-telling.

With just one look, I knew that I had a fortune-telling ANT infestation. Then, just like I tell my patients, I told myself to talk back to my thoughts.

Okay, if I forget my name, I have my driver's license in my pocket and can look it up.

I don't usually stutter, but if I do, all the stutterers out there watching will have a doctor they can relate to.

And as for people thinking I'm stupid, I reminded myself of the 18/40/60 rule, which says when you are eighteen you worry about what everybody is thinking of you. At forty you don't give a damn what anyone else thinks. And, at sixty, you realize that nobody has been thinking about you at all. Most people spend their days worrying and thinking about themselves.

This little exercise helped calm me down so I was able to go on TV, and I did fine. I did not forget my name. I didn't stutter. And I did not get any phone calls, letters, or e-mails from two million people telling me I was stupid. The next time I was asked to appear on TV, I was not quite as nervous. And with each subsequent appearance, I became more relaxed. Since that first time, I have appeared on TV more than one hundred times, and it no longer makes me nervous at all. Just think if I had listened to my lying, fortune-telling ANTs and had run out of the studio. I probably never would have accepted another invitation to be on TV, and it would have dramatically changed my life and career in a negative way.

8. Mind reading When you think you know what somebody else is thinking even though they have not told you, and you have not asked them, it is called mind reading. You are probably familiar with these ANTs: "He is looking at my behind—he must think I'm too fat" and "She is gazing into my eyes—she is probably thinking I look too old because I have crow's-feet."

I have twenty-five years of education—mostly in how to diagnose, treat, and help people—and I can't read anyone's mind. I have no idea what they are thinking unless they tell me. A glance in your direction doesn't mean somebody is judging the way you look. He could be looking at your rear end because you just sat on something that stuck to your pants. Or she could be thinking what beautiful eyes you have.

9. Blame Of all the ANTs, this one is the worst. Blaming others for your problems and taking no responsibility for your own successes and failures is toxic thinking. You know the kind of thoughts I'm talking about: "It is your fault I'm out of shape because you will not go with me to exercise"; "It is my mother's fault I'm overweight because she cooks such fattening foods"; or "I only started smoking because you smoke, so it is your fault I have respiratory problems."

One of my patients was a young girl who spent her entire first session blaming other people for all her problems. I had her make a piggy bank and put all of the excuses she used in it. Every time she would blame someone, she would have to put a quarter in the bank. At first, there were a lot of quarters in the bank. I told her that she and I could write a book together called *101 Reasons Why I'm Not Responsible for How My Life Turns Out*. Shortly, she got the message and gave up blaming others.

Whenever you begin a sentence with "It is your fault . . ." it ruins your life. These ANTs make you a victim. And when you are a victim, you are powerless to change your behavior. In order to have the best body possible, you have to change your behavior, so kill the blame ANTs.

> ### ACTION STEP
> Beware of the blame ANTs. Quit blaming others and take responsibility for your actions. If you are smoking, it is because you made the choice to start, and you can make the choice to quit.

CHANGE YOUR THINKING, CHANGE YOUR BRAIN AND BODY

When you learn to challenge and correct negative, lying thoughts, you take away their power to control you and your body. Instead, by taking control of your thinking, you also take control of your actions and behaviors so you can have the body you want. By changing your thinking, you can make yourself thinner, healthier, and happier. Here is a concept I use with many of my patients to help them take charge of their thinking.

Develop an ANTeater in your brain that can eat up all the negative thoughts that come into your head and mess up your efforts to have a better body. Teach your ANTeater to talk back to the pesky ANTs so you can free yourself from negative thoughts. Whenever you feel mad, sad, nervous, or frustrated, write out your thoughts and the ANT species, then write down what your ANTeater would say to that ANT to kill it. As soon as you write down the truth, it diffuses any negative feelings, and you start to feel better. Look at the following chart for examples of how to talk back to your ANTs.

ANT	Species	ANTeater
I ate a cookie. Now my diet is ruined.	All or nothing	I enjoyed the cookie and will eat fewer calories at dinner to make up for it.
I know I'm going to get Alzheimer's disease.	Fortune-telling	I don't know that. If I take care of my brain health now, I may not get it.
It is your fault.	Blame	I need to take responsibility for my own actions and behaviors.

ANT THERAPY FOR A BETTER BODY

The concept of changing your thinking to change your behavior is rooted in a proven, brain-enhancing technique called cognitive therapy or therapy to counteract your automatic negative thoughts. Used to help patients overcome all sorts of unwanted behaviors, cognitive therapy can also be beneficial in helping you get a better body. That is the premise of *The Beck Diet Solution,* a great book by Dr. Judith S. Beck. In this work, Beck shows how cognitive therapy can help with diet and weight loss by teaching you to "train your brain to think like a thin person." The simple act of thinking the way a thin person thinks helps you behave like a thin person. And that behavior is what will help you lose weight.

Think Like a Thinner Person

"I went to a party last night and ate a lot of guacamole and chips; today, I weigh one pound more. I will try to eat better today."

"I can't resist Mrs. Field's cookies. When I go to the mall, I will avoid the food court so I'm not tempted to buy any."

"When I feel stressed, I will take a warm bath or walk around the block instead of reaching for the candy bowl."

"I'm going to tell my mother how much I love her famous cheese soufflé but that I won't be eating it this time because I'm trying to watch my weight. That way, she will not be insulted and I will not feel guilty when I don't have any at our family dinner."

"Those bagels in the break room look really good, but I just ate breakfast so I'm not going to eat one."

"As a child, I was taught to clean my plate, so I'm going to put a smaller portion of food on my plate. [Or, I'm going to use smaller plates.]"

ACTION STEP

Change your thinking so you start thinking like a younger person, a more fit person, a more energetic person, a healthier person, or a thin person. Your thoughts will translate into actions, and those actions will cause your body to transform into what you have always wanted.

Think Like a More Youthful-Looking Person

"Just because I'm going out to dinner does not mean I have to drink alcohol, which dehydrates my skin and makes it look dull."

"I'm going to avoid places where people are smoking because I don't want to be tempted to smoke."

"I'm not going to stay out really late because I want to look refreshed in the morning."

"It is just as easy to put on moisturizer that has sunscreen in it, and it protects my skin from sun damage."

"No matter how old I am, I can always improve the appearance of my skin by taking care of it."

"Instead of stressing out about work, I'm going to spend five minutes meditating."

Think Like a Healthier Person

"Getting good sleep is a priority for me because it helps keep me from getting sick."

"I'm going to talk to my doctor about what I can do to prevent serious illnesses."

"If I feel under the weather or think I might have a mental health problem, I'm going to seek help from a professional rather than wait for the condition to worsen."

"I always feel so much better after I exercise, so I'm going to get up and do it even though I feel tired this morning."

"I like having a healthy body, and I want to keep it that way, so I'm going to stay away from sports that are not brain safe and play tennis or table tennis instead."

THE WORK: A SIMPLE BUT EFFECTIVE WAY TO KILL ANTS

One of my favorite books, *Loving What Is,* comes from my friend Byron Katie. In this very wise book, Katie, as her friends call her, describes an amazing transformation that took place in her own life. At the age of forty-three, Katie, who had spent the previous ten years of her life in a downward spiral of rage, despair, and suicidal depression, woke up one morning to discover that all those horrible emotions were gone. In their place were feelings of utter joy and happiness. Katie's great revelation, which came in 1986, was that it is not life that makes us feel depressed, angry, abandoned, and despairing; rather, it is our thoughts that make us feel that way. This insight led Katie to the notion that our thoughts could just as easily make us feel happy, calm, connected, and joyful.

It also led her to realize that our minds and our thoughts affect our bodies. "The body is never our problem. Our problem is always a thought that we innocently believe," she wrote in her book *On Health, Sickness, and Death.* In the same book, she also wrote, "Bodies don't crave, bodies don't want, bodies don't know, don't care, don't get hungry or thirsty. It is what that mind attaches—ice cream, alcohol, drugs, sex, money—that the body reflects. There are no physical addictions, only mental ones. Body follows mind. It doesn't have a choice."

Katie wanted to share her revelation with others to help them end their suffering by changing their thinking. She developed a simple method of inquiry—the Work—to question our thoughts. The Work is simple. It consists of writing down any bothersome, worrisome, or negative thoughts, then asking ourselves four questions and doing a turnaround. The goal of the Work isn't pie-in-the-sky positive thinking; it is accurate thinking. The four questions are these:

1. Is it true? (Is the negative thought true?)
2. Can I absolutely know that it is true?
3. How do I react when I think that thought?
4. Who would I be without the thought? Or how would I feel if I didn't have the thought?

After you answer the four questions, you take your original thought and turn it around to its opposite, and ask yourself whether the opposite of the original thought that is causing your suffering is not true or even truer. Then turn the thought around and apply it to yourself (how does the opposite of the thought apply to me personally?). Then turn the thought around to the other person, if the thought involves another person (how does the opposite apply to the other person?).

I have done the Work myself, and it helped me get through a very painful period of grief. When I did the Work, I immediately felt better. I was more relaxed, less anxious, and more honest in dealing with my own thoughts and emotions. Now I always carry the four questions with me, and I use them a lot in my practice and with my friends and family. Here are some examples of how to use the four questions to kill the ANTs that are keeping you from having a body you love.

Do the Work for Weight Loss

Gina was hoping to shed twenty pounds before her wedding, so she changed her diet three months before the big day. After the first two weeks, she lost a few pounds and was feeling good about herself. But after the third week, she stepped on the scale and saw that she had gained a pound even though she was following her nutrition plan. She thought to herself, "I will never lose the weight in time for my wedding." Here is how she worked on that thought.

Negative thought: "I will never lose weight in time for my wedding."

Question #1: Is it true that you will not lose weight in time for the wedding?
"Yes," she said.

Question #2: Can you absolutely know that it is true that you will not lose the weight in time for the wedding?
Initially she said yes, she would not lose the weight. Then she thought about it and said, "Well, maybe I will. I lost weight the first two weeks. Maybe this is just a temporary setback, and I will lose a few more pounds next week."

Question #3: How do you feel when you have the thought "I will never lose weight in time for my wedding"?
"I feel frustrated, and I feel like a failure. I'm afraid that I will be fat on my wedding day, and that I won't fit in my dress. I'm worried that people will not think I'm a beautiful bride."

Question #4: Who would you be without the thought "I will never lose weight in time for my wedding"?
She thought about it for a moment, then said, "I would just be happy that I'm getting married."

Turnaround: What is the opposite thought of "I will never lose weight in time for my wedding"?
Gina thought about it and said that if she continued to follow her diet, "I will lose weight in time for my wedding." Then she felt a renewed energy to keep watching what she ate rather than giving up on her diet.

Do the Work for Better Skin

Negative thought: "I'm over fifty, so there is nothing I can do to prevent wrinkles."

Question #1: Is it true that there is nothing you can do?
"Yes, because I already have wrinkles."

Question #2: Can you absolutely know that it is true that being over fifty makes you incapable of preventing wrinkles?
"No. I mean, I already have some wrinkles, but new wrinkles could be prevented."

Question #3: How do you feel when you have the thought?
 "I feel sad, old, and unattractive."

Question #4: Who would you be or how would you feel without the thought?
 "I would feel like I have more control over how I look."

Turnaround: "There is something I can do to prevent wrinkles."
 Next, find examples to support that thought. "I could stop smoking, try to get more sleep, and start wearing sunscreen. That could help."

Do the Work for Sugar Addiction

Negative thought: "I can't get through the day without eating chocolate."

Question #1: Is that true?
 "Yes."

Question #2: Can you absolutely know that it is true? Would you die if you did not eat chocolate one day?
 "No, of course I would not die."

Question #3: How does that thought make you feel?
 "It makes me feel bad, because I know that eating too much chocolate is making me fat, and that makes me hate my body."

Question #4: Who would I be without that thought?
 "I would feel a whole lot better because I could lose some weight, which would improve my self-esteem."

Turnaround: "I can get through the day without eating chocolate."

Do the Work for Your Health

Negative thought: "My dad had a heart attack at age sixty, so I know that I'm going to have one then, too."

Question #1: Is it true?
 "Yes, it is hereditary."

Question #2: Can you absolutely know that it is true?
 "No, I can't. My dad smoked, never did any exercise, ate a terrible diet, and never went to the doctor. I don't smoke, and if I eat right, exercise, and take medication to lower my cholesterol, I can probably prevent or at least delay heart disease."

Question #3: How do you feel when you have this thought?
 "I feel really stressed out and scared."

Question #4: How would you feel without the thought?

"I wouldn't be so worried, so I would probably be able to sleep better."

Turnaround: "I don't know that I'm going to have a heart attack."

Is this thought true or truer than the original thought? "This thought is true." At this point, if the turnaround does not make sense, and your original thought really is true, you either have to let go of the thought and live with it or do something about it. The goal is not to delude yourself, but to be honest with yourself.

Do the Work for Your Memory

Negative thought: "My memory is awful. I'm sure I'm developing Alzheimer's disease."

Question #1: Is it true that your memory is that bad?

"Yes."

Question #2: Can you absolutely know that it is true 100 percent of the time?

"No, I remember most things, but I feel like I'm forgetting things more often now. Although I have been under a lot of stress lately, and that is when I tend to forget things."

Question #3: How do you feel when you have the thought?

"I feel scared and worried that I won't be able to take care of myself, I will have to be put in a nursing home, and I will lose all my family and friends."

Question #4: How would you feel without the thought?

"I would feel a lot better."

Turnaround: "My memory isn't awful, and I'm not developing Alzheimer's disease."

Is this true or truer than the original statement? "Probably. I should probably check with my doctor to test my memory."

HOW TO GET YOUR UNCONSCIOUS BRAIN TO WORK ON YOUR BODY

Your brain is an amazingly powerful organ, and it can make happen what it sees. If it sees fear, your whole body will feel afraid. Seeing yourself as old, fat, wrinkled, or demented causes increased stress and cortisol production, which will affect your health, your weight, your skin, and your mind in a destructive way. If your brain sees joy, your whole body will feel lighter, healthier, and happier. Negative thoughts can make negative things happen, while positive thoughts can help you reach your health goals.

Physicians have known for centuries that your mind and brain can play a crucial role in your health. Until a hundred years ago, the history of medical therapeutics was largely that of the doctor-patient relationship and the "placebo effect" (placebos being inert substances that have no known physiologic effect on the problem). Actually, most of the treatments by physicians in times past would have been more harmful than beneficial to the patient if it weren't for the belief in the healing power of the physician. The benefits of the placebo effect are determined by the expectations and hopes shared by the patient and the doctor.

Although a placebo is a substance that is considered pharmacologically inert, it is by no means "nothing." It is a potent therapeutic tool—on average about one-half to two-thirds as powerful as morphine in relieving severe pain. It is now recognized that one-third of the general population are placebo responders in clinical situations relating to pain, whether the pain is from surgery, heart disease, cancer, or headache. It is very clear that placebo responses are not simply a result of the patient fooling or tricking himself out of the pain. Placebo administration can produce real physiologic changes. Some of the physiologic pathways through which the placebo effects work have been identified.

In a study done by a University of California research team, it was found that administering naloxone, a drug that neutralizes morphine, could actually block the placebo effect of pain relief in dental patients. From this study and others, it has become clear that the belief in pain relief stimulates the body to secrete its own pain-relieving substance, called endorphins, which act in the same manner as morphine except that they are much more potent. In a recent study, doctors at Houston's Veterans Affairs Medical Center performed arthroscopic knee surgery on one group of patients with arthritis, scraping and rinsing their knee joints. On another group, the doctors made small cuts in the patients' knees to mimic the incisions of a real operation and then bandaged them up. The pain relief reported by the two groups was identical. In a brain imaging study, researchers found that when a placebo worked for depressed patients, brain function also changed in a positive way. Change your beliefs, change your brain, change your body.

Tell your brain what you want and match your behavior to get it. If your mind takes what it sees and makes it happen, it is critical to visualize what you want and then match your behavior to get it. Too many people are thrown around by the whims of the day, rather than using their prefrontal cortex to focus on what they want and then following through on their goals.

As successful athletes visualize their success before a game, you must do the same thing to harness the power of your brain for your body. Too often, people who see themselves as fat and sick actually get their unconscious mind to collaborate on making them fat and sick. If you see yourself as fat, your brain will continue to do what it takes to make you fat. If you see yourself as healthy and trim, your brain will help you accomplish your goal for a better body.

> ### ACTION STEP
>
> To harness the power of your brain in order to enhance your physical body and health, do these four things:
> 1. Clearly define the body you want. Write it down.
> 2. Spend a few minutes each day visualizing your healthy body.
> 3. Put up pictures in your home or at work of when you were your healthiest.
> 4. Ask yourself every day if your behavior is getting you the body you want.

The ANT Solution

Happiness Robbers	Happiness Boosters
Distorted thinking	Accurate thinking
All or nothing	Balanced thinking
Always thinking	Honesty and flexibility
Focusing on the negative	Focusing on the positive
Thinking with your feelings	Thinking with logic
Guilt beating	Using "shoulds" only when they serve you
Labeling	Avoid labeling self or others
Fortune-telling	Being curious about the future in a positive way
Mind reading	Asking for clarification when needed
Blaming	Avoiding blaming self or others, taking responsibility for changing
Never reflecting on your thinking	Using the Work to question your own thoughts whenever you feel sad, mad, or nervous
Thinking like a fat (sick or old) person	Thinking like a thin (healthy or young) person
Visualizing failure	Visualizing success

14

THE PASSION SOLUTION

Make Love to Recharge
Your Brain and Body

Sex . . . what else is free, fun, low calorie, and exercise?
—Barbara Wilson, M.D.,
neurologist and pain specialist

The symbol for love is a heart. "I love you with all my heart." "I give my heart to you." "My heart ACHES when you are gone." How silly, because most of love really happens in the Jell-O–like mass of tissue between your ears. But it just doesn't sound very romantic to say: "I love you with all my brain." "I give my brain to you." That sounds like a weird science experiment. Or, "My brain aches when you are gone."

It is your brain that is the organ of loving, learning, and behaving, and as such, at about three pounds, your brain is the largest sex organ in your body. And in this case, *size* really does matter. Research clearly tells us that being in a loving, healthy, affectionate relationship helps you be happier, live longer, have a better body, and even help to protect you from depression and memory problems. Having a healthy sex life is a key to having a better brain and body.

WHO WANTS TO LIVE TO A HUNDRED?

In August 1982, during my internship year on the sterile surgical floor at the Walter Reed Army Medical Center in Washington, D.C., Jesse was discharged from the hospital. He had been admitted for an emergency hernia operation two weeks earlier and there had been some minor complications. I remember

Jesse so vividly now because he was one hundred years old but talked and acted like a man thirty years younger. Mentally, he seemed every bit as sharp as any patient I had talked to that year or since. He and I developed a special bond, because unlike the surgery interns who spent a maximum of five minutes in his room each day, I spent hours over the course of his hospitalization talking to him about his life. The other interns were excited to learn about the latest operating techniques. I was interested in Jesse's story, and I wanted to know about Jesse's secrets for longevity and happiness.

Jesse had his one hundredth birthday in the hospital, and it was quite an event. His wife, actually his second one who was three decades younger, planned the event with the nursing staff. There was great love, playfulness, and physical affection between Jesse and his wife. Clearly, they still had the "hots" for each other.

Just before his discharge from the hospital, he saw me at the nurses' station writing notes. He enthusiastically waved me over to his room. His bags were packed and he was dressed in a brown suit, a white shirt, and a blue beret. He looked deeply into my eyes as he quietly asked me, "How long, Doc?"

"How long what?" I answered.

"How long before I can make love to my wife?"

I paused and he continued in a hushed voice, "You want to know the secret to live to a hundred, Doc? Never miss an opportunity to make love to your wife. How long should I wait?"

A slow smile came over my face. "I think a week or so and you should be fine. Be gentle at first." Then I gave him a hug and said, "Thank you. You have given me hope for many years to come."

Science finally caught up to Jesse twenty-five years later. Now there is a wealth of research connecting healthy sexual activity to longevity, as well as physical and mental health. While there are many well-known ingredients to a long life—good genes, a positive outlook, a curious mind, and exercise—frequent sexual activity is one of them too. In this chapter, I will illustrate the link between sexual frequency, sexual enjoyment, longevity, and mental and physical health.

> ### ACTION STEP
>
> If you want to live longer, get sick less often, feel more joy, experience less pain, and have better fertility, have more sex (preferably with a loving and committed partner).

HEALING: SEX IS ONE OF THE BEST MEDICINES

Many studies have investigated the relationship between healthy sexual activity and physical health. The potential dangers of sexual activity, including sexually transmitted diseases and unplanned pregnancies, have been widely reported, and rightly so. However, less publicized studies suggest that thoughtful sexual activity with a committed partner improves well-being by enhancing longevity, immune system function, joy, pain management, and sexual and reproductive health. These studies illustrate that sexual activity may be a preventive measure against the two leading causes of death in the United States: heart disease and cancer. Below are some of the ways sex can improve your health.

Longevity

Learning how to enhance the largest sex organ in the body (the brain) and using it well to intimately connect with others may add years to your life and is likely to make you much happier. Serious research on sexuality began in the United States in the 1950s by Alfred Kinsey. He reported that sex reduces stress, and that people who have fulfilling sex lives are less anxious, less violent, and less hostile. Current research bears this out, as physical touch increases the hormone oxytocin, which boosts trust and lowers cortisol levels, the hormone of chronic stress.

In a study done at Duke University, researchers followed 252 people over twenty-five years to determine the lifestyle factors important in influencing life span. Sexual frequency and past and present enjoyment of intercourse were three of the factors studied. For men, frequency of intercourse was a significant predictor of longevity. While frequency of intercourse was not predictive of longevity for women, those who reported past enjoyment of intercourse had greater longevity. This study suggested a positive association between sexual intercourse, pleasure, and longevity.

In 1976, research was published in *Psychosomatic Medicine* that concluded that an inability to reach orgasm may have a negative impact on women's hearts. Only 24 percent of women in the healthy control group reported sexual dissatisfaction, while 65 percent of the women who had heart attacks reported trouble with sex. In this study, the two most common causes of dissatisfaction in women were due to impotence and premature ejaculation in their husbands. Sexual health is not just an individual issue. It affects both parties' satisfaction and overall health.

A Swedish study found increased risk of death in men who gave up sexual intercourse earlier in life. The research was done on four hundred elderly men and women. At age seventy, they were given a survey of their sexual activity and then followed over time. Five years later, the death rates were significantly higher among the men who ceased sexual activity at earlier ages.

ACTION STEP

For men, studies show that engaging in sex two, three, or more times per week can lower the risk for heart attack, stroke, and death.

A daring group of researchers from Queens University in Belfast, Ireland, included a question about sexual activity in a long-term study of health. The authors studied nearly a thousand men between the ages of forty-five and fifty-nine living in or near Caerphilly, Wales. They recorded the frequency of sexual intercourse each week and within that month. The researchers divided the men into three groups: high orgasm frequency (those who had sex twice or more a week), an intermediate group, and low orgasm frequency (those who reported having sex less than monthly). The men were monitored again ten years later. Researchers found that the *death rate from all causes for the least sexually active men was twice as high as that of the most active group.* The death rate in the intermediate group was 1.6 times greater than that for the active group.

Many questions come to mind with this type of study, such as "Is it the orgasm that is healing? Or the touch and physical and emotional connection that comes with intercourse? Does poor health decrease sexual activity? Do other factors such as lack of exercise, alcohol, and/or depression cause both poor health and less sexual activity?" The researchers found that the robustness of their findings persisted even after adjusting for differences in age, social class, smoking, blood pressure, and evidence of existing coronary heart disease at the initial interview. This suggests a more likely protective role of sexual activity.

The researchers wrote, "The association between frequency of orgasm and mortality in the present study is at least—if not more—convincing on epidemiological and biological grounds than many of the associations reported in other studies and deserves further investigation to the same extent. Intervention programs could also be considered, perhaps based on the exciting, 'At least five a day' campaign aimed at increasing fruit and vegetable consumption—although the numerical imperative may have to be adjusted."

ACTION STEP

Looking for a physical activity that
burns calories, provides health
benefits, and is a lot of fun?
Sex is the answer.

In a 2001 follow-up study, this same research group found that having sex three or more times a week reduced the risk in males of having a heart attack or stroke by half. If a drug company came up with a medicine that performed as well, their stock would soar through the roof on Wall Street. Coauthor of the study Shah Ebrahim, Ph.D., underscored the results by saying, "The relationship found between frequency of sexual intercourse and mortality is of considerable public interest." There is truth to the saying that an apple a day keeps the doctor away. It may also be true that an orgasm a day keeps the coroner away.

Weight Loss, Overall Fitness

One of the most compelling benefits of sex comes from studies of aerobic fitness. It has been estimated that the act of intercourse burns about 200 calories, the equivalent of running vigorously for thirty minutes. Most couples average about twenty-four minutes for lovemaking. During orgasm, both heart rate and blood pressure typically double, all under the influence of oxytocin. Muscular contractions during intercourse work the pelvis, thighs, buttocks, arms, neck, and thorax. *Men's Health* magazine has gone so far as to call the bed the single greatest piece of exercise equipment ever invented.

More Youthful Appearance

Regular orgasms can even help you look younger. According to research done by David Weeks, a clinical neuropsychologist at the Royal Edinburgh Hospital, making love three times a week in a stress-free relationship can make you look ten years younger. Dr. Weeks studied more than 3,500 men and women between the ages of 18 and 102. He concluded that genetics were only 25 percent responsible for how young we look—the rest is due to behavior. In his study, a panel of judges viewed the participants through a one-way mirror and then guessed the age of each subject. A group of men and women whose ages were underestimated by seven to twelve years were labeled superyoung. Among these "superyoung" people, one of the strongest correlates of youthful appearance was an active sex life. They reported having sex at least three times per week, in comparison with the control group's average of twice a week. The superyoung were also found to be more comfortable and confident regarding their sexual identity.

Dr. Weeks, whose findings are published in *Superyoung: The Proven Way to Stay Young Forever,* says this is partly because sexual activity in women helps to trigger the production of a human growth hormone that helps them maintain their youthful looks. Sexual activity also pumps oxygen around the body, boosting the circulation and the flow of nutrients to the skin. Moreover, being in a sexual relationship can in itself be a good incentive to look after your appearance and stay in shape.

Higher Youth Hormone Levels (DHEA, Estrogen, and Testosterone)

Dr. Winnifred Cutler, a specialist in behavioral endocrinology, reported that women who enjoy regular sex had significantly higher levels of estrogen in their blood than women experiencing either infrequent sex or no sex at all. The benefits of estrogen include a healthy cardiovascular system, lower bad cholesterol, higher good cholesterol, increased bone density, and smoother skin. There is also growing evidence that estrogen is beneficial to brain function, as noted earlier. (See Chapter 7, "The Hormone Solution," and Chapter 12, "The Memory Solution.")

Another important hormone that seems to be affected by sexual activity is DHEA. Before orgasm, the level of DHEA spikes in the body to several times higher than normal. DHEA is believed to improve brain function, balance the immune system, help maintain and repair tissue, promote healthy skin, and possibly improve cardiovascular health.

Testosterone is increased through regular sexual activity. Testosterone can help strengthen bones and muscles, and is also beneficial to a healthy heart and brain. The risk for Alzheimer's disease is twice as high for people with lower testosterone levels. Low testosterone levels are also associated with a low libido. From this connection one could imply that if you are not interested in sex, your memory may be in jeopardy as well.

Boosted Immune Function

According to gynecologist Dr. Dudley Chapman, orgasms boost infection-fighting cells by up to 20 percent. Psychologists at Wilkes University in Pennsylvania found that students who had regular sexual activity had one-third higher levels of immunoglobulin A (IgA), an antibody that boosts the immune system and can help fight colds and flu. In one study it was reported that women who perform oral sex on their mates are less likely to suffer from preeclampsia, a condition that causes a dangerous spike in women's blood pressure during pregnancy. Plus, sperm carries TGF beta, a molecule that can boost the activities of her natural killer cells, which attack the rogue cells that give rise to tumors.

A study from the Institute for Advanced Study of Human Sexuality conducted by Dr. Ted McIlvenna looked at the sex lives of ninety thousand American adults and found that sexually active people take fewer sick leaves and enjoy life more.

Potential Cancer-Fighting Agent

A study conducted by Graham Giles from Australia concluded that the more often men ejaculate between the ages of twenty and fifty, the less likely they are to develop prostate cancer. A study published by the *British Journal of Urology International* asserted that men in their twenties can reduce by one-third their chance of getting prostate cancer by ejaculating more than five times a week.

Researchers have suggested that sexual expression may lead to a decreased risk of cancer because of the increase in levels of oxytocin and DHEA, which are associated with arousal and orgasm in women and men. A 1989 study found increased frequency of sexual activity correlated with a reduced incidence of breast cancer among women who had never had a child. The study examined fifty-one French women who were diagnosed with breast cancer less than three months prior to the interview. They were matched with ninety-five controls. A higher risk of breast cancer also correlated with lack of a sex partner and rare sexual intercourse, defined as less than once a month.

Better Sexual and Reproductive Behavior

Research done by Dr. Winnifred Cutler indicated that women who have intercourse with a male partner at least once a week are likely to have more regular menstrual cycles than women who are celibate or who have infrequent sex. In same-sex couples, women who engaged in sexual activity at least three times per week also had more regular cycles. In her "White Paper for Planned Parenthood," Dr. Cutler reported that sexual and reproductive health of both women and men is influenced by their sexual activity. She reports that regular sex can have positive effects on reproductive health. Here are several examples.

Fertility Frequent sexual activity may enhance fertility. Studies of menstrual cycle variability and frequency of intercourse have demonstrated that regular intimate sexual activity with a partner promotes fertility by regulating menstrual patterns.

> ### ACTION STEP
> Before you opt for expensive fertility treatments, try having more sex.

Menstrual cycle regularity A series of studies found that women who engaged in intercourse at least once a week had cycle lengths that were more regular than those of women who had sex sporadically or who were celibate.

Relief of menstrual cramps Nine percent of 1,900 women stated that they masturbated in the previous three months to relieve menstrual cramps.

Pregnancy A review of fifty-nine studies that were written between the years 1950 and 1996 concluded that sexual activity during pregnancy does not harm the fetus, as long as there are no other risk factors involved, such as sexually transmitted diseases. In addition, some research has shown that sexual activity throughout pregnancy may serve as protection against early delivery, especially during the third trimester (between the twenty-ninth and thirty-sixth weeks). Of more than 1,800 women, excluding those who could not have sex for medical reasons, preterm delivery was significantly reduced in the women who had intercourse late in their pregnancy.

Healthy prostate The prostate gland is responsible for producing some of the secretions in semen; sometimes the prostate becomes inflamed and painful (prostatitis). In single men who had prostatitis, over 30 percent who masturbated more frequently reported marked or moderate improvement of their symptoms. In addition, there is a suggestion that frequent ejaculation may help prevent chronic nonbacterial infections of the prostate.

Better Sleep
Sexual release can help people go to sleep. Orgasm causes a surge in oxytocin and endorphins that may act as a sedative. One study found that 32 percent of 1,866 U.S. women who reported masturbating in the previous three months did so to help go to sleep. As most women know, men often go to sleep shortly after having sex.

Pain Relief

Studies have shown that orgasms can help treat some types of pain. Research by Beverly Whipple and Barry Komisaruk of Rutgers University, New Jersey, found that through regular orgasm women had higher pain thresholds when suffering from conditions ranging from whiplash to arthritis. Immediately before orgasm, levels of the hormone oxytocin surge to five times their normal level. This in turn releases endorphins, which alleviate the pain. In women, sex also promotes the production of estrogen, which can reduce the pain of PMS.

Dr. Whipple's research identified the female G-spot, the vaginal "on switch" for female arousal, on the front inside wall of the vagina, opposite the clitoris. She showed that gentle pressure to this area raised pain thresholds by 40 percent and that during orgasm women could tolerate up to 110 percent more pain. In brain imaging research to understand this finding, Dr. Whipple found that during peak arousal, the painkilling center deep in the brain is activated. Signals from this part of the brain give orders to the body to release endorphins and corticosteroids. These chemicals help to temporarily numb the pain from many different causes. Activating this region also has a calming effect and can reduce anxiety.

Migraine Relief

Research suggests that when your partner says, "Not tonight, honey, I have a headache," you can help her with a loving roll in the sack. A study from the Southern Illinois University School of Medicine found that having an orgasm could help alleviate the pain from migraines. Of the fifty-two migraine sufferers used in the study, sixteen reported considerable relief after an orgasm and another eight had their headaches completely gone. Since 2001, a couple of case studies reported that orgasm did help them with pain relief. An earlier study of eighty-three women who suffered from migraine headaches showed that orgasm resulted in at least some relief for more than half of them. Using orgasm to help alleviate migraine pain is not as reliable as prescription medications, but it does work much faster, is cheaper, has fewer side effects, and is more fun.

Treatment of Depression

Orgasms can also have an antidepressant effect. Orgasms cause intense increased activity in the deep limbic parts of the brain, which settle down after sex. Antidepressants tend to calm activity in the limbic parts of the brain as well. People who engaged in regular sexual activity experience less depression, and orgasm frequency may be one reason why.

ACTION STEP

If you have symptoms of depression, regular sexual activity may help alleviate them.

When a man has an orgasm, an area in the limbic system, called the meso-diencephalic junction, is activated. Cells in the region are known to produce some of the pleasure chemicals discussed earlier. At the same time, researchers have shown that the amygdala, a fear center in the brain, becomes less active in men's brains during sex. The region also is involved in vigilance, so animals and people may need to shut down that part of the brain to avoid getting distracted during sex. Calming the fear center might also help with a man's sense of commitment. Prostaglandins, fatty acids found in semen, are absorbed by the vagina and may have a role in modulating female hormones and moods.

Gordon Gallup, a psychologist at the State University of New York Albany, headed a study that found women whose male partners did not use condoms were less subject to depression than those whose partners did. One theory put forth was that prostaglandin, a hormone found in semen, may be absorbed in the female genital tract, thus modulating female hormones.

Other research has indicated that high sexual activity is associated with lower risk and incidence of depression and suicide. A Canadian study that examined the correlation between sexuality and mental health found that celibacy was correlated with high scores on depression and suicidality indexes.

Improved Sense of Smell

After sex, production of the hormone prolactin surges. This, in turn, causes stem cells in the brain to develop new neurons in the brain's olfactory bulb, its smell center, improving one's sense of smell.

The Key to Health

Regular sexual contact, especially with a committed partner, helps to keep your body and brain healthy. Do not use excuses, such as you are too tired or too busy for physical affection. Also, try to avoid spending too much time at work at the exclusion of social endeavors. A lack of relationships sets up humans to be depressed or to seek pleasure through solitary sexual activities, such as on the Internet, or to turn to drugs, alcohol, gambling, or other addictions, which are not good for the brain. Men and women need touching, eye contact, and sexual connection to stay healthy. When you feel loved, nurtured, cared for, supported, and intimate, you are much more likely to be happier and healthier. You have a much lower risk of getting sick and, if you do, a much greater chance of surviving.

Happiness

There is happy news for people who have more activity in the bedroom than in their bank accounts. After evaluating the levels of sexual activity and happiness in sixteen thousand people, Dartmouth College economist David Blanchflower and Andrew Oswald of the University of Warwick in England found that sex so positively influenced happiness that they estimated increasing intercourse from once a month to once a week is equivalent to the happiness generated by getting an additional $50,000 in income for the average American.

In addition, they reported that despite what most people think, people who make more money do not necessarily have more sex. There was no difference, in their study, between sexual frequency and income levels. The happiest people in the study were married people who had, on average, 30 percent more sex than single folks. The economists estimated that a lasting marriage equated to the happiness generated by an extra $100,000 annually, while divorce depleted an estimated $66,000 annually worth of happiness. Taking care of your marriage can save you lots of money.

SUMMARY OF SOME OF THE HEALTH BENEFITS OF REGULAR SEXUAL CONTACT FOR WOMEN

- More regular menstrual cycles
- Lighter periods
- Better memories
- Better bladder control
- Reduced stress
- Increased youth-promoting hormone DHEA
- Weight control—sex burns about 200 calories per half hour; yoga, 114; dancing (rock), 129; walking (3 mph), 153; weight training, 153.
- More fertile menstrual cycles
- Better moods
- Pain relief
- Fewer colds and flu
- Staying in shape
- Increased testosterone and estrogen

SUMMARY OF SOME OF THE HEALTH BENEFITS
OF REGULAR SEXUAL CONTACT FOR MEN

- Increased heart rate variability (a sign of heart health and a calmer mind)
- Improved heart cardiovascular function (three times a week decreases risk of heart attack or stroke by half)
- Higher testosterone levels (stronger bones and muscles)
- Improved prostate function
- Improved sleep

TREATING LOW LIBIDO

As you can see, scientific research demonstrates a positive correlation between regular sexual activity and physical and mental health. I gave a lecture on this topic to the Samueli Women & Wellness Conference in Southern California and a married woman came up to me afterward and said that she would rather be doing anything than having sex. She asked me what should she do, as she did not want to die early.

I replied, "There are many ways to stay healthy and live a long life, such as a healthy diet, exercise, mental exercise, supplements, and having an optimistic outlook, but I would hate to see you miss out on the added benefit of a healthy sex life for you and your husband. Low libido is often associated with low testosterone levels, low estrogen levels, depression, a conflicted marriage, or past emotional trauma. Finding and fixing the problem may give you many rewards."

USE YOUR BRAIN TO IMPROVE
YOUR BODY'S SEXUAL RESPONSE

In my book *The Brain in Love*, I wrote about Tantric sexual practices, and was fascinated by the concept, which involves using the mind—the brain, that is—to enhance sexual response and intimacy. I wanted to experience it for myself and thought it would be a wonderful way to enhance my relationship with my wife, Tana. Finding someone whom my wife and I both trusted enough to discuss such personal things took quite a bit of research. In the end, TJ Bartel, an advanced certified Tantra educator, became our teacher. Our experience with him was amazing and transformative. It deepened our relationship in ways we couldn't even have imagined. TJ was such a wonderful teacher that I felt as if I had to share his knowledge with everyone I knew.

One of the basic beliefs of Tantra is that everybody has energy—in particular, sexual energy—within their body and that everybody has the potential to channel that energy within the body and direct it to others. By using your brain, you can learn to harness your sexual energy and circulate it throughout your body to heighten your body's response, intensify the lovemaking experience, and increase the healing power of sex.

When I first heard about moving energy, I thought, "What the heck does that mean? How do you move energy?" But there are many practices in both Eastern and Western religions that practice this. Meditation is a way to move energy. What we see in our brain imaging work is that when people pray or meditate, they dramatically move the energy in their brain to the most human, thoughtful part of the brain. I once did a brain imaging study with a professor from the University of California, Irvine, on qigong, which is the practice of mastering your energy within yourself and directing it to others in a healing way. The results were astounding. We found that the qigong master was able to direct energy at other people and immediately change their brainwave patterns and increase blood flow to their brain.

For most people, sexual activity is a time when they turn off their brain and focus on the feelings in their body. But with Tantric sex, you use your brain to control and enhance what your body is feeling for the ultimate brain-body connection. If you would like to learn more about Tantric sex and how to move sexual energy, check out my book *The Brain in Love* or the six-audio CD set I did with TJ Bartel called *Create More Passion Tonight*. They are both available at www.amenclinics.com.

SUPPLEMENTS THAT MAY INSPIRE PASSION

The following supplements can fuel passion and increase your enjoyment of sexual activity. For more information on these supplements, see Appendix C, "The Supplement Solution," or visit www.amenclinics.com.

- Fish oil is a wonderful supplement to enhance your love life. It helps with mood and joint pain, so you may be happier, less irritable, and subsequently feel more sexual, plus be more limber.
- If you tend to be anxious and worried, 5-HTP can help to boost serotonin and give you more emotional freedom and energy to put toward your sex life.

- If you tend to have low energy and feel negative, SAMe may help to boost your energy and mood, and it also helps with joint pain.
- Ginkgo biloba boosts blood flow to all organs in the body.
- Panax ginseng can increase energy, decrease stress, and improve endurance.

SEXY FOODS TO TRY FOR MORE PASSION

- Almonds enhance phenylethylamine (PEA), a chemical that boosts the alerting response in the brain that something fun is about to happen.
- Apples sweeten the breath.
- Asparagus, rich in vitamin E, is essential for hormone building.
- Avocados have PEA, B_6, and potassium.
- Bananas contain the bromelain enzyme, which is believed to improve male libido.
- Cabbage helps to increase circulation.
- Celery contains androsterone, a hormone released by male sweat that turns women on.
- Chili peppers have capsaicin, which stimulates nerve endings and raises heart rate.
- Chocolate increases PEA and theobromine, a substance similar to caffeine.
- Cheese actually contains more PEA than chocolate.
- Eggs have B vitamins that help balance hormones.
- Figs are high in amino acids that increase libido.
- Garlic contains allicin, an ingredient that increases blood flow to the sexual organs.
- Nutmeg significantly increases sexual activity in rats, so if you are married to a rat, it may be helpful. . . .
- Oysters are high in zinc, which helps produce testosterone and dopamine for stimulation.

The Passion Solution

Passion Robbers	Passion Boosters
Any brain problems	Effectively treating any brain problems
Lack of sleep	Adequate sleep (at least seven hours)
Hormonal fluctuations	Balanced hormones
Alcohol	Freedom from alcohol
Depression	Journaling when sad or anxious, treatment
Negative thinking	Kill the ANTs (automatic negative thoughts)
Chronic pain	Natural pain relief (SAMe, fish oil, 5-HTP)
	Sexy scents for men: lavender, pumpkin pie, black licorice, doughnuts, orange, cheese pizza, roast beef, cinnamon buns
	Sexy scents for women: baby powder, cucumber, black licorice, lavender, pumpkin pie
	Scents for relaxation (for those who need calm before sex): sandalwood, marjoram, lemon, chamomile, bergamot
	Scents for stimulation (for those who need to be activated before sex): jasmine, ylang-ylang, rose, patchouli, peppermint, clove

15

THE BRAIN HEALTH SOLUTION

Treat Brain Disorders to Protect
Against Physical Illnesses

Having a great brain is essential to having a great body.

Your brain and your body are totally connected to each other. Mental (brain) health illnesses, such as depression, bipolar disorder, anxiety disorders, obsessive-compulsive disorders, schizophrenia, grief, posttraumatic stress disorder, substance-abuse problems, eating disorders, and gambling addictions all take a very real toll on your body and how you look and feel. These disorders are intensely stressful, rob you of sleep, alter your appetite, and increase your wrinkles and fat. It is essential to treat these brain health problems as early as possible so they do not make you look and feel old. In this chapter, I will give you a brief overview of the common mental health problems and some ideas on when and how to seek help.

MOOD DISORDERS

Depression

Depressive disorders have been associated with heart disease, immune system dysfunction, and Alzheimer's disease. In Chapter 8, "The Heart Solution," you saw how depression lowers survival rates among heart attack patients. The same thing occurs in cancer patients. A review of twenty-six studies involving more than nine thousand cancer patients revealed that death rates among those diagnosed with minor or major depression were 39 percent higher than in those who weren't depressed. The physical toll of depressive disorders is easy to see on the faces and posture of those who suffer with them.

Barbara, a fifty-two-year-old bookkeeper, wife, and mother of two, was referred to me because she was tired all the time. Her family physician ruled out the physical causes of fatigue and thought she was overstressed. Additionally, she had trouble concentrating at work and experienced difficulty sleeping. Her sex drive was gone, her appetite was poor, and she had no interest in doing things with her family. Barbara would start to cry for no apparent reason, and she even began to entertain desperate thoughts of suicide. Barbara was depressed.

Depression is a series of common mental illnesses. Studies reveal that at any point in time, about 6 percent of the population will have a significant depression. Only 20 to 25 percent of these people ever seek help. This is unfortunate, because depression is a very treatable problem.

The following is a list of symptoms commonly associated with depression:

Sad, blue, or gloomy mood
Low energy, frequent fatigue
Lack of ability to feel pleasure in usually pleasurable activities
Irritability
Poor concentration, distractibility, or poor memory
Suicidal thoughts, feelings of meaninglessness
Feelings of hopelessness, helplessness, guilt, and worthlessness
Changes in sleep, either poor sleep with frequent awakenings or increased sleep
Changes in appetite, either marked decreased or increased
Social withdrawal
Low self-esteem

In evaluating all psychiatric problems, it is helpful to take a bio/psycho/social approach to understanding them.

Biological factors There are several important biological factors to look for in depression.

It is important to consider the family history. We know there is often a genetic link to depression, and it often runs in families where there has been alcohol abuse.

It is also important to evaluate patients from a medical point of view, as there are a number of illnesses that can cause depression. These include thyroid disease, infectious illnesses, cancer, and certain forms of anemia. A heart attack, stroke, or brain trauma can also leave a person vulnerable to depression.

Periods of dramatic hormonal shifts (postpartum or menopause) often precipitate problems with depression.

Additionally, certain medications can cause depression. Most notable among these are birth control pills, certain blood pressure or cardiac medications, steroids, and chronic pain-control medicines.

In evaluating depression, it is essential to take a thorough alcohol and drug abuse history. Chronic alcohol or marijuana use often causes depression, while amphetamine or cocaine withdrawal is often accompanied by serious suicidal thoughts.

Psychological factors The psychological factors to look for in depression include

Major losses, such as the death of a loved one; the breakup of a
   romantic relationship; or the loss of a job, self-esteem, status, health,
   or purpose
Multiple childhood traumas, such as physical or sexual abuse
Negative thinking that erodes self-esteem and drives mood down
Learned helplessness—the belief that no matter what you do, things won't
   change. This comes from being exposed to environments where you are
   continually frustrated from reaching your goals.

Social factors The social factors or current life stresses to evaluate in depression include

Marital problems
Family dysfunction
Financial difficulties
Work-related problems

In Barbara's case, her physical examination was normal, but her mother had periods of depression, and she had an aunt who killed herself. Psychologically, she had a very critical father and subsequently was extremely self-critical herself. Socially, her marriage had been difficult for the past several years, and she was often fighting with her teenage daughter.

The best results in treating any emotional illness occur with a bio/psycho/social approach. Barbara was placed on antidepressant supplements and learned to be significantly less critical of herself. We also spent time working on her marriage and her relationship with her teenage daughter. In ten weeks,

ACTION STEP

Don't ignore symptoms of depression. It can sabotage your efforts to get the body you want.

she felt more energetic and was able to concentrate. Her mood was good. She slept well, and her appetite returned. She also got along better with her spouse and daughter.

Depression is a very treatable illness. We have much better treatments than we did in 1980. Early detection and treatment from a bio/psycho/social perspective is important to a full and complete recovery. From a biological standpoint, we think of medication or supplements and proper diet and exercise. Exercise has been found in some studies to be as effective as medication but cheaper and with fewer side effects (most side effects of exercise are positive). Psychotherapy has also been found to be helpful in treating depression. The two best-studied forms of psychotherapy for depression are cognitive therapy, which teaches patients to counteract the negative thoughts that invariably surface with depression, and interpersonal psychotherapy, which teaches patients to have more effective relationships.

In treating depression, it is often best to take a comprehensive approach that includes several or all of these methods. However, many people look solely to antidepressants to lift the symptoms of depression. The use of antidepressant medication in the United States doubled from 1996 to 2005, according to a study in the *Archives of General Psychiatry*. In 1996, about 13 million people (about 6 percent of the population) were prescribed an antidepressant. That number soared to 27 million people (more than 10 percent of the population) by 2005. The study reported that less than 32 percent of the people being treated with antidepressants see a mental health professional for treatment. Instead, they are receiving a prescription from a general practitioner. In addition, it found that the use of psychotherapy among people being treated with antidepressants has decreased 10 percent.

These trends concern me. Through our brain imaging work at the Amen Clinics, we have identified seven different subtypes of depression, and each one requires individualized treatment. Prescribing antidepressants as a one-size-fits-all treatment doesn't work and could be dangerous for some people. In addition, psychotherapy is a proven technique that has been found helpful in the treatment of depression. Plus, antidepressant medications come with a host of unwanted side effects. In many cases, I recommend trying natural therapies first, including getting daily exercise, practicing positive thinking, and taking fish oil supplements.

Bipolar Disorder

Another type of mood disorder is called bipolar disorder, where people cycle between two poles. There may be periods of depression that alternate with periods of high, manic, irritable, or elated moods. Mania is categorized as a state distinct from one's normal self, where a person has greater energy, racing thoughts, more impulsivity, a decreased need for sleep, and a sense of grandiosity. It is often associated with periods of hypersexuality, hyperreligiosity, or spending sprees. Sometimes it is also associated with hallucinations or delusions.

In treating the depressive part of the cycle, both pharmaceutical and supplement antidepressants have been known to stimulate manic episodes. It is important to vigorously treat this disorder, as it has been associated with marital problems, substance abuse, and suicide. The stress that comes from marital strife and the effects of alcohol or drug abuse can take a toll on your physical health and appearance.

Here is a list of symptoms often associated with bipolar disorder:

- Periods of abnormally elevated, depressed, or anxious mood
- Periods of decreased need for sleep, feeling energetic on dramatically less sleep than usual
- Periods of grandiose notions, ideas, or plans
- Periods of increased talking or pressured speech
- Periods of too many thoughts racing through the mind
- Periods of markedly increased energy
- Periods of poor judgment that leads to risk-taking behavior (separate from usual behavior)
- Periods of inappropriate social behavior
- Periods of irritability or aggression
- Periods of delusional or psychotic thinking

Bipolar disorder used to be called manic-depressive illness and is thought to be the more classic form of this disorder. In recent years, a milder form of the disorder called Bipolar II has been described that is associated with depressive episodes and milder "hypomanic" issues.

The treatment for bipolar disorder, both I and II, is usually medication, such as lithium or anticonvulsants such as Depakote or Lamictal. In recent years, there is literature to suggest that high doses of omega-3 fatty acids—found in fish or flaxseed oil—can also be helpful.

Anxiety Disorders

There are four common types of anxiety disorders that can affect people's brains and bodies in a negative way: panic disorders, agoraphobia, obsessive-compulsive disorders, and post-traumatic stress disorders. I will briefly discuss each of these and their treatments.

Panic Disorder

All of a sudden, your heart starts to pound. You get this feeling of incredible dread. Your breathing rate goes faster. You start to sweat. Your muscles get tight, and your hands feel like ice. Your mind starts to race about every terrible thing that could possibly happen, and you feel as though you are going to lose your mind if you don't get out of the current situation. You have just had a panic attack. Panic attacks are one of the most common brain disorders, and they have a powerful effect on the body. It is estimated that 6 to 7 percent of adults will suffer from recurrent panic attacks at some point in their lives. They often begin in late adolescence or early adulthood but may spontaneously occur later in life. If a person has three attacks in a three-week period, doctors make a diagnosis of a panic disorder.

In a typical panic attack, a person has at least four of the following twelve symptoms:

Shortness of breath
Heart pounding
Chest pain
Choking or smothering feelings
Dizziness
Tingling of hands or feet
Feeling unreal
Hot or cold flashes
Sweating
Faintness
Trembling or shaking
A fear of dying or going crazy

When the panic attacks first start, many people end up in the emergency room because they think they are having a heart attack. Some people even end up being admitted to the hospital.

Anticipation anxiety is one of the most difficult symptoms for a person who has a panic disorder. These people are often extremely skilled at predicting the worst in situations. In fact, it is often the anticipation of a bad event that brings on a panic attack. For example, you are in the grocery store and worry that you are going to have an anxiety attack and pass out on the floor. Then, you predict, everyone in the store will look at you and laugh. Pretty quickly, the symptoms begin. Sometimes a panic disorder can become so severe that a person begins to avoid almost any situation outside of their house—a condition called agoraphobia (see below).

Panic attacks can occur for a variety of different reasons. Sometimes they are caused by medical illnesses, such as hyperthyroidism, which is why it is always important to have a physical examination and screening blood work. Sometimes panic attacks can be brought on by excessive caffeine intake or alcohol withdrawal. Hormonal changes also seem to play a role. Panic attacks in women are seen more frequently at the end of their menstrual cycle, after having a baby, or during menopause. Traumatic events from the past that somehow get unconsciously triggered can also precipitate a series of attacks. Commonly, there is a family history of panic attacks, alcohol abuse, or other mental illnesses.

On SPECT scans, we often see hyperactivity in the basal ganglia, or sometimes temporal lobe problems. Psychotherapy and the use of supplements, such as GABA, B_6, magnesium, and kava kava, are my preferred treatments and work by balancing brain function. Medications can be helpful. Unfortunately, the most helpful medications are also addictive, so care is needed.

Agoraphobia

The name *agoraphobia* comes from a Greek word that means "fear of the marketplace." In behavioral terms, it is the fear of being alone in public places. The underlying worry is that the person will lose control or become incapacitated, and no one will be there to help. People afflicted with this phobia begin to avoid being in crowds, in stores, or on busy streets. They are often afraid of being in tunnels, on bridges, in elevators, or on public transportation. They usually insist that a family member or a friend accompany them

ACTION STEP

If you have panic attacks, get a checkup. They can be caused by certain medical conditions.

> ### ACTION STEP
> The supplements 5-HTP and St. John's wort increase serotonin and calm the anterior cingulate gyrus (the brain's gear shifter) and may ease symptoms of agoraphobia and OCD.

when they leave home. If the fear establishes a foothold in the person, it may affect his or her whole life. Normal activities become increasingly restricted as the fears or avoidance behaviors dominate.

Agoraphobic symptoms often begin in the late teen years or early twenties, but I have seen them start when a person is in their fifties or sixties. Often, without knowing what is wrong, people will try to medicate themselves with excessive amounts of alcohol or drugs. This illness occurs more frequently in women, and many who have it experienced significant separation anxiety as children. Additionally, there may be a history of excessive anxiety, panic attacks, depression, or alcohol abuse in relatives.

Agoraphobia often evolves out of panic attacks that seem to occur "out of the blue," for no apparent reason. These attacks are so frightening that the person begins to avoid any situation that may be in any way associated with the fear. I think these initial panic attacks are often triggered by unconscious events or anxieties from the past. For example, I once treated a patient who had been raped as a teenager in a park late at night. When she was twenty-eight, she had her first panic attack while walking late at night in a park with her husband. It was the park setting late at night that she associated with the fear of being raped and which triggered the panic attack. Agoraphobia is a very frightening illness to the patient and his or her family. With effective, early intervention, however, there is significant hope for recovery.

The scan findings and treatment are similar to those for people with panic disorder. The one difference is that people with agoraphobia often have increased anterior cingulate gyrus activity and get stuck in their fear of having more panic attacks. Getting stuck in the fear often prevents them from leaving home. Using medications, such as Prozac and Lexapro, or supplements, such as 5-HTP and St. John's wort, is often helpful.

Obsessive-Compulsive Disorder

The hallmarks of obsessive-compulsive disorder (OCD) are recurrent thoughts that seem outside a person's control or compulsive behaviors that a person knows make no sense, but he feels compelled to do anyway. The obsessive thoughts may involve violence (such as killing one's child), contamination (such as becoming infected by shaking hands), or doubt (such as the worry of having hurt someone in a traffic accident even though no such accident occurred). Many efforts are made to suppress or resist these thoughts, but the more a person tries to control them, the more powerful they can become.

The most common compulsions involve hand-washing, counting, checking, and touching. These behaviors are often performed according to certain rules in a very strict or rigid manner. For example, a person with a counting compulsion may feel the need to count every crack on the pavement on their way to work or school. What would be a five-minute walk for most people could turn into a three- or four-hour trip for the person with OCD. Many of these types of behaviors can stand in the way of your efforts to get a better body.

They have an urgent internal sense of "I have to do it." A part of the individual generally recognizes the senselessness of the behavior and doesn't get pleasure from carrying it out, although doing it often provides a release of tension. Over the years, I have treated many people with OCD, the youngest of whom was five years old. He had a checking compulsion and had to check the house locks at night as many as twenty to thirty times before he could fall asleep. The oldest person I treated with this disorder was eighty-three. She had obsessive sexual thoughts that made her feel dirty inside. It got to the point where she would lock all her doors, draw all the window shades, turn off the lights, take the phone off the hook, and sit in the middle of a dark room trying to catch the abhorrent sexual thoughts as they came into her mind.

On SPECT studies, we often see excessive activity in the basal ganglia and anterior cingulate gyrus. Behavior therapy can be helpful and has been shown to improve brain function. Using medications, such as Prozac and Lexapro, or supplements, such as 5-HTP and St. John's wort, to increase serotonin and calm these parts of the brain is often helpful.

Post-traumatic Stress Disorder

Joanne, a thirty-four-year-old travel agent, was held up in her office at gunpoint by two men. Four or five times during the robbery, one of the men held a gun to her head and said he was going to kill her. She graphically imagined her brain being splattered with blood against the wall. Near the end of this fifteen-minute ordeal, they made her take off all her clothes. She pictured herself being brutally raped by them. They left without touching her, but locked her in a closet.

Since that time, her life had been thrown into turmoil. She felt tense and was plagued by flashbacks and nightmares of the robbery. Her stomach was in knots, and she had a constant headache. Whenever she went out, she felt panicky. She was frustrated that she could not calm her body—her heart raced, she was short of breath, and her hands were constantly cold and sweaty. She hated how she felt, and she was angry about how her nice life had turned into a nightmare. What was most upsetting to her were the ways that the robbery affected her marriage and her child. Her baby picked up the tension and was very fussy. Every time she tried to make love with her husband, she began to cry and get images of the men raping her.

Joanne had post-traumatic stress disorder (PTSD), a brain reaction to severe traumatic events such as a robbery, rape, car accident, earthquake, tornado, or even a volcanic eruption. Her symptoms are classic for PTSD, especially the flashbacks and nightmares of the event.

Perhaps the worst symptoms, however, come from the horrible thoughts about what never happened, such as seeing her brain splattered against the wall and being raped. These thoughts were registered in her subconscious as fact, and until she entered treatment, she was not able to recognize how much damage they had been doing to her. For example, when she imagined that she was being raped, a part of her began to believe that she actually was raped. The first time she had her period after the robbery she began to cry, because she was relieved she was not pregnant by robbers, even though they never touched her. A part of her even believed she was dead, because she had so vividly pictured her own death. A significant portion of her treatment was geared to counteract these erroneous subconscious conclusions.

Without treatment, PTSD can literally ruin a person's life. The most effective treatment is usually psychotherapy. One type of psychotherapy that I think works especially well for PTSD is called eye movement desensitization and reprocessing (EMDR). Depending on the severity of PTSD, certain types of medications and supplements can also be helpful.

DRUG AND ALCOHOL ADDICTION AND ABUSE

Many people use alcohol or drugs to medicate underlying brain systems that are misfiring. Downers, such as alcohol, marijuana, sedatives, and painkillers, are used to calm hyperactive brain systems. Uppers, such as cocaine and methamphetamine, are used to stimulate underactive areas of the brain. The problem is that most of these substances are addictive and cause damage to the brain and body. Sometimes the damage is permanent.

Substance abuse has a serious negative impact on health. The list of health problems from alcohol and drugs fills volumes of books. Here are just some of the many physical effects of alcoholism:

- Increased risk for heart disease, stroke, and cancer
- Liver inflammation, which can lead to cirrhosis
- Erectile dysfunction
- Stomach problems
- Nutritional deficiencies

> **ACTION STEP**
> Go through the following list of symptoms of excessive alcohol or drug use and check off those that apply to you. This will give you an idea if this area is a problem for you or someone you know.

In addition, alcohol and drug use impair your memory and judgment, preventing you from making the best decisions for your overall health and increasing the likelihood of engaging in bad brain habits.

Denial is frequently strong in substance abusers. The person with the problem is usually the last one to recognize that a problem exists. Alcohol- and drug-related problems are similar in many ways. I have chosen to lump these two groups together for simplicity.

Note: Alcohol includes any beverage or medication that contains any alcohol—from beer to wine to hard liquor, or even some cough preparations. Drugs include any mind-altering substances that produce stimulant, depressant, or euphoric effects—amphetamines, barbiturates, marijuana, cocaine, heroin, PCP, and so on.

LIST OF EXCESSIVE ALCOHOL- OR DRUG-USE SYMPTOMS

___ Increasing consumption of alcohol or drugs, whether on a regular or sporadic basis, with frequent and perhaps unintended episodes of intoxication

___ Use of drugs or alcohol as a means of handling problems

___ Obvious preoccupation with alcohol or drugs and the expressed need to have them

___ Gulping of drinks or using large quantities of drugs

___ The need for increasing quantities of alcohol or the drug to obtain the same "buzz"

___ Tendency toward making alibis and weak excuses for drinking or drug use

___ Needing to have others cover for you, either at work or at home

___ Refusal to concede what is obviously excessive consumption and expressing annoyance when the subject is mentioned

___ Frequent absenteeism from the job, especially if occurring in a pattern, such as following weekends and holidays (Monday-morning "flu")

___ Repeated changes in jobs, particularly if to successively lower levels or employment in a capacity beneath ability, education, and background

___ Shabby appearance, poor hygiene, and behavior and social adjustment inconsistent with previous levels or expectations

___ Persistent vague body complaints without apparent cause, particularly those of trouble sleeping, abdominal problems, headaches, or loss of appetite

___ Multiple contacts with the health care system

___ Persistent marital problems, perhaps multiple marriages

___ History of arrests for intoxicated driving or disorderly conduct

___ Unusual anxiety or obvious moodiness

___ Withdrawal symptoms on stopping (tremors, feeling extremely anxious, craving drugs or alcohol, vomiting, etc.); an alcoholic or drug abuser has usually tried to stop many times but was unable to withstand the symptoms of withdrawal.

___ Hearing voices or seeing things that aren't there is not uncommon.

___ Blackouts (times you cannot remember)

___ Memory impairment

___ Drinking or using drugs alone; early-morning use; secretive use

___ DENIAL in the face of an obvious problem

If you checked any of these symptoms, you or your loved one may be abusing drugs or alcohol.

My favorite definition of an alcoholic or drug addict is anyone who has gotten into trouble (legal, relational, or work related) while drinking or using drugs, then continues to use them. They did not learn from the previous experience. A rational person would realize that he or she has trouble handling the alcohol or drugs and would stay away from them. Unfortunately, many people with these problems have to experience repeated failures because of the substance use, and thus hit "rock bottom" before treatment is sought.

There has been a very helpful trend in medicine over the last ten years to classify alcoholism and excessive drug use as illnesses, instead of morally weak behavior. The American Medical Association, the World Health Organization, and many other professional groups regard these as specific disease entities.

Untreated, these diseases progress to serious physical complications that often lead to death. Here are some important facts you need to know about alcohol and drug abuse:

ACTION STEP

If you or a loved one is using drugs or alcohol excessively, first admit that you have a problem, then seek professional help.

- Addictions often run in families. The more relatives a person has who are alcoholics or addicts, the more likely the person is or will become dependent on these chemicals. As a rule of thumb: one parent = 25 percent chance; two parents or one parent and one sibling = 50 percent chance; three or more family members = 75+ percent chance.
- Alcoholism or drug addiction shortens life expectancy by an estimated ten to fifteen years.
- Alcoholism and drug addictions occur in about fifteen million Americans. If this problem applies to you, you are not alone.
- There is no typical person with alcoholism or drug addictions. These diseases affect people in all socioeconomic classes.
- Drunken driving or driving under the influence of drugs is responsible for well over 50 percent of the highway traffic fatalities.
- Alcoholism and drug addictions are treatable. Treatment for alcohol or drug abusers and their families is widely available today in all parts of the country.

In treating substance abuse, it is important to recognize and treat any underlying cause of the problem, such as unrecognized depression, bipolar disorder, anxiety disorders, or ADD. New medications have been developed that have been found helpful in alleviating withdrawal symptoms and decreasing cravings for the substances. Psychotherapy and support groups are often helpful.

ATTENTION DEFICIT DISORDER

Do you often feel restless? Have trouble concentrating? Have trouble with impulsiveness, either doing or saying things you wish you hadn't? Do you fail to finish many projects you start? Are you easily bored or quick to anger? If the answer to most of these questions is yes, you might have attention deficit disorder (ADD).

ADD is the most common brain problem in children, affecting 5 to 10 percent of them in the United States, and one of the most common problems in adults. The main symptoms of ADD are a short attention span, distractibility, disorganization, procrastination, and poor internal supervision. It is often, but not always, associated with impulsive behavior and hyperactivity or restlessness. Until recently, most people thought that children outgrew this disorder during their teenage years. For many, this is false. While it is true that the hyperactivity lessens over time, the other symptoms of impulsivity, distractibility, and a short attention span remain for most sufferers into adulthood. Current research shows that 60 to 80 percent of ADD children never fully outgrow this disorder.

Over the years, I have seen thousands of children who had ADD. When I meet with their parents and take a good family history, I find that there is about an 80 percent chance that at least one of the parents also had symptoms of ADD as a child and may, in fact, still be showing symptoms as an adult. Many of the parents were never diagnosed. Not infrequently, I learn of ADD in adults when parents tell me that they have tried their child's medication (not something I recommend) and found it to be very helpful. They report it helped them concentrate for longer periods of time, become more organized, and be less impulsive.

Common symptoms of the adult form of ADD include poor organization and planning, procrastination, trouble listening carefully to directions, and excessive traffic violations. Additionally, people with adult ADD are often late for appointments, frequently misplace things, may be quick to anger, and have poor follow-through. There may also be frequent, impulsive job changes and poor financial management. Substance abuse, especially alcohol or amphetamines and cocaine, and low self-esteem are also common. There is often an inability to stick with diet and exercise programs.

Many people do not recognize the seriousness of this disorder and just pass off these kids and adults as lazy, defiant, or willful. Yet ADD is a serious disorder. Left untreated, it affects a person's self-esteem, social relationships, ability to learn and work, and ability to be as healthy as possible. Several studies have shown that ADD children use twice as many medical services as non-ADD kids, 52 percent of untreated adults abuse substances, and teens and adults with ADD have more traffic accidents.

Many adults tell me that when they were children, they were in trouble all the time and had a real sense that there was something very different about them. Even though many of the adults I treat with ADD are very bright, they are frequently frustrated by not living up to their potential.

From our research with SPECT scans, it is clear that ADD is a brain disorder, but not one simple disorder. I described six different types of ADD in my book *Healing ADD*. The most common feature among the six types of ADD is decreased activity in the prefrontal cortex with a concentration task. This means that the harder a person tries, the less brain activity they have to work with. Many people with ADD self-medicate with stimulants, such as caffeine,

nicotine, cocaine, or methamphetamine, to increase activity in the PFC.
They also tend to self-medicate with
conflict-seeking behavior. If they can get
someone upset, it helps to stimulate
their brain. Of course, they have no idea
that they do this. I call it unconscious,
brain-driven behavior. But if you are
around ADD people long enough, you
will see and feel the conflict-seeking behavior.

> **ACTION STEP**
>
> To try to alleviate ADD symptoms
> naturally, exercise at an intense level
> every day and eat a low-carbohydrate,
> high-protein diet.

The best treatment for ADD depends on the type of ADD a person has. See
my book *Healing ADD* for a complete description of types and treatments.
Sometimes medications or supplements are helpful, but sometimes they can
make things worse if they are not right. When correctly targeted, ADD is a
highly treatable disorder in both children and adults. Don't let pride get in
the way of getting the help you need. In order to get the body you want, you
need a great brain and you have to admit when your brain needs help.

SEEKING PROFESSIONAL HELP

Even after doing all of the brain-body–healthy strategies in this book, some
people will still need to seek professional help. Some people will need psychotherapy; some will need medication; others will need more directed guidance with supplements or other alternative treatments. In lecturing around
the world, I am frequently asked the following questions: When is it time to
see a professional about my brain? What to do when a loved one is in denial
about needing help? How do I go about finding a competent professional?

When Is It Time to See a Professional About My Brain?

This question is relatively easy to answer. People should seek professional help
for themselves or a family member when their behaviors, feelings, thoughts, or
memory (all brain functions) interfere with their ability to reach their potential in their relationships, work, academics, or health. If you are experiencing
persistent relationship struggles (parent-child, sibling, friends, romantic), it is
time to get help. If you have ongoing work or school problems related to your
memory, moods, actions, or thoughts, it is time to get professional help. If your
impulsive behavior, poor choices, or anxiety are causing consistent monetary
problems or health problems, it is time to get help. Many people think they

cannot afford to get professional help. I think it is usually much more costly to live with brain problems than it is to get appropriate help.

Pride and denial can get in the way of seeking proper help. People want to be strong and rely on themselves, but I am constantly reminded of the strength it takes to make the decision to get help. Also, getting help should be looked at as a way to get your brain operating at its full capacity.

Marian came to see me for mood swings and work-related problems. Even though she was very competent, her behavior at work often caused problems with her coworkers. When her boss suggested she see me, she resisted. There was nothing wrong with her, she thought, it was everyone else. One day, after exploding at a coworker, she realized it was, at least partly, her fault and agreed to come for help. She resisted because she did not want to be seen as weak or defective. The brain SPECT scan helped her to see that her brain needed to be balanced. With the appropriate help, she got better and didn't have to suffer from mood swings, and she and her coworkers all suffered less stress as a result of her better-balanced brain.

What to Do When a Loved One Is in Denial About Needing Help

Unfortunately, the stigma associated with a "psychiatric illness" prevents many people from getting help. People do not want to be seen as crazy, stupid, or defective and do not seek help until they (or their loved one) can no longer tolerate the pain (at work, in their relationships, or within themselves). Most people do not see psychiatric problems as brain problems, but rather as weak-character problems. Men are especially affected by denial.

Here are several suggestions to help people who are unaware or unwilling to get the help they need. Try the straightforward approach first (but with a new brain twist). Clearly tell the person what behaviors concern you, and explain to them that the problems may be due to underlying brain patterns that can be easily tuned up. Tell them help may be available—help not to cure a defect but rather help to optimize how their brain functions. Tell them you know they are trying to do their best, but their behavior, thoughts, or feelings may be getting in the way of their success (at work, in relationships, or within themselves). Emphasize better function, not defect.

Give them information. Books, videos, and articles on the subjects you are concerned about can be of tremendous help. Many people come to see us because they read a book, saw a video, or read an article. Good information can be very persuasive, especially if it is presented in a positive, life-enhancing way.

When a person remains resistant to help, even after you have been straightforward and given them good information, plant seeds. Plant ideas about getting help and then water them regularly. Drop an idea, article, or other information about the topic from time to time. If you talk too much about getting help, people become resentful and to spite you won't get help—especially the overfocused types. Be careful not to go overboard.

Protect your relationship with the other person. People are more receptive to people they trust than to people who nag and belittle them. Work on gaining the person's trust over the long run. It will make them more receptive to your suggestions. Do not make getting help the only thing that you talk about. Make sure you are interested in their whole lives, not just their potential medical appointments.

Give them new hope. Many people with these problems have tried to get help, and it did not work or it even made them worse. Educate them on new brain technology that enables professionals to be more focused and more effective in treatment efforts.

There comes a time when you have to say enough is enough. If, over time, the other person refuses to get help, and his or her behavior has a negative impact on your life, you may have to separate yourself. Staying in a toxic relationship is harmful to your health, and it often enables the other person to remain sick as well. Actually, I have seen that the threat or act of leaving motivates people to change, whether it is about drinking, drug use, or treating ADD. Threatening to leave is not the first approach I would take, but after time, it may be the best approach. Realize you cannot force a person into treatment unless they are dangerous to themselves, dangerous to others, or unable to care for themselves. You can only do what you can do. Fortunately, there is a lot more we can do today than even ten years ago.

Finding a Competent Professional Who Uses This New Brain Science Thinking

At Amen Clinics, Inc., we get many calls and e-mails a week from people all over the world looking for competent professionals in their area who think in ways similar to the principles outlined in this book. Because our approach is on the edge of what is new in brain science, other professionals who know and practice this information may be hard to find. However, finding the right professional for evaluation and treatment is critical to the healing process. The right professional can have a very positive impact on your life. The wrong professional can make things worse.

There are a number of steps to take in finding the best person to assist you. Get the best person you can find. Saving money up front may cost you in the long run. The right help is not only cost effective but saves unnecessary pain and suffering, so don't rely on a person simply because they are on your managed-care plan. That person may or may not be a good fit for you. Search for the best. If he or she is on your insurance plan—great, but don't let that be the primary criteria. Once you get the names of competent professionals, check their credentials. Very few patients ever check a professional's background. Board certification is a positive credential. To become board certified, physicians must pass additional written and oral tests. They have had to discipline themselves to gain the skill and knowledge that was acceptable to their colleagues. Don't give too much weight to the medical school or graduate school that the professional attended. I have worked with some doctors who went to Yale or Harvard who did not have a clue on how to appropriately treat patients, while other doctors from less prestigious schools were outstanding, forward thinking, and caring. Set up an interview with the professional to see whether or not you want to work with him or her. Generally you have to pay for their time, but it is worth spending the money to get to know the people you will rely on for help.

Many professionals write articles or books or speak at meetings or local groups. If possible, read the work of or hear the professional speak. By doing so, you may be able to get a feel for the kind of person they are and their ability to help you. Look for a person who is open-minded, up-to-date, and willing to try new things. Look for a person who treats you with respect, who listens to your questions and responds to your needs. Look for a relationship that is collaborative and respectful. I know it is hard to find a professional who meets all of these criteria and who also has the right training in brain physiology, but these people can be found. Be persistent. The caregiver is essential to healing.

Make sure to get your brain tuned up and any brain problems treated in order to be your best self, both physically and emotionally.

The Brain Health Solution

Brain Health Robbers	Brain Health Boosters
Depression	Medication, supplements, exercise, enriched diet, psychotherapy
Bipolar disorder	Medication, supplements, fish oil
Panic disorder	Treating medical conditions, reducing caffeine, eliminating alcohol, balancing hormones, GABA, B_6, magnesium, kava kava
Agoraphobia	Medications, supplements
Obsessive-compulsive disorder	Medication, behavior therapy, supplements such as 5-HTP, St. John's wort
PTSD	Psychotherapy, EMDR, supplements
Alcohol/drug abuse	Treating underlying conditions, psychotherapy, support groups, medication to ease withdrawal symptoms
ADD	Medication, supplements, intense exercise, low-carb/high-protein diet

16

CHANGE YOUR BRAIN, CHANGE YOUR BODY, CHANGE OTHER PEOPLE'S BODIES

How Your Brain Influences the Physical and Mental Health of Others

Attitudes are contagious. Are yours worth catching?
—Dennis and Wendy Mannering

My father, who avoided doctors for most of his life, used to say "I give heart attacks, I don't get them." He prided himself on being fiercely independent, not letting anyone ever tell him what to do. He flourished his whole life, owning a very successful chain of grocery stores for more than fifty years, and he was the longtime chairman of the board of Unified Grocers, one of the largest independent grocery wholesale companies in the world. Growing up with him as a father for me personally was a challenge. The "I give heart attacks, I don't get them" attitude was the opposite of my natural personality, which was more like my mother's father, of being a helper and peacemaker. I often found myself tense around Dad yet still wanting to please him. The reactions in my body were directly connected to my dad's brain.

My dad was also the type of person who always said "No" to any question that was asked.

"Can I go here?"

"No."

"Do you think I should do this?"

"No."

"Would you like to go with me?"

"No."

"Can I help you?"

"No."

I remember when I was recruiting adults for one of our healthy studies, I asked him to be scanned for us, his first response was, "No." Actually, it took me twelve years of asking him to finally get a picture of his brain. When I saw it, the scan helped to explain a lot of frustration in my life. He had a lot of activity in the anterior cingulate gyrus, the brain's gear shifter. People who have too much activity in this part of the brain tend to be argumentative and reflexively say no. It can make their loved ones just a bit crazy. Seeing the scan helped me relax and know it wasn't always me.

Balance Your Brain, Be Sexier

Laura and I have been friends since childhood. She was a beautiful girl growing up and turned many heads of the boys we both knew. For some reason, unbeknownst to me, Laura never did it for me romantically. I adored her, but just not in that way. Years later we continued to stay in touch and my feelings never changed.

Then one day, her beauty radiated and I found myself drawn to her in a way that was very unusual. My heart beat faster when I was with her, my thoughts wandered into areas they had never wandered before. What was different? I wondered. It all seemed weird. Then it became clear. She told me that she had suffered from a lifelong anxiety disorder and that she finally found the strength to get it treated. She was taking an antidepressant medication and a group of natural supplements, and she had been seeing a psychotherapist. Her anxiety was down and her level of happiness and joy were up.

When Laura's brain was changed, the look and appeal of her body changed as well, and subsequently, she changed my body's reaction to her. Fortunately for me, my prefrontal cortex works well and I could just notice and enjoy the feeling without jeopardizing my marriage. This story highlights a critically important point that extends the main theme of the book:

> *When you change your brain,*
> *you change your body, and subsequently*
> *you change other people's bodies as well.*

Intuitively, we know this is true.

- Take the angry boss at work. Many of his or her employees will experience physical stress symptoms as a result of the troubled behavior. I have seen this time and again among my patients.

- When your wife or daughter is going through the worst part of her menstrual cycle, the levels of stress everyone in the family feels tend to increase.
- When your husband is going through job stress, with the difficult boss mentioned above, you feel it as well.
- Research tells us that mothers of children who have ADD or autism experience many stress symptoms and there is a higher incidence of depression and divorce in these families.

One reason to take great care of your brain is that its health has a tremendous impact on the health of those you love. People are contagious.

OPTIMIZING YOURSELF TENDS TO ENHANCE THOSE AROUND YOU

When Dr. Irwin Goldstein, an expert in sexual medicine, presented his research findings to a scientific meeting, he said: "It is rare for me to stand in front of an audience and say, 'This is a manuscript that has changed my life.' But this one has done that." The study, published in the *Journal of Sexual Medicine,* seemed obvious. The results showed that females in committed relationships with men who were treated with an impotence drug (Levitra) had better sex. But the women didn't just like sex better, they liked it better because their bodies worked better. Lubrication was better. Orgasms were more intense. They lusted more. The women's bodies reacted as if *they* were receiving the drug. So a drug they didn't even take affected their bodies. "Her physiology is linked to his," Goldstein says. "Men share problems with women, and the solutions. . . . It totally intrigues me. I can change someone's physiology without treating them. It is the wildest thing!" In fact, the better a man's response to the drug, the better her response to him.

"Entanglement" is a physics concept. Subatomic particles have "partners"—other subatomic particles—with which they can be entangled, sometimes over great distances. If you change one particle, the change affects the other one with which it is entangled. Dr. Goldstein's study is a strong indicator that humans can be entangled. We change when we fall in love, we become one unit, at least sexually. The two shall become one, as it says in the Bible. "There are no other physiologic abilities of men and women that are shared, and that is what is so fascinating about these data," Goldstein says. He also says there is some evidence that when he successfully treats women suffering from dyspareunia, or pain with intercourse, their men get better erections and have more sexual satisfaction. Goldstein suspects that male partners of women with low libido have poorer erections and that if those women could be treated, the men would improve too.

Whether you know it or not, you have a significant impact on those around you. Taking care of your own brain allows you to take better care of those you love.

When I was in my psychiatric residency program learning marriage and family therapy, I often heard that it takes two people to change a relationship. Years later I found out that this "common sense" rule is actually wrong. It often takes just one person to change a relationship. Think with me. . . . I know I can go home tonight and make my wife smile just by the comments I make, such as

"Hi, honey, I missed you today."
"Hi, baby, is there anything I can do to help you tonight?"
"Hi, sweetheart, you look great."
"Hello, my love, how was your day?"

I also know I can make Tana scream at me. Particularly if I say thoughtless things like,

"Hey, what did you do all day?"
"Don't you ever get anything done?"
"Why do I have to do everything myself?"
"Take that dress off, it looks terrible."

How my own brain works will have an important impact on how Tana's brain and body work. The same thing is true in your relationships. When you change your brain and change your body in a positive way, you will encourage the brains and bodies of those you love to work right as well.

This phenomenon was one of the main reasons I became a psychiatrist. Unlike giving people antibiotics or performing surgery, where you just fix the immediate problem, I realized in medical school that if I helped my patients feel, think, and act better, it not only helped them become happier, more effective people, it also dramatically helped their interactions with their spouses, their children, and even their grandchildren. I loved the possibilities of helping people across generations.

Of course, when my father found out that I wanted to be a psychiatrist, he asked me why I didn't want to be a real doctor. My body reacted in a stressed way, for feeling I was disappointing him. I was smart enough to know it was my life and not his, and I have loved nearly every day as a psychiatrist. Funny, many years later my dad has become one of my best referral sources. When one of his supervisors was having family problems, he called me up and asked me to see him, because he didn't want his valued employee to quit. With patience, even the tough brains can come around.

APPENDIX A

15 IMPORTANT NUMBERS
I NEED TO KNOW

Here are some important numbers you need to know in order to maintain a healthy brain and body. Some of these have been discussed throughout the book, and some are new here. Simple calculators are found online at www.amenclinics.com/cybcyb.

1. **Body mass index (BMI).** Weight in pounds $\times$ 703/height in inches^2

2. **Daily caloric needs to maintain current body weight.** To find out your basic calorie needs without exercise, which is referred to as your resting basal metabolic rate (BMR), fill out the following equation:

- Women: 655 + (4.35 $\times$ weight in pounds) + (4.7 $\times$ height in inches) − (4.7 $\times$ age in years)
- Men: 66 + (6.23 $\times$ weight in pounds) + (12.7 $\times$ height in inches) − (6.8 $\times$ age in years)

Take that number and multiply by it by the appropriate number below.

- 1.2 if you are sedentary (little or no exercise)
- 1.375 if you are lightly active (light exercise/sports 1–3 days a week)
- 1.55 if you are moderately active (moderate exercise/sports 3–5 days a week)
- 1.75 if you are very active (hard exercise/sports 6–7 days a week)
- 1.9 if you are extra active (very hard exercise/sports and a physical job or strength training twice a day)

3. **Average daily calories you consume** (don't lie to yourself). It would be very instructive for you to keep a log.

4. **Desired weight.** Set a realistic goal for your weight and match your behavior to reach it.

5. **Number of fruits and vegetables you eat a day.** Strive for between 7 and 10 servings per day to lower your risk for cancer.

6. **Number of hours you sleep at night.** Don't fool yourself into thinking you need only a few hours of sleep. Here are the average sleep requirements by age according to the National Sleep Foundation and the National Institute of Neurological Disorders and Stroke:

Age Range	Number of Hours of Sleep
1–3 years old	12–14 hours
3–5 years old	11–13 hours
5–12 years old	10–11 hours
13–19 years old	9 hours
Adults	7–8 hours
Seniors	7–8 hours

7. **Vitamin D level.** Have your physician check your 25-hydroxy vitamin D level, and if it is low, get more sunshine and/or take a vitamin D supplement.

Low = < 30
Optimal = between 50 and 90
High = > 90

8. **Thyroid.** Have your doctor check your free T3 and TSH levels to check for hypothyroidism or hyperthyroidism and treat as necessary to normalize.

9. **C-reactive protein.** This is a measure of inflammation that your doctor can check with a simple blood test. Elevated inflammation is associated with a number of diseases and conditions and should prompt you to eliminate bad brain habits.

10. **Homocysteine level.** This is another marker of inflammation.

11. **Hg A1C.** This test shows your average blood sugar levels over two to three months and is used to diagnose diabetes and prediabetes. According to Lab Tests Online, normal results for a nondiabetic person are in the range of 4 to 6 percent. Numbers higher than that may indicate diabetes.

12. **Fasting blood sugar.** This test usually requires that you fast for about eight hours prior to having your blood drawn. It evaluates your blood sugar levels solely for the day when you have your blood drawn. Here is what the levels mean, according to the American Diabetes Association:

Normal: 70–99 mg/dL
Prediabetes: 100–125 mg/dL
Diabetes: 126 mg/dL or higher

13. **Cholesterol.** Make sure your doctor checks your total cholesterol level as well as your HDL (good cholesterol), LDL (bad cholesterol), and triglycerides (a form of fat). According to the American Heart Association, optimal levels are as follows:

Total cholesterol: less than 200
HDL: 60 or higher
LDL: less than 100
Triglycerides: less than 150

14. **Blood pressure.** Have your doctor check your blood pressure at your yearly physical or more often if it is high. Here is how to interpret the numbers, according to the American Heart Association:

Below 120 over 80: optimal
120–139 over 80–89: prehypertension
140 (or above) over 90 (or above): hypertension

15. **Know how many of the twelve most common preventable causes of death you have . . . then decrease them.**

1. Smoking
2. High blood pressure
3. BMI indicating overweight or obese
4. Physical inactivity
5. High fasting blood glucose
6. High LDL cholesterol
7. Alcohol abuse (accidents, injuries, violence, cirrhosis, liver disease, cancer, stroke, heart disease, HTN)
8. Low omega-3 fatty acids
9. High dietary saturated fat intake
10. Low polyunsaturated fat intake
11. High dietary salt
12. Low intake of fruits and vegetables

APPENDIX B

AMEN CLINICS ABBREVIATED BRAIN SYSTEMS
Questionnaire*

Dr. Amen's *Change Your Brain, Change Your Body* Abbreviated Questionnaire is a great start to helping you evaluate the health and well-being of your brain. Plus, it will lead you to specific parts of the book and specific supplements that may be most helpful for you. For an expanded and a continually updated version of the questionnaire, go online at www.amenclinics.com/cybcyb.

Think of this tool as the beginning of optimizing the brain-body connection. For many years Dr. Amen realized that not everyone is able to get a brain scan to check on the health of his or her brain. So, in order to bring the life-changing information that he has learned through his imaging work to the most people, he has developed a series of questionnaires to help predict the areas of strengths and vulnerabilities of the brain.

A word of caution is in order. Self-report questionnaires have advantages and limitations. They are quick and easy to score. On the other hand, people filling them out may portray themselves in a way they want to be perceived, resulting in self-report bias. For example, some people exaggerate their experience and mark all of the symptoms as frequent, in essence saying, "I'm glad to have a real problem so that I can get help, be sick, or have an excuse for the troubles I have." Others are in total denial. They do not want to see any personal flaws and they do not check any symptoms as significantly problematic, in essence saying, "I'm okay. There's nothing wrong with me. Leave me alone." Not all self-report bias is intentional. People may genuinely have difficulty recognizing problems and expressing how they feel. Sometimes family members or friends are better at evaluating a loved one's level of functioning than a person evaluating himself or herself. They may have noticed things that their loved one hasn't.

* Copyright © 2010 Daniel Amen, M.D. For the full version, go online to www.amenclinics .com/cybcyb.

Questionnaires of any sort should never be used as the only assessment tool. Use this one as a catalyst to help you think, ask better questions, and get more evaluation if needed. Always discuss any recommendations with your personal physician or health-care provider, especially if you are taking any medications, such as for your heart, blood, or blood pressure, or for anxiety, depression, or pain.

AMEN CLINICS ABBREVIATED BRAIN SYSTEMS
Questionnaire

Please rate yourself on each of the symptoms listed below using the following scale.

0	1	2	3	4	NA
Never	Rarely	Occasionally	Frequently	Very Frequently	Not Applicable/ Known

_____ 1. Trouble sustaining attention or being easily distracted

_____ 2. Struggle with procrastination until I "have" to do something

_____ 3. Lacks attention to detail

_____ 4. Difficulty delaying what you want, having to have your needs met immediately

_____ 5. Trouble listening

_____ 6. Feeling restless

_____ 7. Blurts out answers, interrupts frequently

_____ 8. Makes decisions impulsively

_____ 9. Excitement seeking

_____10. Needs caffeine, nicotine, or sugar in order to focus

_____11. Gets stuck on negative thoughts

_____12. Worries excessively

_____13. Tendency toward compulsive or addictive behaviors

_____14. Holds grudges

_____15. Upset when things do not go your way

_____16. Upset when things are out of place

_____17. Tendency to be oppositional or argumentative

_____18. Dislikes change

_____19. Needing to have things done a certain way or you become very upset

_____20. Trouble seeing options in situations

_____21. Feeling sad

_____22. Being negative

_____23. Feeling dissatisfied

_____24. Feeling bored

_____25. Low energy

_____26. Decreased interest in things that are usually fun or pleasurable

_____27. Feelings of hopelessness, helplessness, worthlessness, or guilt

_____28. Crying spells

_____29. Chronic low self-esteem

_____30. Social isolation

_____31. Feelings of nervousness and anxiety

_____32. Feelings of panic

_____33. Symptoms of heightened muscle tension, such as headaches or sore muscles

_____34. Tendency to predict the worst

_____35. Avoid conflict

_____36. Excessive fear of being judged or scrutinized by others

_____37. Excessive motivation, trouble stopping work

_____38. Lacks confidence in abilities

_____39. Always watching for something bad to happen

_____40. Easily startled

_____41. Temper problems

_____42. Short fuse

_____43. Irritability tends to build, then explodes, then recedes, often tired after a rage

_____44. Unstable or unpredictable moods

_____45. Misinterprets comments as negative when they are not

_____46. Déjà vu (feelings of being somewhere you have never been)

_____47. Often feel as though others are watching you or out to hurt you

_____48. Dark or violent thoughts that may come out of the blue

_____49. Trouble finding the right word to say

_____50. Headaches or abdominal pain of uncertain origin

_____51. Forgetfulness

_____52. Memory problems

_____53. Trouble remembering appointments

_____54. Trouble remembering to take medications or supplements

_____55. Trouble remembering things that happened recently

_____56. Trouble remembering names

_____57. It is hard for me to memorize things for school, work, or hobbies

_____58. I know something one day but do not remember it the next day

_____59. I forget what I am going to say right in the middle of saying it

_____60. I have trouble following directions that have more than one or two steps

_____61. Tend to be clumsy or accident prone

_____62. Walk into furniture or walls

_____63. Trouble with coordination

_____64. Poor handwriting

_____65. Trouble maintaining an organized work area

_____66. Multiple piles around the house

_____67. More sensitive to noise than others

_____68. Particularly sensitive to touch or tags in clothing

_____69. Trouble learning new information or routines

_____70. Trouble keeping up in conversations

AMEN CLINICS ABBREVIATED BRAIN SYSTEMS
Questionnaire

Answer Key

Place the number of questions you, or a significant other, answered "3" or "4" in the space provided.

_____ 1–10 Prefrontal cortex (PFC) problems (see page 21 for more information)

- PFC supplements: Dr. Amen's Focus and Energy Solution or Dr. Amen's ADD Solution, plus Dr. Amen's Omega Solution fish oil
- PFC meds: For ADD, stimulants, such as Adderall, Ritalin, or Stratterra

5 questions = Highly probable
3 questions = Probable
2 questions = May be possible

_____ 11–20 Anterior cingulate gyrus (ACG) problems (see page 22 for more information)

- ACG supplements: Dr. Amen's Serotonin Mood Solution plus Dr. Amen's Omega Solution fish oil
- ACG meds: SSRIs, such as Lexapro, Paxil, Zoloft, Celexa, Prozac, and Luvox
- If also low PFC, consider Effexor or Cymbalta

5 questions = Highly probable
3 questions = Probable
2 questions = May be possible

_____ 21–30 Deep limbic system (DLS) problems (see page 22 for more information)

- DLS supplements: Dr. Amen's SAMe Mood Solution plus Dr. Amen's Omega Solution fish oil.
  For cyclic mood changes, fish oil plus Dr. Amen's GABA Calming Solution
- DLS meds: Antidepressants, such as Wellbutrin, SSRIs (if high ACG also present); Effexor or Cymbalta (if high ACG and low PFC also present); for cyclic mood changes, consider anticonvulsants or lithium; for pain, Cymbalta and/or anticonvulsant Neurontin

5 questions = Highly probable
3 questions = Probable
2 questions = May be possible

_____ 31–40 Basal ganglia (BG) problems (see page 22 for more information)

- BG supplements: Dr. Amen's GABA Calming Solution plus Dr. Amen's Omega Solution fish oil
- BG meds: Buspar; anticonvulsants, such as Neurontin; some blood pressure meds, such as propranolol, may help

5 questions = Highly probable
3 questions = Probable
2 questions = May be possible

_____ 41–50 Temporal lobe (TL) problems (see page 22 for more information)

- TL supplements: Dr. Amen's GABA Calming Solution plus Dr. Amen's Omega Solution fish oil
- TL meds: Anticonvulsants, such as Neurontin, Depakote, or Lamictal

5 questions = Highly probable
3 questions = Probable
2 questions = May be possible

_____ 51–60 Memory problems (see Chapter 12, "The Memory Solution," for more information)

- TL Memory supplements: Dr. Amen's Brain Recovery and Memory Solution plus Dr. Amen's Omega Solution fish oil
- TL Memory meds: Namenda, Aricept, Exelon, or Reminyl

5 questions = Highly probable
3 questions = Probable
2 questions = May be possible

_____ 61–70 Cerebellum (CB) problems (see page 23 for more information)

- CB supplements: Dr. Amen's Brain Recovery and Memory Solution plus Dr. Amen's Omega Solution fish oil
- CB meds: Unknown

5 questions = Highly probable
3 questions = Probable
2 questions = May be possible

Combinations

Having more than one system that needs help is common, and it just means that you may need a combination of the interventions listed.

My rule of thumb in our clinics is that if you have a temporal lobe (TL) problem, that gets treated first. If not, anything else you do for the prefrontal cortex (PFC), anterior cingulate gyrus (ACG), or deep limbic system (DLS) may make everything worse for the person.

- It is common to have PFC and ACG problems together, especially in children or grandchildren of alcoholics.
- It is also common to have ACG and deep limbic issues together in worried or obsessive depressions.
- Temper problems may be associated with a combination of TL, PFC, and ACG issues.

It is important to discuss these options with your health-care provider. If he or she does not know much about natural treatments, consult a naturopath or a physician trained in integrative medicine or natural treatments.

APPENDIX C

THE SUPPLEMENT SOLUTION

In treating people, one question I always ask myself is, What would I prescribe if this were my mother, my wife, or my child? More and more, after nearly thirty years of being a psychiatrist, I find myself recommending natural treatments. I am not opposed to medications and I have prescribed them for a long time, but I want you to use all of the tools available, especially if they are effective, less expensive, and have fewer side effects.

One of the cases that got me interested specifically in natural treatments involved my own niece. When she was seven, my sister brought her to see me for problems with moodiness and her temper. I tried her on a number of medications without any success. My sister was calling me upset three times a week. I kept using stronger and stronger medicines. But medications are not without risks and side effects, and when my niece started to gain weight I stopped them and decided to try her on a group of natural supplements that I had heard about from a colleague.

One day about four months later, I realized that I hadn't heard anything from my sister in a long time. So I called her and said, "Hey, don't you love me anymore? How's my niece?"

She said, "Danny, you cannot believe the difference in her. She is so much better. She is calmer, more compliant, and she is getting straight A's in school." The supplements have had long-term benefits for her without any side effects.

Pros and Cons of Supplements

Over time I began to wonder why I didn't start with natural supplements and then use medicines if the supplements didn't work. So, let's talk about the pros and cons of using natural supplements to help the brain. To start, they are often effective. They have dramatically fewer side effects than most prescription medications and they are significantly less expensive. Plus, you never have to tell an insurance company that you have taken them. As awful as it sounds, taking prescription medications can affect your insurability. I know many people who have been denied or made to pay higher rates for insurance because they have taken certain medications. If there are natural alternatives, they are worth considering.

Yet natural supplements also have their own set of problems. Even though they tend to be less expensive than medications, they may be more expensive for you because they are usually not covered by insurance. Many people are unaware that natural supplements can have side effects and need to be thoughtfully used. Just because something is natural does not mean it is innocuous. Both arsenic and cyanide are natural, but that doesn't mean they are good for you. For example, St. John's wort, one of my favorite natural antidepressants, can cause sun sensitivity and it can also decrease the effectiveness of a number of medications such as birth control pills. Oh great! Get depressed, take St. John's wort from the grocery store, now you are pregnant when you don't want to be. That may not be a good thing.

One of the major concerns about natural supplements is the lack of quality control. There is variability and you need to find brands you trust. Another disadvantage is that many people get their advice about supplements from the teenage clerk at the health food store, who may not have the best information. But, even when looking at the problems, the benefits of natural supplements make them worth considering, especially if you can get thoughtful, research-based information.

Every day I personally take a handful of supplements that I know make a significant difference in my life. They have changed the health of my brain, my energy, and my lab values. Many physicians say that if you eat a balanced diet, you do not need supplements. I love what Dr. Mark Hyman wrote in his book *The UltraMind Solution: Fix Your Broken Brain by Healing Your Body First.* He wrote that if people "eat wild, fresh, organic, local, non–genetically modified food grown in virgin mineral- and nutrient-rich soils that has not been transported across vast distances and stored for months before being eaten . . . and work and live outside, breathe only fresh unpolluted air, drink only pure, clean water, sleep nine hours a night, move their bodies every day, and are free from chronic stressors and exposure to environmental toxins," then it is possible that they will not need supplements. Because we live in a fast-paced society where we pick up food on the fly, skip meals, eat sugar-laden treats, buy processed foods, and eat foods that have been chemically treated, we could all use a little help from a multiple vitamin/mineral supplement.

Amen Clinic Supplements

At the Amen Clinics we make our own line of supplements that have taken more than a decade to develop. The reason that I developed this line was I wanted my patients and my own family to have access to the highest-quality research-based supplements available. After I started recommending supplements to my patients, they would go to the supermarket, drugstore, or health food store and have so many choices that they did not know what or how to choose. Plus, there is variability of quality in the supplements available. Another reason I developed my own line was that the Amen Clinics see a high population of people who have attention deficit disorder. I realized if they did not get their supplements as they walked out the door, they would forget about it or procrastinate and not have started them by their next appointment.

Research shows the therapeutic benefit of using supplements in treating mild to moderate depression, insomnia, and cognitive impairment. We strongly recommend that when purchasing a supplement, you consult your health-care practitioner to determine what dosage would be most effective for you. Our website (www.amenclinics.com) contains links to the scientific literature on every product, so you, as a consumer, can be fully informed on the benefits and risks involved. Please remember that supplements can have very powerful effects on the body and caution should be used when combining them with prescription medications.

Here is a list of our supplements and why I recommend them. They are problem focused, evidenced based, and as high quality as possible, while still being affordable.

- **Dr. Amen's Basic Brain Boost:** This supplement contains a high-potency multiple vitamin/mineral supplement, plus nutrients targeted to enhance overall brain function.

- **Dr. Amen's Omega Solution:** High-quality fish oil that contains a balance between EPA and DHA.

- **Dr. Amen's Brain and Memory Recovery Solution:** Contains nutrients targeted to enhance memory and to encourage overall brain healing.

- **Dr. Amen's Sleep Solution:** Proper sleep is a critical component to a brain healthy program. In our formula we use several scientifically based ingredients to enhance restorative sleep.

- **Dr. Amen's Craving Solution:** This solution is formulated to decrease cravings by balancing blood sugar and decreasing compulsive behaviors.

- **Dr. Amen's Serotonin Mood Solution:** This formula is designed to enhance serotonin in the brain to promote a healthy mood.

- **Dr. Amen's Focus and Energy Solution:** This formula was designed to enhance focus and energy.

- **Dr. Amen's SAMe Mood Solution:** This formula is designed to enhance a positive mood and energy.

- **Dr. Amen's GABA Calming Solution:** This GABA-based formula was made to help lower anxiety and stress.

Dr. Amen's Weight-Loss Solutions

Basic Formula—doubles as The Craving Solution
Type 1 The Compulsive Overeater—doubles as Dr. Amen's Serotonin Mood Solution
Type 2 The Impulsive Overeater—doubles as Dr. Amen's Focus and Energy Solution
Type 3 The Impulsive Compulsive Overeater—combines Types 1 and 2
Type 4 The SAD Overeater—doubles as Dr. Amen's SAMe Mood Solution
Type 5 The Anxious Overeater—doubles as Dr. Amen's GABA Calming Solution

Here is a detailed discussion of the supplements discussed in the book in alphabetical order.

ACETYL-L-CARNITINE (ALC)

For focus and energy, ADD

Acetyl-l-carnitine (ALC) is involved in cellular energy production and in removing the toxic accumulation of fatty acids. Its function is to increase energy in the brain, which helps to enhance memory and concentration. ALC has been most studied for its antiaging properties, and research supports the use of acetyl-l-carnitine to slow the decline in cognition, mood, and daily function that occurs with the progression of Alzheimer's disease.

A major cause of aging is deterioration of the energy-producing components of your cells, resulting in reduced cellular activity, the accumulation of cellular debris, and eventually cell death. ALC helps maintain cellular energy metabolism by assisting in the transport of fat through the cell membrane and into the mitochondria within the cell, where fats are oxidized to produce the cellular energy ATP.

ALC is found in the mitochondria, where it helps maintain its energetics and lowers the increased oxidative stress associated with aging. ALC is absorbed into the bloodstream efficiently and is effective at carrying fatty acids across the membrane into the cell, where they are burned as energy and utilized efficiently by the mitochondria. ALC also guards against oxidative damage. Beta amyloid is a principal component of senile plaques and is thought to be central in Alzheimer's disease. ALC appears to exert protective effects against beta-amyloid neurotoxicity and oxidative stress. In my practice, I have found that it can boost focus in ADD patients.

The typical recommended adult dosage is 500 mg twice a day.

ALPHA-LIPOIC ACID (ALA)
For hormones (insulin), skin, cravings and will power

Alpha-lipoic acid is made naturally in the body and may protect against cell damage in a variety of conditions. There is strong evidence that alpha-lipoic acid may help treat type 2 diabetes and nerve damage. In a number of studies, it has also been found to be helpful for skin issues. In 2003, researchers reported in the *British Journal of Dermatology* that in a randomized, placebo-controlled, double-blind study, a cream containing 5 percent alpha-lipoic acid demonstrated significant improvement in facial skin aging. Alpha-lipoic acid also has very good scientific evidence that it helps balance blood sugar, which can help with cravings.

The typical recommended adult dose is 100 mg twice a day.

ASHWAGANDHA
For focus and energy, stress, anxiety, fatigue, passion

Ashwagandha (*Withania somnifera*, Indian ginseng, Indian winter cherry) is a shrub found in India, Nepal, and Pakistan that is commonly used for its sedating properties. The plant itself is an adaptogen, meaning it has the properties that enable the body to better handle stress, anxiety, and fatigue. It helps to rejuvenate and energize the nervous system in addition to increasing physical endurance and restoring sexual health. It also has antioxidant, anti-inflammatory, and antiaging effects. It is well tolerated and few adverse effects have been reported. Because ashwagandha may stimulate thyroid function and it may cause a decrease in blood pressure or lower blood sugar, caution should be used when combining it with hypertensive and diabetic medications.

We recommend 125 mg twice a day. (In capsule form, one can use 1–6 g daily.)

B VITAMINS

For craving and willpower, weight, stress, heart, focus and energy, anxiety, immune system

B vitamins play an integral role in the functioning of the nervous system and help the brain synthesize neurotransmitters that affect mood and thinking. This makes them especially effective in controlling stress. When you are faced with stressful situations or thoughts, the B vitamins are typically the first to be depleted. If you have a B-vitamin deficiency, your ability to cope with stress and anxiety is lowered.

Vitamin B_6 (pyridoxine) is a water-soluble vitamin essential in the metabolism of amino acids, glucose, and fatty acids and is important in the production of neurotransmitters (serotonin, epinephrine, norepinephrine, and GABA). It is required by the nervous system and is needed for normal brain function as well as DNA synthesis. It is hard to find a molecule in our bodies that doesn't rely on vitamin B_6 for its production. It's involved in more than one hundred crucial chemical reactions in our bodies.

B_6 is required for the production of hemoglobin, the compound in red blood cells that transports oxygen and carbon dioxide. It increases the amount of oxygen carried in our blood, helping overcome fatigue. It helps maintain a healthy immune system and calms anxiety. B_6 also helps in processing carbohydrates for energy. Food sources of vitamin B_6 include fortified cereals, beans, meat, poultry, fish, and some fruits and vegetables.

Vitamin B_3 (niacin) was first isolated in the laboratory in the 1930s during research studies done on tobacco; hence niacin or "nicotinic acid." Niacin is important in energy production. It plays an important role in converting fats, proteins, carbohydrates, and starches into energy you can use. It also helps to eliminate toxic chemicals from the body and has been shown to increase the level of HDL (good cholesterol). Niacin helps to increase blood flow near the skin. Higher doses may cause skin flushing in some people, characterized by a red and itchy face and neck that lasts a few minutes. A form of niacin called niacinamide causes little or no flushing. Food sources of niacin include meat and dairy products, leafy vegetables, broccoli, tomatoes, avocados, nuts, and whole grains.

One study showed that high homocysteine levels—associated with increased risk for coronary artery disease, stroke, and dementia—could be treated with folic acid (1 mg), vitamin B$_{12}$ (400 mcg), and vitamin B$_6$ (10 mg).

The typical recommended adult dosage is 100 percent of the B vitamins every day. Make sure you take at least 400 mcg of folate and 500 mcg of B$_{12}$ per day.

CHOLINE

For memory

Choline is a nutrient essential to the structure and function of all cells. It is a precursor molecule involved in the synthesis of the neurotransmitter acetylcholine, which is important for normal brain function. Those deficient in acetylcholine may develop Alzheimer's disease and dementia; therefore, choline supplementation may be helpful in preventing the onset of these neurological disorders. Choline is also involved in producing the cell membrane phospholipids phosphatidylcholine and sphingomyelin. Considering that the breakdown of cell membranes leads to neuronal death, replenishing these vital components of the membrane is a proactive step you can take to help prevent Alzheimer's disease. Food sources of choline include egg yolk, liver, peanuts, fish, milk, and cauliflower. Generally, up to 3 g of choline daily is well tolerated, but possible side effects may include nausea, diarrhea, dizziness, sweating, and hypotension.

The recommended dosage is 300–1,200 mg daily.

CHROMIUM PICOLINATE

For craving and willpower, weight, hormones (insulin), some forms of depression

Chromium picolinate is a nutritional supplement used to aid the body in the regulation of insulin, which enhances its ability to efficiently metabolize glucose and fat. There is a strong link between depression, decreased insulin sensitivity, and diabetes. Supplementation with chromium picolinate has been shown to effectively modulate carbohydrate cravings and appetite, which is beneficial to managing both diabetes and depression.

I often recommend chromium picolinate to help with insulin regulation and to control carb cravings. In a well-designed study, 600 mcg of chromium picolinate was beneficial for patients with atypical depression (the type of depression where people gain weight, rather than lose weight), especially those with carbohydrate cravings.

The typical recommended adult dosage is 200–600 mcg a day.

COCOANOX
For craving and willpower, immune system, and heart

Cocoanox is a cocoa flavonoid from the cacao bean, which is derived from the *Theobroma cacao* tree. Cocoa flavonoids contain antioxidant, anti-inflammatory, and immune-stimulating effects. They function as a free-radical scavenger, binding to highly reactive molecules and neutralizing them to prevent cell damage. Cocoa flavonoids have been shown to promote heart health by inhibiting the oxidation of LDL cholesterol, a step that commonly leads to atherosclerosis. It may lead to increased blood flow to the brain and lower blood pressure. The polyphenol profile of cocoanox is 45 percent.

The recommended dosage is 8 mg twice a day.

DHEA
For weight, hormones (adrenal fatigue, testosterone), depression, passion

DHEA is one of the most abundant hormones in the body, second only to cholesterol. DHEA, if low, is an important supplement to counteract adrenal fatigue. According to the NaturalStandard.com website, there is good scientific evidence supporting the use of DHEA in the treatment of adrenal insufficiency, depression, and obesity. Supplementing with DHEA has good scientific evidence that it is helpful for weight loss in certain patients. It is usually well tolerated. Acne and facial hair are common side effects, as it increases the body's testosterone levels. To avoid getting acne or facial hair, many doctors prescribe a metabolite of DHEA called 7-keto-DHEA; it is more expensive, but if acne and facial hair are an issue, it is worth it.

The main worry about DHEA by some professionals is that it will partly convert itself into sex hormones such as testosterone and estrogens. This seems to be an obvious advantage for healthy people, looking to combat age-associated hormonal decline. Unfortunately, this means advising people who are at risk for hormonally dependent cancers (prostate, breast, ovarian) against taking DHEA. For these, 7-keto-DHEA is a good solution.

DHEA supplementation is not recommended for children, adolescents, or pregnant or nursing women. Androgenic effects including acne, hair loss, and a deepening of the voice have been reported in women. If this occurs, discontinue DHEA immediately.

The typical recommended adult dosage is 25–50 mg daily. DHEA is banned by the International Olympic Committee, the National Collegiate

Athletic Association, the NFL, and other sports organizations for its performance-enhancing properties.

DL-PHENYLALANINE
For craving and willpower, weight, focus and energy, skin, depression

This is an essential amino acid (cannot be produced by the body) and thus must be obtained through the diet. Phenylalanine is used in different biochemical processes to produce the neurotransmitters dopamine, norepinephrine, and epinephrine. There is evidence that phenylalanine can increase mental alertness and release hormones affecting appetite. There have been reports that L-phenylalanine can promote high blood pressure in those predisposed to hypertension. Monitoring in the first few months on phenylalanine can detect blood pressure increases in the minority of people who will have this symptom. Phenylalanine can promote the cell division of existing malignant melanoma cells. If you have melanoma, or any other form of cancer for that matter, avoid phenylalanine. Persons who have PKU (phenylketonuria) cannot use phenylalanine. This includes those born with a genetic deficiency that prevents them from metabolizing phenylalanine.

There is also good scientific evidence that phenylalanine may be helpful for vitiligo, a chronic and relatively common skin disorder that causes depigmentation in patches of skin. It occurs when the cells responsible for skin pigmentation die or become unable to function.

The typical recommended starting dose for adults is 500 mg a day, slowly working up to 1,500 mg a day.

DMAE
For skin, memory, ADD

Also known as deanol, DMAE is an analog of the B vitamin choline. DMAE is a precursor of the neurotransmitter of acetylcholine, and it has strong effects on the central nervous system. DMAE is commonly used to increase the capacity of neurons in the brain and is also thought to have antiaging properties. Often DMAE is used to treat children with attention deficit disorder (ADD) because it is known to decrease aggression and to increase attention span and memory abilities.

DMAE's antiaging effects have recently been demonstrated in a placebo-controlled trial. In this study, a 3 percent DMAE facial gel was applied daily for sixteen weeks. Deanol-infused topical gel was found to be safe and effective in the mitigation of forehead wrinkles and fine lines around the eyes. It also improved lip shape, fullness, and the overall appearance of skin. When treatment stopped, the effects were not reversed. The possible benefits of DMAE in dermatology include anti-inflammatory effects, increases in skin firmness, and improvements in facial muscle tone. There were few adverse effects compared to placebo treatment, and DMAE use was shown to be safe for up to a year. There are also reports that lipofuscin (age spots) can be decreased by DMAE use.

The typical recommended adult dosage of DMAE is 300–500 mg daily.

FISH OIL
For cravings and willpower, weight, nutrition, skin, hormones, heart, focus and energy, exercise, immune system, sex, depression, bipolar disorder

Fish oil, a great source of omega-3 fatty acids, has been the focus of many research studies. The two most studied fish oils are eicosapentaenoic acid (EPA) and docosahexaenoic acid (DHA). DHA is a vital component of cell membranes, especially in the brain and retina. DHA is critical for normal brain development in fetuses and infants and for the maintenance of normal brain function throughout life. DHA appears to be a major factor in the fluidity and flexibility of brain cell membranes, and it could play a major role in how we think and feel.

Fish oil appears to have mood-stabilizing properties when used in the treatment of bipolar disorder. On SPECT scans, bipolar disorder shows overall increased activity in the brain, and EPA and DHA tend to calm down these overactive brain signals.

Fish oil has been found to have many positive effects on health in general as well. It lowers triglyceride levels and has anti-inflammatory, anti-arrhythmic, immune-enhancing, and nerve-cell–stabilizing properties. In addition, it helps to maintain normal blood flow, as it lowers the body's ability to form clots.

In a landmark study published in the journal *Lancet,* researchers followed more than eleven thousand subjects who had suffered a heart attack within three months of entering the trial. The trial, which lasted forty-two months, found a reduction in risk for cardiac death in the subjects who took fish oil and vitamin E. It is believed that the antiarrhythmic effect of the fish oil was responsible for the lowered risk. The study suggests that up to twenty lives per thousand post–heart attack patients could be saved by consuming daily doses of less than 1 g of EPA and DHA. As I always say, what's good for your heart is good for your brain.

A number of studies report that taking fish oil and boosting omega-3 fatty acids helps to raise heart rate variability (HRV), which is good for both brain and heart health. There is also strong scientific evidence that omega-3 fatty acids may reduce high cholesterol and triglycerides in the blood, decrease the risk of sudden cardiac death, and decrease blood pressure. Other studies have shown that fish oil can help reduce joint pain and stiffness in rheumatoid arthritis sufferers.

Fish oil is often helpful for your skin. It has anti-inflammatory properties, helps depression, and improves heart function—all things that will help your skin look younger and more vibrant. It may help ease symptoms associated with hormonal changes, such as during perimenopause and menopause. Fish oil may also improve focus and concentration in people with ADD. For over-focused or obsessive ADD symptoms, include more DHA; for inattentive or low-energy ADD symptoms, include more EPA. Most people do best on a combination of DHA and EPA.

The typical dosage of fish oil is 1–2 g a day for prevention and 4 to 6 g a day to treat illness. I often recommend 2–4 g a day for adults.

FLAXSEED OIL
For hormones (perimenopause, menopause)

Like fish oil, flaxseed oil is a rich source of essential fatty acids and has been found to ease symptoms associated with perimenopause and menopause. Vegetarians may prefer to take flaxseed oil rather than fish oil.

The typical recommended adult dosage is 1,000 mg (1 g) up to twice a day (7.2 g of flaxseed oil is equivalent to 1 g of fish oil).

GABA
For craving and willpower, weight, stress, anxiety, some forms of depression

Gamma-aminobutyric acid (GABA) is an amino acid that also functions as a neurotransmitter in the brain. GABA is reported in the herbal literature to work in much the same way as antianxiety drugs and anticonvulsants. It helps stabilize nerve cells by decreasing their tendency to fire erratically or excessively. This means it has a calming effect for people who struggle with temper, irritability, and anxiety, whether these symptoms relate to anxiety or to temporal lobe disturbance.

The typical recommended adult dosage ranges from 100 to 1,500 mg daily for adults and from 50 to 750 mg daily for children. For best effect, GABA should be taken in two or three doses a day.

GINKGO BILOBA
For memory, focus and energy, passion

The prettiest brains I have seen are those on ginkgo. Ginkgo biloba, from the Chinese ginkgo tree, is a powerful antioxidant that is best known for its ability to enhance circulation, memory, and concentration. Consider taking ginkgo if you suffer from low energy or decreased concentration.

The best-studied form of ginkgo biloba is a special extract called EGB 761, which has been studied in blood-vessel disease, clotting disorders, depression, and Alzheimer's disease. A 2000 comparison of all the published, placebo-controlled studies longer than six months for ginkgo biloba extract, EGB 761, versus Cognex, Aricept, and Exelon showed they all had similar benefits for mild to moderate Alzheimer's disease patients.

The most widely publicized U.S. study of ginkgo biloba appeared in the *Journal of the American Medical Association* in 1997 and was conducted by Dr. P. L. Le Bars and colleagues from the New York Institute for Medical Research. EGB 761 was used to assess the efficacy and safety in Alzheimer's disease and vascular dementia. It was a fifty-two–week, multicenter study with patients who had mild to severe symptoms. Patients were randomly assigned to treatment with EGB 761 (120 mg per day) or placebo. Progress was monitored at twelve, twenty-six, and fifty-two weeks, and 202 patients finished the study. At the end of the study, the authors concluded that EGB was safe and appears capable of stabilizing and, in a substantial number of cases, improving the cognitive performance and the social functioning of demented patients for six months to one year. Although modest, the changes induced by EGB were objectively measured and were of sufficient magnitude to be recognized by the caregivers.

Consider taking ginkgo if you are at risk for memory problems or stroke, or if you suffer from low energy or decreased concentration. There is a small risk of bleeding in the body, and the dosages of other blood-thinning agents being taken may sometimes need to be reduced.

The typical adult dose is 60–120 mg twice daily.

GLYCINE
For craving and willpower, obsessive-compulsive disorder

Glycine is also an inhibitory neurotransmitter, which means it calms brain activity. It is an important protein in the brain, and recent studies have demonstrated its effectiveness in the treatment of obsessive-compulsive disorder and in reducing pain.

The typical adult dose is 500 mg daily.

GRAPE SEED EXTRACT
For skin, heart, memory

Grape seed extract comes from grape seeds that are waste products of the wine and grape juice industry. These seeds contain flavonoids and oligomeric proanthocyanidins (OPCs). Grape seed extract is known as a powerful antioxidant. Studies have shown that the antioxidant power of OPCs is twenty times greater than vitamin E and fifty times greater than vitamin C. Extensive research suggests that grape seed extract is beneficial in many areas of health because of its antioxidant effect to bond with collagen, promoting youthful skin, elasticity, and flexibility.

Other studies have shown that proanthocyanidins help to protect the body from sun damage; to improve vision; to improve flexibility in joints, arteries, and body tissues such as the heart; and to improve blood circulation by strengthening capillaries, arteries, and veins. There is strong scientific evidence it helps with skin edema, venous insufficiency, and varicose veins.

It is also often found in products used to enhance brain function. In a 2009 study, grape seed extract was found to decrease beta-amyloid plaque formation, the plaques commonly associated with Alzheimer's disease, by more than one-third in the brains of mice with Alzheimer's disease.

The typical adult dose of grape seed extract is 50–100 mg daily.

GREEN TEA LEAF EXTRACT
For focus and energy, weight, heart, anxiety, immune system

Made from the dried leaves of *Camellia sinensis,* green tea leaf extract is an evergreen shrub. It has been used as a remedy for many ailments, including anxiety, cancer prevention, and cardiovascular health, for the prevention of cold and flu, and for weight loss. The green tea component *epigallocatechin gallate* (EGCG) is a potent free-radical scavenger. Included in the extract is L-theanine, which has been scientifically proven to bring the brain into an alpha wave state, which means it induces relaxation and reduces feelings of anxiety but also increased concentration and energy.

The typical adult dose is 200–300 mg of green tea leaf extract capsules daily for cancer prevention and possible effects on weight loss. Up to three cups a day of green tea can be consumed for health benefits, but caution should be used with pregnant women as green tea does contain caffeine.

5-HTP

For craving and willpower, weight, hormones (adrenal fatigue, PMS, leptin and ghrelin), sleep, stress, exercise, sex, insomnia, brain disorders (agoraphobia, obsessive-compulsive disorder)

The amino acid 5-HTP is a building block for serotonin, and using this supplement is another way to increase cerebral serotonin, which may help control stress and improve sleep. There are several reasons why 5-HTP may be a better sleep aid than L-tryptophan. It is a step closer than L-tryptophan in the serotonin production pathway, is more widely available than L-tryptophan, and is more easily taken up in the brain. Seventy percent of 5-HTP is taken up into the brain, compared to only 3 percent of L-tryptophan. In addition, 5-HTP is about five to ten times more powerful than L-tryptophan. A number of double-blind studies have shown 5-HTP is as effective as antidepressant medication. In my experience, I have found it to be very helpful for some people as a sleep aid.

5-HTP boosts serotonin levels in the brain and helps to calm anterior cingulate gyrus hyperactivity (greasing the cingulate, if you will, to help with shifting of attention). For people who can't seem to turn off their brains at bedtime, or who have anxious thoughts that keep them awake, 5-HTP may help. The most common side effect of 5-HTP is an upset stomach, although it is usually very mild. To avoid an upset stomach, start by taking small doses of 5-HTP and gradually increase the dosage as you get used to it. Taking it with food can also help. Because 5-HTP increases serotonin, you should not take it with other medications that increase serotonin, such as St. John's wort, L-tryptophan, or prescribed antidepressants, unless you are closely supervised by your physician.

The typical adult dose of 5-HTP is 50–100 mg two or three times daily with or without food.

HUPERZINE A

For memory

Huperzine A is a remarkable compound that has been studied in China for nearly twenty years. It appears to work by increasing the availability of acetylcholine, a major memory neurotransmitter in the brain, and preventing cell damage from excitotoxins. It has been shown to be effective in improving patients who suffered cognitive impairment due to several different types of dementia, including Alzheimer's disease and vascular dementia. Since 1991, it has been studied as a treatment for the prevention of Alzheimer's disease and can be considered safe to use as an alternative or adjunct to medication in the treatment of AD.

Huperzine A has also been found to help learning and memory in teenagers. Researchers divided thirty-four pairs of junior high school students complaining of memory problems into a huperzine A group and a placebo control group. The huperzine A group was given two (50 mcg) capsules of huperzine A twice a day, while the placebo group was given two capsules of placebo (starch and lactose inside) twice a day for four weeks. At the end of the trial, the huperzine A group's memory abilities were significantly superior to those of the placebo group. Those with seizure disorders, cardiac arrhythmias, asthma, or irritable bowel syndrome should avoid huperzine A. Possible side effects include gastrointestinal effects, dizziness, blurred vision, slow heart rate, arrhythmias, seizures, and increased urination. Use of huperzine A with acetylcholinesterase inhibitors or cholinergic drugs may produce additive effects, so caution should be used.

The typical adult dose is 50–100 mcg twice a day and 200–400 mcg daily if cognitive impairment is already noted.

INOSITOL
For craving and willpower, weight

Inositol is a sugar that is considered part of the B vitamin family. It is a natural chemical found in the brain that is reported to help neurons use serotonin more efficiently. It is important in the maintenance of cell membranes, the breakdown of fat, hair growth, and the regulation of estrogen and insulin. Preliminary studies demonstrate its efficacy in treating those with obsessive-compulsive disorder, panic disorder, anxiety, depression, and other psychiatric disorders. It also functions to neutralize free-radical activity, thereby protecting neurons and promoting brain health. There is good scientific evidence showing that it also helps with weight loss.

The typical adult dose is 500 mg twice a day. Scientific studies have shown 12–18 g of inositol daily has beneficial effects in the treatment of depression, anxiety, panic disorder, and obsessive-compulsive disorder.

IODINE
For weight, hormones (thyroid), focus, and energy

Iodine is a mineral found mainly in the thyroid gland. The thyroid gland uses iodine to produce other hormones within the body. Weight gain, fatigue, and an intolerance of cold are symptoms of an iodine deficiency.

The typical adult dose is 150 mg a day.

KAVA KAVA
For hormones (leptin and ghrelin), sleep, panic disorder

A search of the medical literature on kava kava supplementation found seventeen studies for anxiety and insomnia on approximately 1,400 patients. Of the seventeen studies, fifteen were positive. In my experience, kava kava can help with sleep and can have a calming effect on anxiety and irritability. It can also help with weight loss, by balancing the appetite hormones leptin and ghrelin, which are regulated during sleep.

Several years ago I went through a painful time of grief. For the first time in my life, I experienced panic attacks and had trouble sleeping. Of all the supplements I tried, kava kava helped me the most. Kava kava is recommended by some alternative-medicine practitioners to promote healthy sleep, calm anxiety, and reduce the physical and emotional effects of stress. Kava kava is thought to work by enhancing the production of GABA in the brain. It comes from the root of a South Pacific pepper tree and is widely used as a social and ceremonial drink in the Pacific Islands. The herb is so widely used that it is thought to be, in part, responsible for the laid-back island lifestyle.

Kava kava works quickly and is well suited for short-term sleeping problems, such as when you can't sleep the night before a big test or presentation. It is associated with minimal morning-after effects, leaving people feeling rested and alert after waking. My patients have reported the following relief after taking kava kava: being relaxed without feeling drugged, less muscle tension, a sense of peace and contentment, increased sociability, and an initial alertness followed by a feeling of drowsiness.

It is not the type of supplement, like fish oil, that you should take every day. At most use it for three weeks, then take a week off. Kava kava use on a daily basis may harm the liver. Kava kava has known adverse interactions with alcohol, barbiturates, MAO inhibitor antidepressants, benzodiazepines, other tranquilizers and sleeping pills, anticoagulants, antiplatelet agents including aspirin, antipsychotics, drugs used for treating Parkinson's disease, and drugs that suppress the central nervous system. Kava kava can exacerbate Parkinson's disease and increase muscle weakness and twitching. Women who are pregnant or breastfeeding should not take kava kava. Do not take kava kava if you are going to drive.

The typical adult dose is 150–300 mg one to three times daily as needed for anxiety or nervousness, or just at bedtime for sleep, standardized to contain 30 to 70 percent kavalactones. Most clinical trials have used the German kava extract WS 1490.

L-GLUTAMINE
For craving and willpower

L-glutamine is an amino acid that is important in the synthesis of the excitatory neurotransmitter glutamate and the inhibitor neurotransmitter GABA. It is also a nutrient for the brain, as it is used for energy if the brain does not have enough glucose to function. Supplemental glutamine has been used in the treatment of ADD, anxiety, and depression. It has been shown to decrease carbohydrate cravings.

The typical adult dose is 500 mg three to four times a day.

L-THEANINE
For craving and willpower, stress, focus and energy, anxiety, some forms of depression

L-theanine is an amino acid mainly found naturally in the green tea plant. It has been shown to penetrate the brain and produce significant increases in the neurotransmitters serotonin and/or dopamine concentrations. These findings led to recent studies investigating the possibility that L-theanine might induce relaxation and relieve emotional stress. When researchers tested the effects of L-theanine on a small group of volunteers, they found that it resulted in significantly increased production of alpha brain-wave activity, which they viewed as an index of increased relaxation. Pregnant women and nursing mothers should avoid L-theanine supplements.

The typical adult dose is between 50 and 200 mg, as necessary. L-theanine is available in some green tea preparations. The amino acid constitutes between 1 percent and 2 percent of the dry weight of green tea leaves.

L-TRYPTOPHAN

For craving and willpower, weight, hormones (leptin and ghrelin), sleep, exercise

L-tryptophan is an amino acid building block for serotonin, and taking L-tryptophan supplements increases cerebral serotonin. Serotonin is a neurotransmitter that plays an important role in sleep as well as a number of other functions. L-tryptophan is a naturally occurring amino acid found in milk, meat, and eggs. It is very helpful for some patients in improving sleep, decreasing aggressiveness, and stabilizing mood. The high doses of L-tryptophan found in turkey may explain why we get sleepy after devouring a big Thanksgiving meal.

L-tryptophan was taken off the market more than a decade ago because a contaminated batch from one manufacturer caused a rare blood disease and a number of deaths. L-tryptophan itself actually had nothing to do with these deaths. L-tryptophan was reapproved by the Food and Drug Administration several years ago and is currently available again. One of the problems with dietary L-tryptophan is that a significant portion of it does not enter the brain, but rather is used to make proteins and vitamin B_3. This necessitates taking large amounts of tryptophan. Scientific evidence also shows that L-tryptophan can help people lose weight.

The typical adult dose is 1,000–3,000 mg taken at bedtime.

L-TYROSINE

For craving and willpower, weight, focus and energy

This amino acid is important in the synthesis of brain neurotransmitters. It is the precursor to the brain neurotransmitters (epinephrine, norepinephrine, and dopamine), which are critical for balancing mood and energy. It is also helpful in the process of producing thyroid hormones, which are important in metabolism and energy production. A sluggish thyroid can have significant effects on brain health. The beneficial effect of tyrosine supplementation is that an efficiently functioning thyroid will not only result in a better-functioning brain, but will also help in weight loss.

Tyrosine supplementation has been shown to improve cognitive performance under periods of stress and fatigue. Stress tends to deplete the neurotransmitter norepinephrine, and tyrosine is the amino acid building block to replenish it. Tyrosine should not be taken with MAO and tricyclic antidepressants, when a cancerous melanoma is present, with a history of cancerous melanoma, or with elevated blood pressure.

The typical adult dose is 500–1,500 mg two to three times a day. It is best taken on an empty stomach with water or juice.

MAGNESIUM
For craving and willpower, weight, focus and energy, anxiety, panic disorder

Magnesium, needed for more than three hundred biochemical reactions in the body, is a mineral that is essential to good health. It has been shown to be helpful in calming anxiety and balancing the brain's pleasure centers, which can help reduce cravings. Magnesium is also important in energy production and assists in calcium and potassium uptake in the body. A deficiency in magnesium can lead to irritability and nervousness. Supplementing the body with magnesium can help with mood and muscle weakness. In combination with vitamin B_6, it has been shown to reduce the hyperactivity seen in children with ADD.

The typical adult dose is 400–1,000 mg daily, divided into three doses. It is best to take with calcium, as these minerals work synergistically. Magnesium is usually half of your total calcium intake.

MELATONIN
For hormones (female hormones, leptin and ghrelin), sleep

Melatonin is a hormone made in the brain that helps regulate other hormones and maintains the body's sleep cycle. Darkness stimulates the production of melatonin, while light decreases its activity. Exposure to too much light in the evening or too little light during the day can disrupt the production of melatonin. Jet lag, shift work, and poor vision are some of the conditions that can disrupt melatonin production. Some researchers think that being exposed to low-frequency electromagnetic fields (from common household appliances) may disrupt melatonin levels.

Research suggests that taking melatonin may help sleep patterns in shift workers or those with poor vision. One study found that melatonin helps prevent jet lag, particularly in people who cross five or more time zones. Melatonin has been found to be more effective than placebo in decreasing the time required to fall asleep, increasing the number of hours sleeping, and improving alertness. Melatonin may be helpful for children with learning disabilities who suffer from insomnia. And although taking melatonin does not help the primary symptoms of ADD, it does seem to help the sleep disturbances common in these children.

One study of postmenopausal women found that melatonin improved depression and anxiety. Studies of people with depression and panic disorder have shown low levels of melatonin. People who suffer winter blues or seasonal affective disorder (SAD) also have lower-than-normal melatonin levels. Melatonin causes a surge in the neurotransmitter serotonin, which may help explain why it is helpful in both sleep and depression.

Melatonin is also involved in the production of female hormones and influences menstrual cycles. Researchers also consider melatonin levels to be involved in aging. Melatonin levels are highest when we are children and diminish with age. The lower levels of melatonin may help explain why older adults tend to get less sleep.

Melatonin is a strong antioxidant, and there is some evidence that it may help strengthen the immune system. It has also been shown to have powerful neuroprotective effects both as an antioxidant and in the prevention of plaque formation as observed in Alzheimer's disease. The benefit to taking melatonin as opposed to other sleep aids is that it is both safe and nonaddictive.

The best approach for dosing melatonin is to begin with very low doses. In children, start with 0.3 mg a day and raise it slowly. In adults, start with 1 mg an hour before bedtime. You can increase it to 6 mg.

MULTIVITAMINS
For nutrition, skin, immune system

I recommend taking a daily multiple vitamin/mineral complex to all of my patients. Studies have reported that they help prevent chronic illness. The American Medical Association recommends a daily vitamin for everybody because it helps prevent chronic illness. In addition, people with weight-management issues often are not eating healthful diets and have vitamin and nutrient deficiencies.

N-ACETYL-CYSTEINE
For craving and willpower

NAC is an amino acid that is needed to produce glutathione, a very powerful antioxidant. NAC binds to and removes dangerous toxic elements within the cells, making it a molecule critical to brain health. NAC is used by the liver and the lymphocytes to detoxify chemicals and other poisons. In addition, NAC is a vasodilator, working to relax blood vessels and allow for more oxygen delivery within the body. Recently, NAC has been studied as a treatment for drug addiction, as it functions to restore levels of the excitatory neurotransmitter glutamate in the reward center of the brain. Studies have shown that NAC supplementation can be effective in the treatment of OCD, depression in those with bipolar disorder, and schizophrenia. New scientific research supports the efficacy of NAC for the reduction of cocaine cravings. It may also be helpful in reducing food cravings.

The typical adult dose is 600–1,200 mg twice a day.

PANAX GINSENG
For weight, stress, memory, exercise, hormones (insulin), focus and energy, antiaging, immune system, passion

This is considered to be a rejuvenation herb. Research supports that it is an antioxidant that protects cells from the free-radical damage associated with aging as well as boosting energy levels. Ginseng also has research suggesting it helps to increase endurance and stamina and improve the immune system.

Panax ginseng is a plant with fleshy roots that typically grows in cooler climates—such as the northern hemisphere of eastern Asia, Korea, and Russia—and is used in the treatment of weakness and fatigue. The active components are ginsenosides (2.6 to 6.6 percent of the dry weight of the root), which also regulate blood glucose and blood pressure. Ginsenosides are unique to *Panax* species and are believed to be responsible for its antioxidant, anti-inflammatory, and immunostimulant properties. Ginsenosides have also been found to reduce food intake, fat composition, and serum leptin levels, which helps with weight loss. Panax ginseng is considered an adaptogen, meaning that it aids the body's ability to handle stress. It has also been shown to improve cognitive performance in healthy adults and those with dementia, and it has been shown to improve physical performance during endurance exercise. Clinical studies support the use of Panax ginseng as a way to maintain blood glucose and insulin levels in type 2 diabetes and as a treatment for erectile dysfunction. Yet it is most widely known as a stimulant that promotes energy, improves circulation, and speeds recovery after illness.

Panax ginseng is well tolerated, but caution should be used when taking warfarin (Coumadin), as its effects can be additive. Ginseng may cause hypoglycemic activity, so caution should be used when taking it with insulin or medications for hypoglycemia. Side effects include insomnia, nausea, diarrhea, euphoria, headaches, and issues with regulating blood pressure.

The typical adult dose is 200 mg a day of the standardized extract, containing 4 to 7 percent of ginsenosides.

PHOSPHATIDYLSERINE (PS)
For weight, hormones (adrenal fatigue), memory

Phosphatidylserine (PS) is a naturally occurring nutrient that is found in foods such as fish, green leafy vegetables, soy products, and rice. PS is a component of cell membranes. As we age, these membranes change in composition. There are reports of the potential of PS to help improve age-related declines in memory, learning, verbal skills, and concentration. PS is essential to brain health by maintaining neurons and neuronal networks so that the brain can continue to form and retain memories.

PET studies of patients who have taken PS show that it produces a general increase in metabolic activity in the brain. In the largest multicenter study to date of phosphatidylserine and Alzheimer's disease, 142 subjects aged forty to eighty were given 200 mg of phosphatidylserine per day or placebo over a three-month period. Those treated with phosphatidylserine exhibited improvement on several items on the scales normally used to assess Alzheimer's status. The differences between placebo and experimental groups were small but statistically significant.

The types of symptoms that improved in placebo-controlled studies of cognitive impairment or dementia include loss of interest, reduced activities, social isolation, anxiety, memory, concentration, and recall. Milder stages of impairment tend to respond to PS better than more severe stages. With regard to depression in elderly individuals, Dr. M. Maggioni and colleagues studied the effects of oral PS (300 mg/day) versus placebo and noted significant improvements in mood, memory, and motivation after thirty days of PS treatment. Phosphatidylserine can also be helpful for adrenal fatigue.

The typical adult dose is 100–300 mg a day.

PRIMROSE OIL
For hormones (perimenopause, menopause)

Evening primrose is a native North American plant that is also found in other areas of the world. Primrose oil contains gamma-linolenic acid (GLA), an omega-6 essential fatty acid that may alleviate perimenopausal and menopausal symptoms.

The typical adult dose is 1,000 mg (1 g) up to three times daily.

RESVERATROL
For craving and willpower, weight, heart, immune system, anticancer properties

Resveratrol is a phytoalexin, or a chemical that is produced by plants in response to injury or infection. Resveratrol has been shown to have very powerful anticancer, anti-inflammatory, and cardioprotective effects and may be important in extending life span. Resveratrol can be found in red wine, grape skins, chocolate, peanuts, and mulberries. Red wine contains more resveratrol than white wine because it is made from the grape skins, which contain 50–100 mcg resveratrol, while white wine is made only from the juice of the grape, which contains no resveratrol. Scientific studies show that mice given the equivalent of 20 mg of resveratrol per day had significant changes in genes involved in the antiaging process. In addition, it has been shown to reduce amyloid plaque formation, which suggests that resveratrol may be a powerful ally in the fight against Alzheimer's disease and dementia. Side effects of resveratrol include diarrhea, anxiety, and thinning of the blood. Pregnant women and nursing mothers should avoid the use of resveratrol supplements. Caution should be used when taking it with anticoagulant, antihypertensive, and antidiabetic medication.

Recommended dosage is 15 mg twice a day. One glass of red wine is the equivalent of 600–700 mcg, so supplementation is advised in the long run to obtain the most brain-healthy effect. Resveratrol lasts nine hours in the body, so a small dose taken twice a day will maintain the beneficial effects of this powerful antioxidant.

RHODIOLA
For focus and energy, stress, immune system, depression, passion

Rhodiola is an herb that is grown at high altitudes in Asia and Europe. Traditionally, it has been used to fight fatigue, improve memory, and increase attention span. Research has found that it does indeed help prevent fatigue. In addition, scientific evidence points to an ability to fuel sexual energy, boost immunity, and ease depression.

The typical adult dose is 200–600 mg daily for the treatment of fatigue and depression, and it is best taken on an empty stomach. Rhodiola should be taken early in the day, as it may interfere with sleep and it should not be used in individuals with bipolar disorder or those taking hypertensive or hypoglycemic medications.

SAGE

For memory

NaturalStandard.com gives the common herb sage its highest "A level" scientific evidence rating for cognitive improvement. It cites research that has demonstrated that sage can improve memory, confirming centuries-old theories. In the seventeenth century, noted herbalist Nicholas Culpeper wrote that the herb sage could "heal" the memory while "warming and quickening the senses."

Culpeper wasn't the only herbalist (and certainly not the first) to recognize that sage can help improve memory. Now—centuries later—scientists believe they know why. An enzyme called acetylcholinesterase (AChE) breaks down a chemical called acetylcholine, which is typically deficient in Alzheimer's patients. Researchers from the Medical Plant Research Centre (MPRC) at the Universities of Newcastle and Northumbria in the United Kingdom have shown that sage inhibits AChE.

A study conducted by researchers at MPRC demonstrates the possible results of inhibiting AChE. Researchers gave forty-four subjects either sage oil capsules or placebo capsules containing sunflower oil and then conducted word-recall tests. The group that received sage oil turned in significantly better test results than subjects who took placebo. However, researchers say that further tests are needed to fully determine just how far-reaching sage's effect on memory may be.

The typical adult dose for improved mood, alertness, and cognitive performance is 300–600 mg daily of dried sage leaf capsules. Sage can also be used as an essential oil in doses of 25–50 mcL (microliters). Sage should be used cautiously in those with hypertension or those who have seizure disorders.

SAMe

For craving and willpower, weight, focus and energy, sleep, ADD, passion

S-adenosyl-methionine (SAMe) is involved in the production of several neurotransmitters (serotonin, dopamine, epinephrine) and helps the brain to function properly. The brain normally manufactures all the SAMe it needs from the amino acid methionine. When a person is depressed, the synthesis of SAMe from methionine is impaired. People who have a certain type of ADD that is linked with depression may experience an improvement in focus when taking SAMe.

SAMe is also involved in the production of the sleep hormone melatonin and has been found to improve sleep quality. It has also been found to suppress appetite and reduce joint inflammation and pain.

The typical adult dose is 200–400 mg two to four times a day.

SATIEREAL
For craving and willpower, weight, sleep, stress, depression, and mood

Satiereal is a patented product made from the extract of saffron (*Crocus sativus*) and has been shown to have powerful antidepressant effects. Saffron is grown in Iran, Greece, Spain, and Italy and traditionally has been used to ease the digestion of spicy food, to soothe an irritated stomach, and to treat depression. The active ingredients of satiereal include safranal, picrocrocine, and crocine, which work synergistically to help with satiety and to help curb the compulsive desire to eat. Like SSRIs, satiereal works by preventing the reuptake of serotonin, thereby improving mood and well-being. It differs in that a small amount is potent, and it has been shown to be a successful weight-loss aid by reducing appetite and sugar cravings. In clinical trials, satiereal has been shown to be well tolerated with few adverse side effects.

The recommended dosage is 100 mg twice a day.

SELENIUM
For hormones (thyroid)

Selenium is a mineral found in some foods, water, and soil. Selenium has antioxidant properties that help the body prevent damage from free radicals. This mineral regulates thyroid function, strengthens the immune system, and helps prevent heart disease.

The typical adult dose is 80–200 mcg.

ST. JOHN'S WORT
For craving and willpower, weight, stress, agoraphobia, depression, obsessive-compulsive disorder

Saint John's wort (*Hypericum perforatum*) is a plant located in the subtropical regions of North America, Europe, Asia, India, and China and has been used for centuries in the treatment of mood disorders and depression. The biologically active ingredient in Saint John's wort is hypericin, which functions to inhibit the reuptake of various neurotransmitters, including serotonin, dopamine, GABA, and glutamate. The mechanism of action for the supplement St. John's wort is similar to that found in popular antidepressants, including Prozac, Paxil, and Zoloft. These drugs and the herb work to maintain elevated levels of serotonin, which has a mood-enhancing effect.

Stress depletes the brain of serotonin. St. John's wort combats that and may actually be the most potent of all the supplements at increasing serotonin availability in the brain. I have seen dramatic improvement for many of my patients on St. John's wort and have SPECT scan studies of patients before and after treatment with St. John's wort that document its effectiveness. St. John's wort decreases anterior cingulate gyrus hyperactivity (which can make you rigid and stressed out when things don't go your way) for many patients and decreases moodiness.

An unfortunate side effect is that it can also decrease prefrontal cortex activity. One of the women in the study said, "I'm happier, but I'm dingier." We also don't start people with temporal lobe symptoms (anger, epilepsy, memory, hallucinations, and so on) on St. John's wort without first stabilizing the temporal lobes with anticonvulsant medication. An important note is that it has been found to decrease the effectiveness of other drugs, including birth control pills.

The typical dose is 300 mg a day for children, 300 mg twice a day for teens, and 600 mg in the morning and 300 mg at night for adults. Sometimes, the dose may be slowly increased to 1,800 mg for adults. It is important that the preparation of St. John's wort contains 0.3 percent hypericin, one of the active ingredients of St. John's wort.

VALERIAN
For hormones (leptin and ghrelin), sleep, stress

Many patients find valerian to be remarkably helpful as a sleeping aid and stress-relief aid. Valerian is a well-recognized herb with antianxiety properties that is used as a mild tranquilizer, sedative, and muscle relaxant. There are about 150 species of valerian widely distributed in temperate regions of the world. The active ingredient is found in a foul-smelling oil produced in the root of the plant. Throughout history, people have turned to valerian for its unique properties. The ancient Roman physician Galen wrote about the virtues of valerian; in the Middle Ages, medical literature used the term "All Heal" to describe the herb; and valerian has long been a staple of Chinese and Indian medicine. In the United States, valerian was commonly used prior to the development of modern pharmaceuticals.

This centuries-old treatment for insomnia has also been helpful for symptoms of nervousness, stress, and pain. And it has been found to decrease seizure frequency in epileptic patients. Studies have shown valerian to be helpful for many types of anxiety disorders and for people with performance anxiety and those who get stressed in daily situations like traffic. Valerian appears to work by enhancing the activity of the calming neurotransmitter, GABA.

Unlike prescription tranquilizers, valerian has a much lower potential for addiction and has been used to help people who are trying to decrease their use of prescription tranquilizers or sleeping pills. (Anyone using prescription sleeping pills or tranquilizers should decrease or stop their use only under the supervision of a physician.) It may take two to three weeks to start feeling the effects of valerian, so it isn't the best sleep aid for short-term use, such as when you have jet lag. It is better suited for long-term use and has been found to improve deep sleep, which leaves you feeling more rested in the morning. Valerian should not be taken in combination with alcohol, barbiturates, or benzodiazepines, and it is not recommended for use during pregnancy or breastfeeding.

Since valerian promotes sleep, it may also help balance leptin and ghrelin, the appetite hormones that are regulated during sleep.

Valerian is available in capsules, tablets, liquids, tinctures, extracts, and teas. Most extracts are standardized to 0.8 percent valeric acids. The typical recommended adult dosage is 150 to 450 mg in capsules or teas. For children the recommended dosage is 50–100 mg.

VINPOCETINE

For memory

Vinpocetine has been shown in a number of studies to help memory, especially for people who are at risk for heart disease or strokes. It also helps lower high homocysteine levels, which are dangerous to your heart and brain. Vinpocetine is derived from an extract of the common periwinkle plant (*Vinca minor*) and is used in Europe, Japan, and Mexico as a pharmaceutical agent for the treatment of blood-vessel disease in the brain and cognitive disorders. In the United States, it is available as a dietary supplement. It is sometimes called a nootropic, meaning cognition enhancer, from the Greek *noos* for "mind." Vinpocetine selectively widens arteries and capillaries, increasing blood flow to the brain. It also combats accumulation of platelets in the blood, improving circulation. Because of these properties, vinpocetine was first used in the treatment of cerebrovascular disorders and acute memory loss due to late-life dementia. But it also has a beneficial effect upon memory problems associated with normal aging.

There is evidence that vinpocetine may be useful for a wide variety of brain problems. A 1976 study found that vinpocetine immediately increased circulation in fifty people with abnormal blood flow. After one month of taking moderate doses of vinpocetine, patients showed improvement on memorization tests. After a prolonged period of vinpocetine treatment, cognitive impairment diminished significantly or disappeared altogether in many of the patients. A 1987 study of elderly patients with chronic cerebral dysfunction found that patients who took vinpocetine performed better on psychological evaluations after the ninety-day trial period than did those who received a placebo.

More recent studies have shown that vinpocetine reduces neural damage and protects against oxidative damage from harmful beta-amyloid buildup. In a multicenter, double-blind, placebo-controlled study lasting sixteen weeks, 203 patients described as having mild to moderate memory problems, including primary dementia, were treated with varying doses of vinpocetine or placebo. Significant improvement was achieved in the vinpocetine-treated group as measured by "global improvement" and cognitive performance scales. Three 10 mg doses daily were as effective as or more effective than three 20 mg doses daily. Similarly good results were found in another double-blind clinical trial testing vinpocetine versus placebo in elderly patients with blood vessel and central nervous system degenerative disorders. Some preliminary research suggests that vinpocetine may also have some protective effects in both sight and hearing.

Reported adverse reactions include nausea, dizziness, insomnia, drowsiness, dry mouth, transient hypotension, transient fast heart rate, pressure headaches, and facial flushing. Slight reductions in both systolic and diastolic blood pressure with prolonged use of vinpocetine have been reported, as well as slight reductions in blood sugar levels.

The typical adult dose is 10 mg a day.

VITAMIN D
For nutrition, weight, skin, heart, memory, immune system, depression, bipolar disorder

Vitamin D, also known as the sunshine vitamin, is an essential vitamin for brain health, mood, memory, and skin. While classified as a vitamin, it is a steroid hormone vital to health. Low levels of vitamin D have been implicated in depression, bipolar disorder, and memory problems, including Alzheimer's disease. One study in the *Journal of Alzheimer's Disease* found that vitamin D_3, a form of vitamin D, may stimulate the immune system to rid the brain of beta amyloid, an abnormal protein that is believed to be a major cause of Alzheimer's disease. Vitamin D activates receptors on neurons in regions important in the regulation of behavior, and it protects the brain by acting in an antioxidant and anti-inflammatory capacity. Other benefits of vitamin D supplementation include reducing the risk of bone diseases and fractures, improved muscular function, improved metabolic and cardiovascular function, and increased protection from diabetes and cancer. Adequate vitamin D levels are essential for ensuring normal calcium absorption and maintenance of healthy calcium plasma levels. Scientists now feel that supplementation with vitamin D is critical to helping maintain healthy bone remodeling as we age. There is also strong scientific evidence that vitamin D can be helpful for psoriasis, and vitamin D_3 appears to control skin cell growth.

Unfortunately, vitamin D deficiencies are becoming more and more common, in part because we are spending more time indoors and using more sunscreen. Americans over the age of fifty, those living at higher latitudes, those who are obese, and children and teens are at increased risk for vitamin D deficiency. In fact, seven out of ten kids are lacking in the nutrient. A pair of studies in the journal *Pediatrics* found that 7.6 million kids had a vitamin D deficiency and 50.8 million had insufficient amounts.

The American Academy of Pediatrics recently increased their recommendations for children to 400 IUs a day. I recommend that children and adults get their vitamin D levels checked to see what their specific needs should be. My levels were low when they were tested, and I live in Southern California and am an active person. I found that I need to take 5,000 IUs a day. The blood test is called 25-hydroxy vitamin D level. The current scientific literature recognizes that 400 IU daily is well below the physiological needs of most individuals and suggests 2,000 IU of vitamin D daily for the prevention of cancer, heart disease, and osteoporosis.

ZINC
For focus and energy, ADD, passion

Zinc is an essential mineral found in many foods, such as red meat, poultry, beans, nuts, and whole grains. Zinc activates more than one hundred different enzymes in the body, and daily supplementation is important because the body does not store extra zinc. It is involved in numerous bodily processes, including cell division, prostate health, immune function, and wound healing. Zinc deficiency has been linked to mental lethargy. There is good scientific evidence that it may be helpful for children with hyperactivity and impulsivity. Zinc also helps produce testosterone and dopamine for a healthy libido and has been effective in the treatment of eczema and psoriasis, so it is a supplement important in the maintenance of beautiful skin.

The typical adult dosage is 25–80 mg daily, not to exceed 100 mg. Zinc is best taken with food or juice, as it may result in a feeling of nausea on an empty stomach.

NOTE ON REFERENCES
AND FURTHER READING

The information in *Change Your Brain, Change Your Body* is based on more than six hundred sources, including scientific studies, books, interviews with medical experts, statistics from government agencies and health organizations, and other reliable resources. Printed out, the references take up more than one hundred pages. In an effort to save a few trees, I have decided to place them exclusively on the *Change Your Brain, Change Your Body* website. I invite you to view them at www.amenclinics.com/cybcyb.

ACKNOWLEDGMENTS

I am grateful to the host of people who have been instrumental in making this book a reality, especially all of the patients and professionals who have taught me so much about how the brain relates to our bodies. I am especially grateful to my writing partner Frances Sharpe, who was invaluable in the process of designing and completing this book. She is truly a treasure. Also, Dr. Kristen Willeumier, our director of Nutrition and Neutraceuticals at the Amen Clinics, was a wonderful resource for research, collaboration, and encouragement. Amen Clinics, Inc., consultant Paul Roper was also instrumental and inspirational in developing this book. Other staff at Amen Clinics, Inc., as always, provided tremendous help and support during this process, especially my personal assistant Catherine Hanlon, along with Dr. Leonti Thompson, Dr. Joseph Annibali, Dr. Chris Hanks, and Jill Prunella. Dr. Earl Henslin, as always, has been helpful and a joy to have as a friend and mentor. Dr. Manuel Trujillo from New York University was also helpful in reviewing the manuscript and giving me his thoughtful comments. Dr. Angie Meeker was instrumental on advice and guidance for the hormone chapter. TJ Bartel is an amazing Tantra teacher and gave guidance on the passion chapter. As usual, I am grateful to David and Sandy Brokaw of the Brokaw Company, who gave many helpful suggestions. I also wish to thank my amazing literary team at Harmony Books, especially my very thoughtful and patient editor Julia Pastore and my loving publisher Shaye Areheart. I am forever grateful to my literary agent Faith Hamlin—who, besides being one of my best friends, is a thoughtful, protective, creative mentor—along with the whole team at Sanford J. Greenburger Associates for their long-standing love, support, and guidance. And to Tana—my wife, my joy, and my best friend—who patiently listened to me for hours on end and gave many thoughtful suggestions on the book. I love all of you.

INDEX

Acetyl-l-carnitine (ALC), 183, 187, 323–324

Acetylcholine, 138

Acne, 199, 217

Acupuncture, 51

Adderall, 59, 183

Adenosine, 99

Adiponectin, 66

Adrenal fatigue, 148–149

Adrenal glands, 111, 148–149

Adrenaline, 148, 165, 174, 214

Adrenaline-overload anorexic type, 56, 62–63, 79

Advanced glycation end products (AGEs), 134

Aerobic exercise, 110, 112, 114, 119, 120, 122–124

Agave, 98

Aging, brain and, 76

Agoraphobia, 293–294

Alcohol use, 24, 29, 53, 133, 137, 173, 189, 233, 244–245

facts on excessive, 298–299

physical effects of, 297

symptoms of excessive, 297–298

All or nothing thoughts, 259

Alpha-lipoic acid (ALA), 71, 139, 161, 324

Always thinking, 259–260

Alzheimer's disease, 10, 23–26, 65, 67, 89, 91, 99, 111, 140, 150, 151, 158, 159, 162, 172, 185, 203, 237–244, 250–252, 277, 287

exercise and, 113–114

Amen Clinics, Inc., 4, 14, 67, 76, 92, 223, 290, 303

Abbreviated Brain Systems Questionnaire, 30–31, 314–319

supplements, 321–323

American Heart Association, 93

American Journal of Clinical Nutrition, 197

Amygdala, 216, 281

Amyotrophic lateral sclerosis (ALS), 89

Andropause, 135
Anemia, 186
Annals of Internal Medicine, 197
Anorexia nervosa, 22, 23, 107
Anterior cingulate gyrus (ACG), 21–23, 29, 31, 32, 55, 57, 65, 121, 165, 224, 294
Antidepressants, 39, 97, 112, 248, 290
Antioxidants, 242
  benefits of, 100
  exercise and, 115
  foods rich in, 100–102
ANTs (automatic negative thoughts), 9, 26, 48, 61, 62, 67, 73, 149, 256–271
  effects of, 257–258
  talking back to, 263
  types of, 259–263
  The Work and, 266–269
Anxiety, 39, 40, 49, 50, 56, 61, 142, 171, 174–175, 182, 202
  exercise and, 113
  heart rate variability (HRV) and, 168
  types of disorders, 292–296
Anxious overeater type, 56, 61–62, 79
Appetite, 66, 71–72, 153
Arthritis, 97, 98
Artificial sweeteners, 85, 97–98
Ashwagandha, 191, 324–325
Aspartame, 97–98
Asperger's syndrome, 107
Atherosclerosis, 165, 246
Athletes, sleep and, 200–201
Attention deficit disorder (ADD), 6, 26, 40, 49, 55, 58, 59, 91, 106, 171, 182–183, 202
  exercise and, 114
  symptoms of, 299–300
  types of, 300–301

Autism, 107
Automatic negative thoughts (*see* ANTs [automatic negative thoughts])
Autonomic nervous system (ANS), 166–167

B vitamins (*see* Vitamins)
Bargh, John A., 176, 177
Bariatric surgery, 75
Bartel, TJ, 283, 284
Basal ganglia, 17, 21–23, 29, 32, 37–40, 47–48, 61, 65, 121, 224, 230, 293
Basal metabolic rate (BMR), 68
Baumeister, Roy, 42
Beck, Judith S., 264
Benson, Herbert, 225
Berk, Lee, 234
Bieler, Henry, 191
Bike accidents, 125
Bio-identical hormones, 158
Biofeedback, 4, 131, 167, 175–177, 257
Bipolar disorder, 132, 291–292
Birth control pills, 135, 321
Blame, 262–263
Blanchflower, David, 282
Blood flow, 25, 27, 29, 107, 109, 115, 116, 118, 130, 170, 174, 233
Blood sugar levels, 42–43, 65, 66, 82, 89, 96, 104, 161, 172–173, 185–186, 197–198, 312–313
Body mass index (BMI), 64, 65, 67, 68, 198, 311
Brain (*see also* Dopamine; Endorphins; GABA; Serotonin)
  amygdala, 216, 281

anterior cingulate gyrus (ACG), 21–23, 29, 31, 32, 55, 57, 65, 121, 165, 224, 294
ANTs and (see ANTs [automatic negative thoughts])
basal ganglia, 17, 21–23, 29, 32, 37–40, 47–48, 61, 65, 121, 224, 230, 293
cerebellum (CB), 5, 23, 29, 32, 120–121, 227, 239, 258
deep limbic system (DLS), 17, 21–23, 29, 31, 39, 41, 48, 60, 221, 231, 280–281
diagrams of, 21
diet and nutrition and (see Diet and nutrition)
exercise and (see Exercise)
focus and energy and (see Focus and energy)
frontal lobes, 65, 237, 248
healthy, example of, 5–6
heart and (see Heart)
hippocampus, 65, 111, 148–149, 215, 237, 238, 248
hormones and (see Hormones)
hypothalamus, 71, 72
insular cortex, 165
long-term potentiation (LTP) and, 46
memory and (see Memory)
nucleus accumbens, 37–39
occipital lobes, 23, 121
parietal lobes, 21–23, 65, 121, 224, 253
posterior cingulate gyrus, 159
prefrontal cortex (PFC), 6, 9, 16, 19, 21, 23, 24, 29, 32, 37–41, 42–43, 55, 56, 58–60, 76, 97, 110, 121, 189, 199, 224, 236, 271

sexual activity and (see Sexual activity)
skin and (see Skin)
sleep and (see Sleep)
stress and (see Stress)
systems, 20–23
temporal lobes, 19, 21–23, 65, 105, 110, 111, 121, 189, 199, 224, 228, 236, 237, 239, 248, 258, 293
troubled, example of, 6
weight-management issues (see Weight-management issues)
willpower and self-control and, 38–52
Brain-body connection, 3–4
examples of, 7–9
taking advantage of, 10–12
Brain-derived neurotrophic factor (BDNF), 110
Brain envy, 13
Brain imaging, 4–5, 13, 29–30
examples of, 6, 7, 10, 14, 20, 30, 41, 76, 86, 141, 142, 169, 180, 181, 184–186, 204, 228
Brain injury, 6, 9, 18–19, 24, 40, 41, 58, 169–170, 186–187
Brain Research, 111
Brain reserve, 19–20
Brain surgery, 75–76
Braverman, Eric, 161–162
Breast cancer, 116, 158, 251, 278
Breathing exercises, 62, 63, 230
Bright light therapy, 56, 60–61, 211
British Journal of Dermatology, 134
British Journal of Nutrition, 74
British Journal of Sports Medicine, 119
British Journal of Urology International, 278

British Medical Journal, 133
Bryant, Kobe, 81
Buddha, 37
Bulimia, 54, 55, 60, 107

Caffeine, 25, 70, 179–180, 191
    limiting intake of, 85, 99–100
    skin and, 133, 137
    stress and, 233
California Department of
    Education (CDE), 111
Calorie log, 68
Calories, 67, 68–70, 85, 87–89,
    311–312
Carbohydrates, 42, 43, 58, 71, 85,
    92–93, 96, 97, 160, 172, 197
Cardiovascular disease, 172, 246
Cardiovascular exercise, 119
Carlson, Richard, 213
Casein, 107
CAT scans, 5
Celiac disease, 107
Cell phones, 47, 48
Cerebellum (CB), 5, 23, 29, 32,
    120–121, 227, 239, 258
Cerebral vascular disease, 246–247
Chapman, Dudley, 277
Chemotherapy, 188, 245
Chest pain, causes of, 31
Cholesterol, 66–67, 89–90, 144, 146,
    245, 246, 249, 313
Choline, 138, 326
Chromium picolinate, 71, 75,
    326–327
Chronic fatigue syndrome (CFS),
    58, 184–185
Cinnamon, 71, 89, 161
Cocaine, 22, 24, 26, 39, 42, 47, 49,
    93, 245, 296
Cocoanox, 327
Coenzyme Q10, 252

Cognitive therapy, 264–265, 290
Collagen, 116, 130, 136, 137, 139,
    217
Colon cancer, 116
Complex carbohydrates, 92
Compulsive behaviors, 22, 49
Compulsive overeater type, 55,
    57–58, 79, 92
Coordination exercises, 71
Corona radiata, 65
Cortisol, 24, 25, 111, 133, 148, 149,
    165, 174, 191, 214–216, 219,
    231
Cosby, Bill, 53
Cravings, 37–52, 236 (*see also*
    Weight-management issues)
CRON (calorie restriction with
    optimal nutrition), 87
Curcumin, 254
Cutler, Winnifred, 277, 278
Cytokines, 66

Dancing, 71, 121, 238–239
DASH (Dietary Approaches to Stop
    Hypertension) diet, 103
Davis, Anthony, 75
Decaffeinated drinks, 99
Deep brain stimulation, 75–76
Deep limbic system (DLS), 17,
    21–23, 29, 31, 39, 41, 48, 60,
    221, 231, 280–281
Dehydration, 26, 85–86, 134
Dementia, 65, 91, 113–114, 135,
    172, 203, 239, 240, 243, 245,
    247, 249, 251
Depression, 39, 40, 49, 50, 60, 61,
    67, 89, 91, 140, 142, 150, 151,
    164, 182–184
    biological factors and, 288–289
    dementia and, 247–248
    exercise and, 111–112

heart health and, 170, 287
psychological factors and, 289
sexual activity and, 280–281, 283
sleep and, 202
social factors and, 289
symptoms of, 288
treatment of, 289–290
DHEA, 24, 61, 75, 137, 148, 149, 150, 152, 277, 278, 327–328
Diabetes, 25, 64, 65, 66, 93, 115, 117, 160, 162, 172, 202, 236, 248–249
Dickinson, Emily, 236
Diet and nutrition, 11, 27, 81–108, 247
    antioxidants, 100–102
    artificial sweeteners, 85, 97–98
    blood sugar levels and, 42–43, 65, 66, 82, 96, 104, 161, 172–173, 185–186, 189
    caffeine, 25, 70, 85, 99–100
    calories, 67, 68–70, 85, 87–89, 311–312
    carbohydrates, 42, 43, 58, 71, 85, 92–93, 96, 97, 160, 172, 197
    eating disorders, 22, 23, 54, 55, 107
    eleven rules for healthy, 85–107
    fats, 66–67, 85, 89–92, 246
    five truths about foods you eat, 83–85
    focus and energy and, 191
    food allergies, 85, 105–107
    food labels, 94–95, 98, 104
    glycemic index (GI), 95–97, 172
    heart and, 172–173
    salt and potassium intake, 85, 103
    skin and, 134, 137
    snacking, 104
    sugar, 25, 37, 81–82, 85, 90, 93–95, 98, 134, 253
    water consumption, 26, 85–86, 134, 138
Diet programs, 53, 54
Diet sodas, 97
Divorce, 140, 151
DL-phenylalanine, 138, 191, 328
DMAE (deanol), 138, 328–329
Docosahexaenoic acid (DHA), 105
Dopamine, 37, 39, 40, 42, 47, 54–56, 58, 248, 252
    boosting levels of, 49, 59–60
Dossey, Larry, 226
Drug abuse, 24, 245
    facts on excessive, 298–299
    symptoms of, 297–298
Dysthymia, 60

Early Human Development journal, 231
Eating disorders, 22, 23, 54, 55, 107
Ebrahim, Shah, 276
Ecstasy, 24
Eicosapentaenoic acid (EPA), 105
Elastin, 217
Elimination diet, 106, 183
EMDR (eye movement desensitization and reprocessing), 48, 56, 62, 221, 234–235, 296
Emotional memory centers, 38, 40
End of Overeating, The: Taking Control of the Insatiable American Appetite (Kessler), 22, 93
Endorphins, 39, 174, 234, 270, 280
    boosting levels of, 50–51
Energy (see Focus and energy)
Ephedra, 70
Epilepsy, 252–253
Essential fatty acids (EFAs), 91–92
Estradiol, 153, 154, 157, 250, 251

Estriol, 153, 154, 157

Estrogen, 24, 28, 67, 137, 145, 146, 152–154, 156, 157, 185, 250–251, 277, 280, 283

Estrone, 153, 154

Exercise, 62, 63, 67, 109–126, 247
  adolescents and, 117–118
  aerobic, 110, 112, 114, 119, 120, 122–124
  benefits of, 27–28, 43, 48, 50, 59, 71, 109–115
  best kinds of, 119–125
  brain safety and, 124, 125
  as daily habit, 122
  dancing, 71, 121, 238–239
  diabetes and, 248–249
  effects of lack of, 26
  excessive, 107
  excuses and, 125–126
  heart health and, 176
  skin and, 116–117, 134–135, 136
  stress and, 116, 229
  table tennis, 43, 71, 120–121, 124–125
  tennis, 121
  walking, 70–71

Facebook, 47

Fast-food diet, 24–25, 83, 84, 88

Fats, 66–67, 85, 89–92, 246

Fen-phen, 54, 59

Fenfluramine, 54

Fertility
  sexual activity and, 279
  stress and, 219–220

Fish, 91

Fish oil supplement, 27, 74, 92, 102, 105, 126, 129, 138, 172, 176, 183, 187, 284, 291, 329–330

5-HTP (5-hydroxytryptophan), 9, 50, 55, 57, 59, 60, 126, 149, 156, 157, 160, 211, 235, 284, 294, 295, 333

Flaxseed oil, 330

Focus and energy, 11, 179–192
  boosters, 189–192
  diet and nutrition and, 84
  robbers, 182–189, 192
  typical lab panel, 190

Focusing on negative, 260

Folic acid, 250

Food (*see* Diet and nutrition)

Food allergies, 85, 105–107

Food and Drug Administration (FDA), 92

Food journal, 68, 69

Food labels, 94–95, 98, 104

Forgiveness, 168–170

Fortune-telling, 261–262

Frankenfats, 90–91

Free radicals, 100, 115, 242

Frontal lobes, 65, 237, 248

Fruit juice, 95–96

Fruits, antioxidant, 100–102

GABA (gamma-aminobutyric acid), 39, 41, 56, 235, 293, 330–331
  boosting levels of, 50, 62, 63

Gabapentin, 50

Gailliot, Matthew, 42

Gallup, Gordon, 281

Gambling, 47

Gamma-linolenic acid (GLA), 138

Ghrelin, 71, 72, 158–159, 197, 198

Giles, Graham, 278

Ginkgo biloba, 187, 191, 254, 285, 331

Ginseng, 71, 161, 191, 285, 340–341

Glucophage, 144, 161
Glucose, 43, 71, 109, 160, 161, 242, 248
Glutathione, 115
Gluten, 107
Glycation, 134
Glycemic index (GI), 95–97, 172
Glycine, 50, 332
Glycogen, 71, 160
Goldstein, Irwin, 308–309
Golf, 124
Grape seed extract, 139, 332
Gratitude, 28, 48, 61, 227–229, 257
Green tea, 50, 59, 60, 86, 191, 332–333
Grief
    physical effects of, 164–165, 171
    unresolved, 131–132
Guided imagery, 167
Guilt, 60, 260

Hair growth, 132
Hand temperature, 130, 131
Hand-warming techniques, 62, 63, 175–177
Harris Benedict Formula, 68
Headaches
    chronic, 65
    migraine, 280
Healing ADD (Amen), 300, 301
Health bars, 94–95
Heart, 11, 164–178
    autonomic nervous system and, 166–167
    blood flow, 25, 27, 29, 107, 109, 115, 116, 118, 130, 170, 174, 233
    brain-heart connection boosters, 173–178
    brain-heart connection robbers, 170–173, 178

Heart disease, 25, 64, 67, 90, 93, 99, 103, 118, 146, 158, 160, 244, 245–247, 287
Heart rate, 110, 119, 124
Heart rate variability (HRV), 168–170, 257
Helplessness, 60, 183
Heroin, 24, 245
High blood pressure, 64–65, 67, 118–119, 162, 175, 246, 313
High-carbohydrate diets, 58
Hippocampus, 65, 111, 148–149, 215, 237, 238, 248
Homocysteine, 249–250
Honolulu Study of Aging, 119
Hopelessness, 60, 183
Hormone replacement therapy (HRT), 158–159
Hormones, 11, 24, 67, 71–72, 115, 140–163
    adrenaline, 148, 165, 174, 214
    cortisol, 24, 25, 111, 133, 148, 149, 165, 174, 191, 214–216, 219, 231
    defined, 145–146
    DHEA, 24, 61, 75, 137, 148, 149, 150, 152, 277, 278, 327–328
    estrogen, 24, 28, 67, 137, 145, 146, 152–154, 156, 157, 185, 250–251, 277, 280, 283
    ghrelin, 71, 72, 158–159, 197, 198
    hormonal cascade, 146
    human growth hormone, 161–163, 202
    insulin, 71, 115, 160–161
    leptin, 66, 153, 159–160
    melatonin, 61, 72, 115, 132, 160, 211, 252, 338–339

Hormones (*cont.*)
  menopause and, 65, 115, 135,
    142, 145, 153, 157–159, 250,
    251
  myths and misconceptions
    about, 145
  perimenopause and, 115, 135,
    144, 153, 157, 158
  progesterone, 46
  skin and, 135, 137
  testosterone, 24, 28, 135, 137,
    140–141, 144–146, 150–152,
    180–181, 251–252, 277, 283
  thyroid, 24, 140, 141, 145,
    146–148, 185
Hot flashes, 157, 158
Human Brain Mapping journal, 65
Human growth hormone, 161–163,
  202
Human Reproduction journal, 220
Huperzine A, 254, 333–334
Hyman, Mark, 321
Hypertension, 64–65, 67, 118–119,
  162, 175, 246, 313
Hyperthyroidism, 147
Hypnosis, 4, 51, 62, 63, 131
  heart health and, 167, 175
  self-, 62, 63, 211, 232
  sleep and, 209–210
  weight-management issues and,
    67, 73–74
Hypothalamus, 71, 72
Hypothyroidism, 135, 147, 185
Hysterectomy, 157, 158, 251

IGF-1 (insulinlike growth factor-1),
  161–162
Immune system, 217–218, 277–278,
  287
Impulsive-compulsive overeater
  type, 55–56, 59–60, 79

Impulsive overeater type, 55, 58–59,
  79, 92, 102
Inflammation, 66, 82, 93, 99, 117,
  172, 312
Inhalants, 24
Inositol, 50, 334–335
Insular cortex, 165
Insulin, 71, 115, 160–161
Insulin resistance, 66, 144, 160
*International Journal of Cosmetic
  Science*, 136
Interpersonal psychotherapy, 290
Iodine, 335

Jabbari, Bahman, 209
Jackson, Phil, 82
Journal of Adolescent Health, 219
Journal of American College Health,
  206
Journal of Clinical Hypnosis, 167
Journal of Clinical Investigation, 90
Journal of Clinical Oncology, 134
Journal of Immunotoxicology, 217
Journal of Neuroscience, 154
Journal of Psychiatric Research, 189
*Journal of the American Medical
  Association (JAMA)*, 103,
  104–105
Judo, 120
Junk food, 24–25, 83, 84, 88

Katie, Byron, 180, 265–266
Kava kava, 62, 63, 160, 211, 293,
  335–336
Kessler, David, 22, 93
Kinsey, Alfred, 274
Komisaruk, Barry, 280
Kraft Foods, 100

Laaser, Mark, 38
Labeling, 260

Lane, James, 233
Laughter, benefits of, 174, 234
Lavender, 61, 231
Leptin, 66, 71–72, 153, 159–160, 197, 198
Lexapro, 57, 59, 294, 295
L-glutamine, 75, 336
Libido, low, 60, 112, 140, 151, 277, 283
Lifespans, 15
Limbic system (*see* Deep limbic system [DLS])
Long-term memory, 237
Long-term potentiation (LTP), 46
Los Angeles Lakers, 81–82
Los Angeles Times, 81
Love and Survival (Ornish), 165
Loving What Is (Katie), 180, 265–266
L-theanine, 50, 191, 235, 336
L-tryptophan, 33, 49, 50, 57, 58, 111, 160, 211, 337
L-tyrosine, 49, 191, 337–338
Lyme disease, 184–185

Maas, James, 195
Magnesium, 56, 62, 160, 186, 211, 235, 293, 338
Male menopause, 140
Malnutrition, 24–25
Marijuana, 24, 55, 189, 245
Martial arts, 124
Matthews, Dale, 226
McIlvenna, Ted, 278
Medications (*see also* specific medications; Supplements)
depression and, 289
focus and energy and, 188
Meditation, 28, 43, 62, 63, 167, 174, 190–191, 223–226, 284
Meeker, Angie, 162

Melatonin, 61, 72, 115, 132, 160, 211, 252, 338–339
Memory, 11, 135, 140, 142, 151, 162, 236–244
exercise and, 111, 119
medical tests and, 241–242
new learning and, 237–238
risk factors for loss of, 242–244
sleep and, 199–200
supplements for, 254
types of, 237
understanding and treating loss of, 239–241
Mendoza, Ivan, 171
Menopause, 65, 115, 135, 142, 145, 153, 157–159, 250, 251
male, 140
Menstrual cycles, 143, 144, 152–155, 279
Mental disorders, 28, 135, 138
Metabolic syndrome, 67, 160, 219
Metabolism, 117, 147
Methamphetamines, 25, 245, 296
Midlife crisis, 140
Migraine headaches, 280
Mind reading, 262
Minerals, 25, 27, 56, 62, 160, 183, 186, 211, 235, 293, 338, 348–349
Mitral valve prolapse, 171
Model, Douglas, 133
Mold exposure, 187–188
Monounsaturated fats, 91
Mood disorders, 22
agoraphobia, 293–294
bipolar disorder, 132, 291–292
depression (*see* Depression)
obsessive-compulsive disorder, 49, 50, 182, 294–295
post-traumatic stress disorder (PTSD), 62, 135, 209, 221–222, 295–296

Moore, Dudley, 41
Morbid obesity, 64–65
MSG (monosodium glutamate), 105–106
Multiple sclerosis (MS), 89
Multivitamins, 321, 339
Music, 230–231
Myelin, 76, 89
Myelinization, 189

NAC (n-acetyl-cysteine), 48, 75, 339–340
Naltrexone, 51
Naperville, Illinois, 110
National Mortality Followback Survey (1986), 251
Negative thinking patterns (*see* ANTs [automatic negative thoughts])
Nelson, Noelle, 227–228
Neurogenesis, 110
Neurology journal, 118, 203
Neurotransmitters, 38–39
New England Journal of Medicine, 78, 87, 161
Newberg, Andy, 224
Nicotine, 25, 254
Night sweats, 157, 158
Nighttime-eating syndrome, 57
Nitric oxide, 115, 118
Nowak, Lisa, 156
Nucleus accumbens, 37–39
Nutrition (*see* Diet and nutrition)

Obama, Barack, 186
Obesity, 24–27, 61, 162, 173 (*see also* Weight-management issues)
  causes of, 31
  children and, 65
  epidemic of, 64

leptin and, 72
medical conditions associated with, 64–66
morbid, 64–65
Obsessive-compulsive disorder, 49, 50, 182, 294–295
Occipital lobes, 23, 121
Odom, Lamar, 81–83, 93
Oetgen, Bill, 167
Omega-3 fatty acids, 15, 72, 74–75, 91, 105, 134, 176, 292
One-Page Miracle (OPM) exercise, 43–45
Online dating, 47
Orange juice, 95–96
Orgasm, 274–277, 280, 281
Ornish, Dean, 165
Osteoporosis, 116, 162
Oswald, Andrew, 282
Overeating, 90
Oxidative stress, 100
OxyContin, 24, 126
Oxygen, 109, 116, 230, 233, 242, 277
Oxytocin, 278, 280

Pain medications, 126
Panax ginseng, 285, 340–341
Panic disorders/attacks, 113, 292–293
Paoletti, Christine, 144
Parasympathetic nervous system, 166–167
Parietal lobes, 21–23, 65, 121, 224, 253
Parkinson's disease, 40, 49, 99, 203, 209, 239, 240, 242, 244, 245, 252
Passion (*see* Sexual activity)
Pediatrics, 58, 111, 117
Perimenopause, 115, 135, 144, 153, 157, 158

Phelps, Michael, 114
Phentermine, 54, 59
Pheochromocytoma, 149
Phosphatidylserine (PS), 56, 62,
    149, 254, 341
Physical activity (*see* Exercise)
Physical examination, 68
Pituitary gland, 161
Placebo effect, 270
Plaque, 90, 99
PMS (*see* Premenstrual syndrome
    [PMS])
Pollution, skin and, 136
Polycystic ovarian syndrome
    (PCOS), 135, 141, 144, 152
Polyunsaturated fats, 91
Pornography, 47
Post-traumatic stress disorder
    (PTSD), 62, 135, 209, 221–222,
    295–296
Posterior cingulate gyrus, 159
Postmenopause, 157–158
Potassium intake, 85, 103
Power of Now, The (Tolle), 232
Prayer, 62, 63, 223, 226
Prefrontal cortex (PFC), 6, 9, 16, 19,
    21, 23, 24, 29, 32, 37–41, 55,
    56, 58–60, 76, 97, 110, 121,
    189, 199, 224, 236, 271
    boosting, 42–43
Pregnancy, 115, 135, 154–155, 279
Pregnenolone, 146
Premenstrual syndrome (PMS),
    115, 135, 141–142, 153,
    156–157, 280
Prempro, 158
Prescription drugs, 24
Primrose oil, 138, 341
Professional help, 301–304
Progesterone, 24, 46, 154–155, 156
Prolactin, 281

Prostaglandins, 281
Prostate cancer, 278
Prostatitis, 279
Provigil, 183
Prozac, 50, 57, 59, 60, 157, 294, 295
Psychological Bulletin, 217
Psychological Science journal, 116
Psychology & Behavior, 218
Psychoneuroendocrinology journal,
    215
Psychosis, lack of sleep and, 203
Psychosomatic Medicine journal, 274
Puberty, 135
PYY3-36, 72–73

Ratey, John J., 110–111
Relaxation Response, 225–226
Relaxation techniques, 28, 48, 56,
    62, 167
Resistance training, 119–120
Resveratrol, 342
Rhodiola, 59, 191, 342
Ritalin, 39, 49, 57, 59, 60, 183
Runner's high, 50

SAD or emotional overeater type,
    56, 60–61, 79
SAD (seasonal affective disorder),
    56, 60–61, 211
Saffron, 89
Sage, 89, 254, 343
St. John's wort, 50, 57, 235, 294, 295,
    321, 344–345
Salt intake, 85, 103
SAMe (s-adenosyl-methionine), 8,
    9, 49, 56, 61, 126, 183, 191, 285,
    343–344
Satiereal, 344
Saturated fats, 90, 246
Schizophrenia, 132, 248
Scratching, 132

Sears, Barry, 102
Secret Service: National Threat
     Assessment Center on school
     shootings, 112–113
Seizure disorders, 252–253
Selenium, 344
Self-hypnosis, 62, 63, 211, 232
Seligman, Martin, 229
Serotonin, 9, 39, 41–42, 48, 54–56,
     97, 111, 132, 156, 248
   boosting levels of, 49–50, 57–60,
     97, 126, 157
Sexual activity, 11, 28, 29, 272–286,
     308–309
   benefits of, 273–283
   longevity and, 273–276
   sexy food, 285
   skin and, 137
   supplements and, 284–285
   Tantric, 283–284
Sexual dysfunction, 112
Sexual performance, 26
Shechter, Michael, 172
Short-term memory, 237
Simonton, O. Carl, 4
Simple carbohydrates, 92
Skateboarding, 125
Skin, 11, 29, 129–139
   alcohol use and, 133, 137
   birth control pills and, 135
   brain-skin connection, 130–133
   caffeine and, 133, 137
   diet and nutrition and, 134, 137
   exercise and, 116–117, 134–135,
     136
   hormones and, 135, 137
   pollution and, 136
   sexual activity and, 137
   sleep and, 134, 136, 199
   smoking and, 130, 133, 137

stress and, 131, 135, 136, 216–217
sun exposure and, 135–136, 138
supplements for, 138–139
unresolved emotions and,
     131–132, 135
water consumption and, 134, 138
weight-management issues and,
     134, 137
Skin cancer, 134, 135
Skin picking and cutting, 135
Sleep, 11, 195–212
   aids, 58, 62, 63, 208–209, 211
   amount of, 25, 28, 40, 42, 72,
     195–196, 312
   causes of too little, 204–206
   effects of too little, 202–204
   exercise and, 115
   hormones and, 159
   risk factors for poor, 206–207
   sexual activity and, 279
   skin and, 134, 136, 199
   tips for good, 207–208
   weight-management issues and,
     197–199
Sleep apnea, 65, 72, 203–205, 253
Sleep journal, 207, 210
Smoker's face, 133
Smoking, 25, 233, 247, 253–254
   quitting, 43
   skin and, 130, 133, 137
Snacking, 104
Social networking, 26
Sodium, 103
Spark (Ratey), 110–111
SPECT (single photon emission
     computed tomography)
     imaging (*see* Brain; Brain
     imaging)
Spices, 89
Stanley, Edward, 109

Steele, Alicia, 8, 9
Stevia, 98
Stress, 11, 19–20, 213–235
   -management techniques, 67, 73,
     223–235
   adrenal fatigue and, 148
   caffeine and, 233
   common signs and symptoms of,
     222
   dehydration and, 85–86
   events causing, 214–215
   exercise and, 116, 229
   fertility and, 219–220
   focus and energy and, 187, 188
   heart health and, 170
   immune system and, 217–218
   skin and, 131, 135, 136, 216–217
   supplements for, 235
   weight-management issues and,
     62, 218–219, 233–234
Stroke, 65, 67, 91, 93, 103, 118, 158,
   160, 244–247
Sucralose (Splenda), 98
Sugar, 25, 37, 81–82, 85, 90, 93–95,
   98, 134, 253
Suicidal thoughts, 60, 113, 281,
   288
Sun exposure, 135–136, 138
Supplements, 11, 27, 48–50, 67,
   74–76, 320–349
   Amen Clinics, 321–323
   for memory, 254
   pros and cons of, 320–321
   sexual activity and, 284–285
   for skin, 138–139
   for stress, 235
Sweating, 130, 131
Sweeteners, artificial, 85, 97–98
Sympathetic nervous system,
   166–167

Table tennis, 43, 71, 120–121,
   124–125
Tang, Yiyuan, 225
Taste buds, 98
Technology, growth of, 47–48
Television viewing, 26, 118
Telomeres, 216–217
Temporal lobes, 19, 21–23, 65, 105,
   110, 111, 121, 189, 199, 224,
   228, 236, 237, 239, 248, 258,
   293
Tennis, 121
Testosterone, 24, 28, 135, 137,
   140–141, 144–146, 150–152,
   180–181, 251–252, 277, 283
Text messaging, excessive, 26, 47
Thermogenesis, 75
Thinking with feelings, 260
Thyroid, 24, 135, 137, 140, 141, 145,
   146–148, 185
TIMSS (Trends in International
   Mathematics and Science
   Study), 110
Tolle, Eckhart, 232
Topamax, 62
Toxic exposure, 6, 58, 136,
   187–188
Traffic accidents, 204
Trans fats, 90–91
Triglycerides, 67, 144
TSH (thyroid-stimulating
   hormone), 147
Turmeric, 89
Twain, Mark, 179
Twitter, 47

U.S. Centers for Disease Control
   and Prevention, 112
Unsaturated fats, 90, 91
Uterine cancer, 251

Valerian, 62, 63, 160, 211, 235, 345–346
Vegetables, antioxidant, 100–102
Vicodin, 24, 126
Video games, 26, 47, 118
Vinpocetine, 254, 346–347
Visualization, 270–271
Vitamins, 27, 86, 104–105, 325–326
   A, 133
   B$_3$ (niacin), 191, 325
   B$_6$ (pyridoxine), 48, 56, 62, 183, 191, 293, 325
   D, 25, 56, 60, 75, 136, 138, 312, 347–348
Vitiligo, 138
Volunteering, 61

Wain, Harold, 73–74
Walking, 70–71
Water consumption, 26, 85–86, 134, 138
Weeks, David, 276–277
Weight-management issues, 11–12, 53–80, (*see also* Diet and nutrition; Obesity)
   adrenaline-overload anorexic type, 56, 62–63, 79
   anxious overeater type, 56, 61–62, 79
   body mass index (BMI), 64, 65, 67, 68, 198, 311
   calories, 67, 68–70, 85, 87–89, 311–312
   case histories, 53–56
   compulsive overeater type, 55, 57–58, 79, 92
   failure of most approaches, 56–57
   fat, 66–67, 85, 89–92, 246
   friends and family influences on, 77–79

   hormones, 71–72
   hypnosis and, 67, 73–74
   impulsive-compulsive overeater type, 55–56, 59–60, 79
   impulsive overeater type, 55, 58–59, 79, 92, 102
   list of boosters and trimmers, 80
   SAD or emotional overeater type, 56, 60–61, 79
   skin and, 134, 137
   sleep and, 197–199
   stress and, 62, 218–219, 233–234
   supplements and, 67, 74–76
   thirteen tips for healthy weight, 67–76
Weight scale, 69
Wellbutrin (bupropion), 61, 254
Whipple, Beverly, 280
Williams, Lawrence, 176
Willpower, 37–52, 236
Wilson, Barbara, 272
Winfrey, Oprah, 146–147
Working memory, 237
Work, The, 266–269
World Health Initiative Study, 158
Wound-healing process, 116–117, 136

Xanax, 24
Xylitol, 98

Yo-yo dieting, 89, 134
Yoga, 116, 122, 174, 226
Yosipovitch, Gil, 132
YY3-36, 73

Zinc, 183, 348–349
Zoloft, 57, 59, 112, 157
Zone diet, 102

ABOUT THE AUTHOR

Daniel G. Amen, M.D., is a physician, child and adult psychiatrist, brain imaging specialist, and *New York Times* bestselling author. He is the writer, producer, and host of four highly successful public television programs, raising more than $20 million for public television. He is a Distinguished Fellow of the American Psychiatric Association and the CEO and medical director of Amen Clinics in Newport Beach and Fairfield, California; Tacoma, Washington; and Reston, Virginia.

Amen Clinics is the world leader in applying brain imaging science to everyday clinical practice and has the world's largest database of functional scans related to behavior, now totaling more than 55,000.

Dr. Amen is the author of thirty-five professional scientific articles and twenty-four books, including the *New York Times* bestsellers *Change Your Brain, Change Your Life* and *Magnificent Mind at Any Age*. He is also the author of *Healing ADD, Healing the Hardware of the Soul, Making a Good Brain Great,* and *The Brain in Love* and the coauthor of *Healing Anxiety and Depression* and *Preventing Alzheimer's.*

Newsmax publishes Dr. Amen's monthly newsletter.

Dr. Amen has appeared on the *Dr. Oz Show,* the *Today* show, *Good Morning America, The View, Larry King, The Early Show,* CNN, HBO, Discovery Channel, and many other national television and radio programs. His brain imaging work has been featured on *Oprah.* His national public television shows include *Change Your Brain, Change Your Life; Magnificent Mind at Any Age; The Brain in Love;* and *Change Your Brain, Change Your Body.*

A small sample of the organizations and conferences Dr. Amen has spoken for include the National Security Agency (NSA), the National Science Foundation (NSF), Harvard's Learning and the Brain Conference, the Million Dollar Roundtable, Independent Retired Football Players Summit, and the Supreme Courts of Delaware, Ohio, and Wyoming. Dr. Amen has been featured in *Newsweek, Parade* magazine, *The New York Times Magazine, Men's Health,* and *Cosmopolitan.*

Dr. Amen is married, the father of four children, grandfather to Elias, and an avid table tennis player.

AMEN CLINICS, INC.

Amen Clinics, Inc. (ACI), was established in 1989 by Daniel G. Amen, M.D. They specialize in innovative diagnosis and treatment planning for a wide variety of behavioral, learning, emotional and cognitive, and weight problems for children, teenagers, and adults. ACI has an international reputation for evaluating brain-behavior problems, such as attention deficit disorder (ADD), depression, anxiety, school failure, brain trauma, obsessive-compulsive disorders, aggressiveness, marital conflict, cognitive decline, brain toxicity from drugs or alcohol, and obesity. Brain SPECT imaging is performed in the Clinics. ACI has the world's largest database of brain scans for behavioral problems.

ACI welcome referrals from physicians, psychologists, social workers, marriage and family therapists, drug and alcohol counselors, and individual clients.

Amen Clinics, Inc., Newport Beach
4019 Westerly Place, Suite 100
Newport Beach, CA 92660
(949) 266-3700

Amen Clinics, Inc., Fairfield
350 Chadbourne Road
Fairfield, CA 94585
(707) 429-7181

Amen Clinics, Inc., Northwest
3315 South 23rd Street
Tacoma, WA 98405
(253) 779-HOPE (4673)

Amen Clinics, Inc., DC
1875 Campus Commons Drive
Reston, VA 20191
(703) 860-5600
www.amenclinic.com

AMENCLINIC.COM

Amenclinic.com is an educational interactive brain website geared toward mental health and medical professionals, educators, students, and the general public. It contains a wealth of information to help you learn about our clinics and the brain. The site contains more than three hundred color brain SPECT images, thousands of scientific abstracts on brain SPECT imaging for psychiatry, a brain puzzle, and much, much more.

VIEW HUNDREDS OF ASTONISHING COLOR 3-D BRAIN SPECT IMAGES ON

Aggression
Attention deficit disorder, including the six subtypes
Dementia and cognitive decline
Drug abuse
PMS
Anxiety disorders
Brain trauma
Depression
Obsessive-compulsive disorder
Stroke
Seizures